Infectious Diseases:
A Geographic Guide

"Knowledge is little; to know the right context is much; to know the right spot is everything."
Hugo von Hofmannsthal, 1874–1929

Infectious Diseases: A Geographic Guide

Eskild Petersen MD, DMSc, DTM&H
Department of Infectious Diseases
Aarhus University Hospital Skejby
Aarhus, Denmark

Lin H. Chen MD, FACP
Travel Medicine Center
Mount Auburn Hospital and Harvard Medical School
Cambridge, Massachusetts, USA

Patricia Schlagenhauf PhD, FFTM RCPS (Glasg)
University of Zürich Centre for Travel Medicine
WHO Collaborating Centre for Travellers' Health
Zürich, Switzerland

WILEY-BLACKWELL

A John Wiley & Sons, Ltd., Publication

Contents

List of Contributors

Jaffar A. Al-Tawfiq, MD, FACP, FCCP, DTM&H, DipHIC
Consultant Infectious Diseases
Dhahran Health Center
Saudi Aramco Medical Services Organization
Saudi Aramco
Dhahran, Saudi Arabia

Rodrigo Nogueira Angerami, MD, PhD
Infectious Diseases and Epidemiological Surveillance;
Hospital of Clinics,
State University of Campinas;
Campinas, Sao Paolo
Brazil

Ashish Bhalla, MD
Associate Professor,
Department of Internal Medicine,
Post Graduate Institute of Medical Education and Research
Chandigarh
India

Barbra M. Blair, MD
Division of Infectious Diseases,
Mount Auburn Hospital,
Cambridge, Massachusetts
Instructor, Harvard Medical School,
Boston, Massachusetts
USA

Lucille Blumberg, MB,BCh,MMed (Clin Microbiol), ID (SA) FFTM RCP (Glasgow), DTM&H, DOH, DCH
Epidemiology Division (Travel and International Health)
National Institute for Communicable Diseases
Johannesburg
South Africa

Michael G. Bruce, MD, MPH
Arctic Investigations Program,
NCEZID, CDC,
Anchorage, Alaska
USA

Fabio Buelli, MD
Institute for Infectious and Tropical Diseases
University of Brescia

Gerd D. Burchard, MD
Department of Tropical Medicine and Infectious Diseases
University Medical Center Hamburg
Germany

Francesco Castelli, MD, FRCP (London), FFTM RCPS (Glasg)
Professor
Institute for Infectious and Tropical Diseases
University of Brescia,
Italy

Lin H. Chen, MD, FACP
Director of the Travel Medicine Center
Mount Auburn Hospital
Cambridge, Massachusetts
Assistant Clinical Professor,
Harvard Medical School,
Boston, Massachusetts
USA

Peter L. Chiodini, MD, PhD FRCP FRCPath FFTM RCPS (Glasg)
Professor
Department of Parasitology
Hospital for Tropical Diseases, and
London School of Hygiene and Tropical Medicine
London, UK

Francis E. G. Cox, PhD, DSc
Senior Research Fellow
Department of Disease Control
London School of Hygiene and Tropical Medicine
London, UK

Stephan Ehrhardt MD, MPH
Clinical Research Unit
Bernhard Nocht Institute for Tropical Medicine
Hamburg, Germany

Birgitta Evengård, Professor, MD, PhD,
Department of Clinical Microbiology
Division of Infectious Diseases
Umeå University Hospital
UMEÅ
Sweden

Philip R. Fischer, MD, DTM&H
Professor of Pediatrics
Department of Pediatric and Adolescent Medicine,
Mayo Clinic College of Medicine,
Rochester, Minnesota
USA

David O. Freedman, MD
Professor of Medicine and Epidemiology
Director Travelers Health Clinic
William C. Gorgas Center for Geographic Medicine
Division of Infectious Diseases
University of Alabama at Birmingham
Birmingham, Alabama,
USA

Philippe Gautret, MD, PhD, DTMH
Infectious Diseases and Tropical Medicine Unit,
North University Hospital
Marseille
France

Pier Francesco Giorgetti, MD
Institute for Infectious and Tropical Diseases
University of Brescia
Italy

David Harley, BSc, MBBS, PhD, FAFPHM, MMedSc
Associate Professor of Epidemiology
National Centre for Epidemiology and Population Health,
Australian National University,
Canberra
Australia

Christoph Hatz, MD, DrMed, DTM&H
Professor
Swiss Tropical and Public Health Institute
Basel
Universities of Basel and Zürich
Switzerland

Joanna S Herman, MD, MBBS, MSc, MRCP, DTM&H
Department of Parasitology
Hospital for Tropical Diseases
London, UK

Yasuyuki Kato, MD, MPH
Disease Control and Prevention Center
National Center for Global Health and Medicine
Tokyo
Japan

Anders Koch, MD, PhD, MPH
Department of Epidemiology Research,
Statens Serum Institut,
Copenhagen, Denmark
Department of Infectious Diseases,
Copenhagen University Hospital,
Copenhagen, Denmark

Karin Ladefoged, MD, DMSci
Queen Ingrid's Hospital
Nuuk
Greenland

Karin Leder, MD, FRACP, PhD, MPH, DTMH
Associate Professor,
School of Public Health and Preventive Medicine,
Monash University,
Victoria, Australia
Victorian Infectious Disease Service,
Royal Melbourne Hospital,
Victoria
Australia

Eyal Leshem, MD, MFTM RCPS (Glasg)
The Center for Geographic Medicine and Tropical Diseases,
The Chaim Sheba Medical Center, Tel Hashomer and Sackler Faculty of Medicine,
Tel Aviv University,
Israel

Michael Libman, MD
Director, Division of Infectious Diseases, McGill University
Director, J.D. MacLean Centre for Tropical Medicine at McGill University
Department of Microbiology, McGill University Health Centre
Associate Professor of Medicine, McGill University
Montreal
Canada

Rogelio López-Vélez, MD, DTM&H, PhD
Associate Professor, Alcala University
Tropical Medicine & Clinical Parasitology
Infectious Diseases Department
Ramón y Cajal Hospital
Madrid
Spain

Larry I. Lutwick, MD
Director, Infectious Diseases,
VA New York Harbor Health Care System,
Brooklyn, New York, and
Professor of Medicine
State University of New York (SUNY) Downstate Medical School
Brooklyn, New York
USA

Susan MacDonald, MDCM, CCFP, DTM&H
MSc in Infectious Diseases
University Hospital of Northern British Columbia
Northern Health Authority
Prince George, BC
Canada

Lawrence Madoff, MD
Professor
Division of Infectious Diseases and Immunology,
University of Massachusetts Medical School,
Worcester, MA, USA and
ProMED-mail
International Society for Infectious Diseases
Brookline, MA
USA

Audrone Marcinkute, MD
Department of Infectious Diseases, dermato-venerology and microbiology
State Hospital for Tuberculosis and Infectious diseases
Vilnius University
Vilnius
Lithuania

Anthony McMichael, MBBS, PhD, FAFPHM
Professor of Population Health
National Centre for Epidemiology and Population Health,
Australian National University,
Canberra
Australia

Ziad A. Memish, MD, FRCPC, FACP, FIDSA
Assistant Deputy Minister for Preventive Medicine
Ministry of Health
Infectious Diseases Consultant
King Fahad Medical City
Professor, College of Medicine
Al Faisal University
Riyadh,
Kingdom of Saudi Arabia

Marc Mendelson, MD, PhD
Division of Infectious Diseases and HIV Medicine
Department of Medicine
Groote Schuur Hospital,
University of Cape Town,
Cape Town
South Africa

Maria D. Mileno, MD
Division of Infectious Diseases
The Miriam Hospital
Associate Professor of Medicine
Warren Alpert School of Medicine at Brown University
Providence, Rhode Island
USA

Brian T. Montague, DO, MS, MPH
Division of Infectious Diseases
Miriam Hospital, and
Warren Alpert School of Medicine at Brown University,
Providence, Rhode Island
USA

Terri L. Montague, MD
Division of Nephrology and Hypertension
Rhode Island Hospital, and
Warren Alpert School of Medicine at Brown University,
Providence, Rhode Island
USA

Nadjet Mouffok, MD, PhD
Professor of Medicine
Infectious Diseases Department,
Centre hospitalo-universitaire d'Oran
Oran
Algeria

Holly Murphy, MD
Infectious Disease Consultant
CIWEC Clinic Travel Medicine Center &
Patan Academy of Health Sciences
Kathmandu
Nepal

Andreas Neumayr, MD, DrMed, DTM&H
Swiss Tropical and Public Health Institute
Basel
Switzerland

Francesca F. Norman, MBBS, MRCP, BMedSci
Tropical Medicine & Clinical Parasitology
Infectious Diseases Department
Ramón y Cajal Hospital
Madrid
Spain

Prativa Pandey, MD
Medical Director
CIWEC Clinic Travel Medicine Center
Kathmandu
Nepal

Daniel H. Paris, MD, PhD
Mahidol-Oxford Tropical Medicine Research Unit
Faculty of Tropical Medicine
Mahidol University
Bangkok, Thailand, and
Centre for Clinical Vaccinology and Tropical Medicine
Nuffield Department of Clinical Medicine
Churchill Hospital
University of Oxford
United Kingdom

Philippe Parola, MD, PhD
Professor of Medicine
Infectious Diseases and Tropical Medicine Unit, North University Hospital,
WHO Collaborative Centre for Rickettsioses and other Arthropod Borne Bacterial Diseases,
Faculty of Medicine
Marseille
France

Malgorzata Paul
Department and Clinic of Tropical and Parasitic Diseases
University of Medical Sciences
Poznan, Poland

José-Antonio Pérez-Molina, MD, PhD, DTM&H
Tropical Medicine & Clinical Parasitology,
Infectious Diseases Department,
Ramón y Cajal Hospital, Madrid, Spain

Olga Perovic MD, DTM&H, FCPath (MICRO) SA, MMED (WITS)
Microbiology External Quality Assessment Reference Unit
National Institute for Communicable Diseases
Johannesburg
South Africa

Natalia Pshenichnaya
Department of Infectious Diseases
Rostov State Medical University
Rostov-on-Don, Russia

Eskild Petersen, MD, DMSc, DTM&H, MBA, FFTM RCPS (Glas)
Associate Professor
Department of Infectious Diseases
Institute of Clinical Medicine
Aarhus University Hospital Skejby
Aarhus,
Denmark

Giles Poumerol, MD, MPH
International Health Regulations Department
World Health Organization
Geneva, Switzerland

Jana I. Preis MD, MPH
Infectious Diseases,
VA New York Harbor Health Care System,
Brooklyn, New York
Assistant Clinical Professor of Medicine
State University of New York (SUNY) Downstate Medical School
Brooklyn, New York
USA

Julius B. Salamera, MD
Post-Doctoral Fellow in Infectious Diseases
State University of New York (SUNY) Downstate Medical School
Brooklyn, New York
USA

Francisco G. Santos-O'Connor, MD, MSc, DTMH
Specialist in Medical Microbiology
Expert in Epidemic Intelligence
European Centre for Disease Prevention and Control
Stockholm
Sweden

Patricia Schlagenhauf-Lawlor, BSc (Pharm), MPSI, PhD, FFTM RCPS (Glasgow)
Professor,
University of Zürich Centre for Travel Medicine
WHO Collaborating Centre for Travellers' Health
Zürich, Switzerland

Eli Schwartz, MD, DTMH
Professor of Medicine,
The Center for Geographic Medicine and Tropical Diseases,
The Chaim Sheba Medical Center, Tel Hashomer and Sackler Faculty of Medicine,
Tel Aviv University,
Israel

**Marc Shaw, DrPH, FRGS, FRNZCGP, FACTM, FFTM (ACTM),
FFTM RCPS (Glas), DipTravMed**
Associate Professor
School of Public Health
James Cook University
Townsville, Australia, and
WORLDWISE Travellers Health & Vaccination Centres
Auckland
New Zealand

Luiz Jacintho da Silva, MD
Dengue Vaccine Initiative
International Vaccine Institute
Seoul
Republic of Korea

Ashwin Swaminathan, MBBS (Hons), MPH, FRACP
Research Scholar
National Centre for Epidemiology and Population Health,
Australian National University,
Physician, Infectious Diseases & General Medicine Units
Canberra Hospital
Canberra
Australia

Joseph Torresi, MD, MBBS, BMedSci, FRACP,PhD
Associate Professor
Department of Infectious Diseases
Austin Hospital,
Melbourne, and
Department of Medicine, Austin Health
The University of Melbourne
Victoria
Australia

Peter J. de Vries, MD, PhD
Division of Infectious Diseases, Tropical Medicine and AIDS
Academic Medical Center
Amsterdam
the Netherlands

Nicholas J. White, MD, FRS
Professor
Mahidol-Oxford Tropical Medicine Research Unit
Faculty of Tropical Medicine
Mahidol University
Bangkok, Thailand, and
Centre for Clinical Vaccinology and Tropical Medicine
Nuffield Department of Clinical Medicine
Churchill Hospital
University of Oxford
United Kingdom

Annelies Wilder-Smith, MD, PhD, DTM&H, MIH, FAMS
Mercator Professor
Institute of Public Health
University of Heidelberg
Germany

Mary Elizabeth Wilson, MD, FACP, FIDSA
Associate Professor
Global Health and Population
Harvard School of Public Health
Harvard University
Boston, Massachusetts
USA

Foreword

Where have you been? In the world of clinical medicine, this is a critical question that opens a treasure chest or sometimes a Pandora's box of epidemiologic information often leading the infectious disease specialist to a correct diagnosis or intervention that otherwise might not be considered. When this key question is forgotten, a poor or preventable outcome may follow. But what happens when the experienced physician or travel medicine specialist, who unfailingly includes this question in his or her initial assessment, hears a patient respond with a lengthy discussion of a complex itinerary, multiple exposures, or unusual symptoms? Sometimes the destination is not familiar, the exposures trigger a distant memory of "something important" but one cannot recall exactly the connection, or a specific finding can generate a limited differential diagnosis. The physician or travel medicine specialist then attempts to locate the missing information in published papers, books, and online references.

Where are you going? In the pretravel setting, this book is an indispensable reference for travel medicine practitioners advising individual long-term travelers or making recommendations for expatriates who will stay for prolonged periods in a particular geographic area. Long-term travelers have been shown to have a higher risk of acquiring travel-associated illness because of their prolonged exposure, suboptimal adherence to preventive measures, and often a lack of knowledge on risks at the destination. The comprehensive regional disease profile presented in this volume will allow for tailored advice for this important group of travelers.

This book, *Infectious Diseases: A Geographic Guide* by Eskild Petersen, Lin H. Chen, and Patricia Schlagenhauf, admirably fills the need for a single reference structured to assist the travel medicine practitioner to answer these questions.

The book is organized by geographic regions of the world; for example, South Asia, Central Europe, and South America. Each chapter pertaining to a geographic region is then organized into an initial section on important regional infections, a series of very useful and easily scanned tables, a section on antibiotic resistance, a short section on vaccine-preventable diseases in the region, and finally a section on background data from the region. The tables are organized by presenting clinical syndromes, the way we actually encounter patients, subdivided where appropriate into those that usually occur within 4 weeks of exposure and those that occur greater than 4 weeks after exposure. Each table then divides infectious pathogens into those that are frequently encountered, uncommonly encountered, and rarely encountered. The sections on antibiotic resistance are unique and quite useful. This kind of antibiotic resistance information is usually not presented by geographic region but rather by pathogen with a secondary linkage to geographic regions. Having this regional perspective is novel and fits nicely with the evaluation of the ill returned traveler. There are several other very interesting and useful chapters in the introductory and closing sections of the book with inviting titles such as "Historical overview of global infectious diseases and geopolitics," "Detection of infectious diseases using unofficial sources," "Microbes on the move: prevention, curtailment, outbreak," "Diagnostic tests and procedures," "The immunosuppressed patient," "Migration and the geography of disease," and "Climate change and the geographical distribution of infectious diseases."

The editors of this new text are leaders in the field of international travel medicine and have attracted a brilliant and luminous collection of chapter contributors. The regional chapters are written by individuals living in the region or expatriates with long-standing affiliations with the area. The strength of this book is the editorial oversight and vision of the editors who skillfully bring together a very diverse, international team to yield a cohesive, multiauthored, yet well-written textbook.

The global community of the twenty-first century is connected by ever growing bonds of communication, economic growth, shared aspirations, and increasingly, a globalized enterprise of international treaties, agreements, covenants, and structures. Global health is now part of the daily lexicon of universities, governments, and multinational companies. The basis for this explosive growth over the last half century lies in the movement of people from one place to another. The motivation for movement is varied, but the most important questions that a travel medicine practitioner can ask are: *"Where are you going?"* in the pretravel setting or *"Where have you been?"* when seeing the ill returned traveler. *Infectious Diseases: A Geographic Guide* by Eskild Petersen, Lin H. Chen, and Patricia Schlagenhauf will be the first resource most of us reach for when those questions are fielded.

Alan J. Magill MD, FACP, FIDSA
President of the International Society of Travel Medicine (2009–2011)

Infectious Diseases in a Global Perspective

"The microbe is nothing; the terrain everything."

(Louis Pasteur)

We beg to differ with Louis Pasteur regarding this statement! Both the microbe *and* the terrain are important and this book is concerned with both. It is primarily concerned with global disease risk. The increasing mobility and diversity in traveling populations challenge tropical medicine, infectious disease, and travel medicine practitioners, whether they are advising travelers visiting specific destinations or evaluating patients with distinct travel histories.

For the clinician, the book is intended as a guide to generate differential diagnoses in consideration of the geographical history, and in concert with presenting symptoms and duration of illness. Once a diagnosis has been made, classic textbooks on infectious diseases should be consulted for guidelines on specific management and therapy.

For the travel medicine specialist, the book provides information on risks of different diseases in the destination region and will be particularly useful in advising and assessing travelers visiting environments off the beaten path and for travelers visiting friends and relatives in their countries of origin.

The book can also be used by health care personnel from one area of the world practicing medicine in another area as a guide to distinguish the infections that are locally prevalent from those that occur in their home medical environment.

In addition to general background chapters, the book is divided according to United Nations (UN) world regions and addresses geographic disease profiles, presenting symptoms and incubation periods of infections. Geographic childhood vaccination coverage is addressed. Each chapter therefore contains a section on childhood vaccination programs in the countries included in that region.

The important topic of antibiotic resistance is addressed on a regional basis. The distribution of antimicrobial resistance in common bacteria is disparate worldwide, and with the increasing volume of travelers an increasing number will travel with or import multiresistant infections. Recent reports of gram-negative Enterobacteriaceae with resistance to carbapenem conferred by the New Delhi metallo-β-lactamase-1 (NDM-1) and imported into the United Kingdom by "medical tourists" (patients who traveled for medical interventions or operations) sketch a frightening scenario of the ease of the global travel of microbes.

This book has a special focus on immigrants and those visiting friends and relatives. It is estimated that nearly 200 million people are refugees or permanently displaced persons. In Europe alone 30 million inhabitants have an immigrant background of which approximately one-third were born outside the industrialized countries. Individuals migrating from one country to another carry a history of exposures to infections not present in the destination country, and a sensible strategy for evaluating infections in this group requires knowledge of disease patterns in the country of origin, often including childhood immunization coverage. When a diagnosis or presumptive diagnosis is made, knowledge of the susceptibility patterns including those for malaria in the country of origin is crucial to determine the appropriate treatment. Furthermore, exposure earlier in life should be included when diagnostic considerations are made, as tuberculosis, HIV, schistosomiasis, leishmaniasis, and onchocerciasis can remain undiagnosed for up to several decades.

Immigrants obtaining residency status through the UN program for refugees often originate in countries with rudimentary health systems, are torn by civil strife, and have spent years in refugee camps where health care facilities have limited resources. Health problems in this special group require specific knowledge of infections present in the countries of origin and the effect of civil war on the childhood vaccination program or disease control programs. An example is the current epidemic of African trypanosomiasis in the Democratic Republic of Congo, which escalated during the years of civil war with the concomitant breakdown of control programs.

Trypanosomiasis is now as prevalent in the Democratic Republic of Congo as 90 years ago when control measures were originally introduced by the colonial power Belgium. The introduction of Chagas' disease to Europe, in particular Spain, with immigrants from South America is another recent example of how migration can bring a health problem to the new country of residence.

This book also contains a number of fascinating "background and general chapters."

The riveting historical perspective on infectious diseases is key to understanding present-day geopolitics. Another important section addresses infection prevention, outbreak, and the role of the International Health Regulations (IHRs) in the curtailment of disease. Data on disease epidemiology and changing disease patterns are provided by surveillance networks exemplified here by GeoSentinel and ProMED, which publish and rapidly disseminate information to the infectious disease and travel medicine communities. Emerging infections is a key topic in a world where an infected individual can travel halfway around the globe in twelve hours. Newly emerging infections are very likely to emerge from a zoonotic reservoir whenever the contact between humans and the reservoir animal is altered. Another chapter in this book addresses individuals with an impaired immune system who constitute a special risk group including patients with transplants, HIV, and other conditions like immunoglobulin deficiency. These travelers will often have a decreased humoral and cellular immune response to vaccines and may be at higher risk of certain infections at their destination compared to their immunocompetent counterparts.

Climate change will affect the distribution of infectious diseases. Most obvious are the effects on vector-borne infections, where change in temperature, humidity, vegetation, and distribution of the zoonotic reservoirs will influence the distribution of the infections. The recent introduction of Chikungunya virus in Italy, dengue transmission in the south of France, and dengue outbreaks in Key West, Florida, are associated with the recent establishment of *Aedes albopictus* in these regions.

We hope that this book will be a useful aid for those involved in preventing or treating infection and that you, the reader, will enjoy using and browsing this volume. Most of all, we are grateful to all the collaborators worldwide who contributed to this global project and who made it possible.

Eskild Petersen
Aarhus, Denmark

Lin H. Chen
Cambridge, USA

Patricia Schlagenhauf
Zurich, Switzerland

Chapter 1
Historical overview of global infectious diseases and geopolitics

Francis E.G. Cox

Department of Disease Control, London School of Hygiene and Tropical Medicine, London, UK

Over millennia, national boundaries have largely been shaped by the retention or acquisition by discrete populations of strategically important land areas necessary to satisfy their needs for resources such as food, settled agriculture, and trade. Wars and conquest have played important roles in these processes but a number of infectious diseases, including cholera, leprosy, typhoid, typhus, plague, tuberculosis, measles, smallpox, yellow fever, and malaria, have also played their parts in important historical events. This chapter discusses some of the ways in which infectious diseases have influenced the course of history and have changed the political maps of the world.

Introduction

Superimposed upon physical maps of the world are political maps that show not only natural boundaries but also boundaries created by humans through the acquisition of territories by conquest and colonization or subjugation by force. Geopolitics, a term that has had many meanings some politically extreme, is concerned with ". . . power relationships in international politics including, *inter alia*, the acquisition of natural boundaries, the control of strategically important land areas and access to sea routes," Kjellén's original definition that will be adopted here [1,2].

The present-day political maps of the world have been largely determined by military successes and failures and, throughout history, civilian casualties and deaths have been regarded as unfortunate by-products of conflicts. The role played by disease among both armies and civilians is seldom acknowledged despite the fact that in virtually all wars morbidity and loss of life from disease has massively exceeded losses caused by weapons [3,4]. It can, therefore, be argued that disease within the civilian populations during and as an aftermath of conflict has been as important in shaping the political maps of the world as military successes or failures [5].

Most anthropologists agree that our species, *Homo sapiens*, emerged in Africa about 150,000–200,000 years ago and from ca. 70000 BC dispersed in waves throughout the world until by the end of the last ice age, ca. 10000 BC, had occupied most of the inhabitable planet except New Zealand and some other isolated islands [6]. The world population was then about 1 million, and increasing, and discrete populations began to covet territory that others already occupied

---

Infectious Diseases: A Geographic Guide, First Edition.
Edited by Eskild Petersen, Lin H. Chen & Patricia Schlagenhauf.
© 2011 John Wiley & Sons, Ltd. Published 2011 by John Wiley & Sons, Ltd.

leading to conflict and occupancy—the beginnings of geopolitics. Acquisition of territory became more important as the population of the world grew to about 10 million by 3000 BC and nearly 500 million by AD 1500 when the political world as we know it today began to take shape [7]. Nearly all that we know about the epidemiology and effects of infectious diseases dates from about 1500.

The most important diseases in the past, as now, were those caused by microparasites (viruses, bacteria, and protozoa) that multiply within their hosts causing an immediate threat unless brought under control by an immune response. Individuals differ in the degree of susceptibility or resistance to infection and, over time, the more susceptible individuals die out while the more resistant ones pass on their genes; thus, whole populations develop "herd immunity" which protects them against diseases prevalent in their particular communities [8]. When such individuals move into areas where there are infections to which they have not developed herd immunity, they rapidly succumb and, conversely, spread their own infections among the susceptible local inhabitants. This is an oversimplification that takes no account of such factors as the role of nutrition which markedly affects an individual's capacity to resist infection, and it has been argued that improvements in nutrition have, over the centuries, enabled populations to withstand diseases that would have killed their ancestors [9]. This is a study in itself and will not be considered further in this chapter.

Of the 150 common infectious diseases, 28 caused by viruses, 35 by bacteria, and 6 by protozoa are the most serious [10]. Of these, cholera, leprosy, typhoid, typhus, plague, tuberculosis, measles, smallpox, yellow fever, and malaria in particular have markedly affected the course of history. The following sections will discuss, region by region, the ways in which some of these diseases have exerted seismic changes on the history of the world. The topics covered are of necessity selective and for more information, particularly regarding the background, the reader is referred to the following: [2,5,9,11–22] and for historical continuity [23–25] and also, for more information on disease and geopolitics [26].

The Near East and North Africa

Human civilization emerged somewhere between 12,000 and 10,000 years ago in this region and by 2000 BC there were great cities and a population that stretched over Mesopotamia, Egypt, North Africa, and the Mediterranean. For nearly 300 centuries great empires including Babylonian, Phoenician, Persian, Greek, and Roman came and went until the rise of Islam in the seventh century AD. We know from military and civilian records and archeological evidence that several infectious diseases, including tuberculosis, leprosy (brought from India by the troops of Alexander III), typhus, typhoid, and malaria, existed in the region but there appear to have been no epidemics that could have significantly altered the course of history. There is, however, one intriguing possibility. Alexander III (the Great) having amassed a great empire and having conquered the Greek, Persian, Syrian, Phoenician, and Egyptian empires was on the brink of bringing much of Asia and parts of Europe under his control when he died suddenly in 323 BC. Although most commentators believe that he was poisoned some think that he died of typhoid or malaria [27]. After Alexander's death his empire began its terminal decline and, if this decline resulted from his death from an infection, this could well be the earliest documented example of a disease changing the course of history. There is a need for some caution here because many historians believe that his death merely accelerated a process that would inevitably have occurred within the next decade or two.

The rise of Islam, in the seventh century, might also be traced back to the effects of a disease. By AD 632, most of the Arab world had been converted to Islam and the next target for conversion was the Byzantine Empire (the successor of the Roman West, see later) and its capital,

Damascus, which fell after a siege in 634. The origins of this defeat can be traced back to 542 when the "Justinian Plague" (see later) frustrated plans to reunite the Roman Empire after which the Roman and Byzantine armies never recovered and by 634 they were so weakened that Damascus surrendered with hardly a fight. There followed the Islamic golden age during which the religion spread throughout the Mediterranean area and into Spain and southern France. It is tempting to speculate that if the fall of Damascus can be traced back to the Justinian Plague of 542 and had Damascus not fallen the advance of Islam might have been haltered.

Europe

By 7000 BC, farming was established in Europe and for the next 6,000 years people lived as small tribes on farms or small villages. Several infectious diseases must have been prevalent but, because of the scattered nature of the population, it is unlikely that there were any significant epidemics. This situation changed with the development of the first city-states which brought people together in large numbers and witnessed the growth of military expeditionary forces. The first European city-state, Athens, emerged as a major power in about 750 BC and flourished until it was defeated by its rival, Sparta, in the Peloponnesian wars (431–405 BC) after which it fell into decline [28]. The outcome of the wars was determined less by superior military achievements than by the arrival of the "Plague of Athens," from Africa, via Egypt, Libya, and Persia, that killed an estimated quarter to one-third of the population of Athens. The cause was probably louse-borne typhus, for which the crowded and humid conditions were ideal. Measles and smallpox have also been suggested but the actual cause will probably never be known [29].

The next great power to emerge in Europe was the Roman Empire whose influence spread until, by the third century AD, it included nearly all of Western Europe, North Africa, and the Near East [30]. Under a series of ambitious military emperors, however, the empire grew so large that it became almost ungovernable and by the beginning of the fourth century had split into the West centered on Rome and the East centered on Constantinople. By the end of the fifth century the empire had begun to disintegrate and most of the West had succumbed to the Visigoths while the East became the precursor of the Byzantine Empire. In 540 there was one last abortive attempt to restore the old Roman Empire by the Emperor Justinian who by then had regained most of the former Mediterranean possessions and had hoped to regain the more important Eastern section. He was, however, stopped in his tracks by the arrival of the "Plague of Justinian" (541–542), which most experts agree was bubonic plague that had spread from Alexandria to Constantinople, where it killed an estimated 5,000–10,000 people every day. Because of the "plague" Justinian could not raise the armies required for his campaign and abandoned his ambitious plans and this eventually led to the terminal decline of the Roman Empire.

Bubonic plague spread to Western Europe in 547 and continued to recur sporadically for the next 200 years until it virtually disappeared but returned with a vengeance in 1347 as the "Black Death." The origins of this epidemic are obscure but it appears to have emerged in about 1300 along the Caspian Sea and thence to the Crimea and Constantinople by 1346–1347. Beginning insignificantly with the arrival of infected Genoese merchants from the Black Sea to Messina in Sicily, the infection spread with amazing rapidity throughout Europe and in less than 10 years it had reduced the population from about 75 million to less than 50 million. The plague was particularly felt in the great cities of Venice, Florence, Genoa, London, Paris, and Barcelona, some of which lost half their population. Plague also affected even the most remote rural areas taking with it princes, the clergy, and peasants leaving Europe in a state of chaos; agriculture failed and millions who had survived the plague died of starvation. As a result of the plague, the former feudal system fell into abeyance; there was a shortage of labor and peasants realized that the laborer was worth his wage with implications that lasted for centuries. There were also other long-lasting effects including the irrevocable loss of whole villages, migration to larger con-urbations, and a diminution of the authority of Church and State [31]. Plague continued to rumble on in waves across Europe about every 15–20 years from the mid-1550s until the 1670s causing the deaths over half of the inhabitants of many cities and persisted at insignificant levels until about 1800 [32]. Like the Black Death plague in Europe brought with it starvation, and severely curtailed the economies of the countries affected.

The last great epidemic to hit Europe was the 1918 influenza pandemic also known as Spanish flu [33]. The first records are from the United States and Austria in 1917, the rest of Europe in 1918 and worldwide in two waves, the second more virulent than the first. Survivors of the first wave had some protection against the more dangerous form but by the time the pandemic ended in the summer of 1920 it had infected between one-quarter and one-fifth of the world's population and killed 50–100 million people. This epidemic might also have affected the out-come of the final stages of the First World War (1914–1918) as it seems to have adversely affected German and Austrian forces more than the Allies. The impact of this epidemic on the economies of European countries cannot be overestimated and it took decades before its effects wore off and may even have influenced the depression of the 1930s.

The Americas

Nowhere have the effects of infectious diseases on geopolitics been more marked than in the Americas [34]. The first human arrivals came from northern Europe via the Bering Strait where the "cold filter" prevented many Old World diseases from reaching the continent. We know very little about any of the diseases that afflicted these early peoples who had virtually no contact with the wider world. There is evidence of villages and permanent settlements from about 2000 BC and civilizations that rivaled those of Mesopotamia, Egypt, and China existed over 2,000 years ago in present-day Mexico, Peru, and Ecuador. When Europeans first arrived in AD 1500, Central and South America was dominated by two advanced and powerful civiliza-tions, the Aztecs in Mexico and the Incas in Peru and Ecuador, while North America was occupied by scattered and sparsely populated Indian tribes. From the beginning of the sixteenth century, successive waves of small numbers of Spanish troops overcame the vastly superior Inca and Aztec armies. It is not at all clear why they succumbed so easily and although infections played a major role it has been suggested that nutritional, psychological, economic, and reli-gious factors and the fear of disease also contributed to their defeat. Spanish conquistadors introduced smallpox, almost invariably accompanied by measles, to the Caribbean in 1507 and from there it spread as far as Mexico by 1520 causing massive mortality wherever it went and killing between one quarter and one-third of its victims. The pattern was nearly always the same; disease spread ahead of the invading armies causing overwhelming mortality and mor-bidity leaving the dispirited survivors at the mercy of the invaders, thus clearing the whole region and making it available for colonization by generations of Europeans. North America became "virgin territory" ready to be carved up and colonized by Portugal, Spain, Britain, Denmark, France, Sweden, and the Netherlands.

Waves of infected immigrants and slaves added the disease burden, and by the early seven-teenth century smallpox and measles had spread along the coast of North America as far as Massachusetts and by the nineteenth century these diseases had reached the west and had become endemic throughout the Americas. Infectious diseases continued to be significant into the nineteenth century as they spread along the Mississippi as a result of trade and settlement and during the Civil War (1861–1865) the majority of deaths were caused by disease.

One disease in particular played an important role in the later history of North America. Yellow fever, brought from Africa by infected slaves together with its mosquito vector, arrived in Yucatan in 1649 and spread to Cuba, Hispaniola, and across mainland America and in 1793 reached Philadelphia [35]. Philadelphia was then the favored site for the new capital of the United States established in 1783, but epidemics of yellow fever (and dengue) in 1793 and subsequent years were partly responsible for George Washington's decision to found the new capital elsewhere in Washington in 1800 [36]. Meanwhile, in 1800, the Spanish West Indian colony, Haiti, had been seized by the French against the wishes of the local population and the French Emperor Napoleon sent massive reinforcements of French troops to quell any rebellion. This was disastrous for the French who succumbed to yellow fever and out of 40,000 soldiers only 3,000 returned to France. This was a major, but not fatal, setback for Napoleon's ambitions in the New World and in 1802 he sent an army to claim New Orleans for France but 29,000 out of 35,000 soldiers succumbed to yellow fever effectively ending France's claims to New Orleans and French aspirations for New World dominance which had begun in the 1530s. It has even been suggested that were it not for yellow fever Americans would today probably be speaking French [17].

Yellow fever was to have one other major effect on the relationships between France and the United States. In 1879–1889 the French had tried to link the Pacific with the Atlantic via a Panama Canal but had to abandon the scheme partly because of the devastating effects of yellow fever and malaria. Following the discovery by American and Cuban scientists that mosquitoes transmitted yellow fever, the threat of disease was virtually eliminated and work on the Panama Canal was resumed and when it was opened in 1914 it gave the United States unfettered dominance of the whole region [37].

Australasia

It is not certain when humans first arrived in Australia and estimates range from 125,000 to 40,000–50,000 years ago. Written history begins with sporadic visits by Europeans in the early sixteenth century and much of the coastline had been mapped by Dutch explorers by 1650. When the British arrived in 1769 the country was sparsely populated with about 250 well-defined and scattered Aboriginal tribes each with its own culture and language and a total population of about 350,000. Shortly after the colonization of New South Wales in 1788 there was a major and well-documented epidemic of smallpox in Sydney and, thereafter, elsewhere there were sporadic epidemics of smallpox and measles. In 1798 one particularly severe epidemic of smallpox killed 90% of the Darug (also spelled Dharug, Daruk, or Dharuk) tribe in the area now including Sydney [38]. Overall, however, disease played only a minor role in the decline of the aboriginals to about 93,000 in 1900 which was mainly due to deliberate killings, starvation, and forcible resettlement. The aboriginals were largely protected from infectious diseases because their populations were so isolated that infections could not spread easily and contact between Europeans and aboriginals was very limited. In addition, because of the distance from Europe, any smallpox carriers would have either died or recovered by the time their ships reached Australia and from about 1798 many of the immigrants from Europe would have been vaccinated against the disease. Finally, Australia never imported large numbers of slaves together with their infectious diseases from Africa as had occurred in the Americas and bubonic plague did not reach Australia until 1900 [39].

New Zealand was even more fortunate than Australia. The first European contacts occurred in 1672 but it was not until 1679 that there was any significant impact. In 1769 the local, Maori, population was 85,000–110,000 which fell to 70,000 by 1840 mainly due to conflict not disease. The European population was tiny, about 2,000, so presented little or no risk of transmitting disease and by the time that Europeans began to arrive in large numbers between 1850 and 1870 the causes of infectious diseases and means of controlling them were well established. The only significant smallpox epidemic occurred as late as 1913.

The islands of Oceania began to experience European diseases with the increase in explora-
tion, trade, missionaries, and labor movements from 1788 onward. The large number of small
islands meant that epidemics could be serious for a particular population but could not spread
quickly or widely. Following the epidemic in Sydney in 1788, smallpox arrived in some of the
nearby islands and spread throughout Oceania during the nineteenth century reaching Hawaii
in 1853, Papua New Guinea in 1865, and New Guinea in 1870. Tuberculosis reached Fiji in 1791
and measles began to spread from about 1800. In addition to the common European diseases,
malaria and dengue began to spread throughout the region and, with the movement of labor in
the nineteenth century, there were also new importations of infectious diseases including
malaria from Asia and South America.

Infectious diseases in Australia and Oceania played little part in geopolitics, they did not
facilitate colonization nor did they bring about the downfall of governments or powers but did
have a major impact on the economic development of all the countries in the region simply by
their presence.

Sub-Saharan Africa

Hominids emerged in Africa and evolved to become our species, *Homo sapiens*, that now
inhabits the whole of the planet. Little is known about the early history of the inhabitants of
the continent as, apart from one first century AD document, the "Periplus of the Erythrean Sea"
which describes trade routes down the African coast [40], there are no written records until
about AD 1000 when most of the inhabitants of the interior lived in small and isolated communities that were too small to sustain and spread contagious diseases. They did, however,
suffer from mosquito-transmitted malaria and yellow fever. European diseases reached the
African coasts with Portuguese and Arab traders and slavers from the beginning of the sixteenth century and quickly spread inland where they took a disproportionate toll of the
indigenous people who had had no opportunity to build up any herd immunity. Although
smallpox had been present along the coastal regions from the seventh century, the first records
of major epidemics are from the Gulf of Guinea in 1680 and thereafter there are numerous
records from as far south as Cape Town in 1713. This latter epidemic began when a Dutch ship
with infected slaves and colonists landed in the Cape and quickly spread killing about a
quarter of the European settlers. It had a particularly adverse effect on the Khoikhoi (Khoi), a
genetically distinct population of herdsmen who had inhabited and dominated parts of
South West Africa since the fifth century, and killed over 90% of the Khoi who never recovered
from their loss allowing settler farmers to take over the territory that they had held for over
1,000 years.

Sub-Saharan Africa was to experience other disasters and cholera and tuberculosis spread
throughout the country after 1900 and when the 1918 influenza epidemic arrived in Sierra
Leone it quickly spread and killed an estimated 2 million people.

In some ways the presence of malaria and yellow fever protected Africa from military invasion
because European armies suffered huge losses when they penetrated into an interior so hostile
that it permitted little more than the establishment of a few strategically placed forts and
garrisons. Parts of West Africa became known as the "white man's grave" and until about 1900 it
was believed that there was something about Africa itself that made it inimical to Europeans.
The presence of African diseases prevented or delayed major projects such as the building of
roads and railways leaving some to wonder if, after the ending of the slave trade, Africa was
worth the effort of colonizing which had been so easy in the Americas and Australasia.
Nevertheless, what has become known as the "scramble for Africa" began followed by the
partitioning of Africa between the European powers in 1884–1886.

Colonization did have some beneficial effects on Africa. Toward the end of the nineteenth century herds of cattle were succumbing to a wasting disease called nagana while humans were suffering and dying from a condition known as sleeping sickness. British colonial scientists and doctors unraveled the mysteries of these two diseases, which were found to be caused by protozoan parasites, trypanosomes [41]. This led to measures for the control of these diseases and made it safer for Europeans and Africans to keep their cattle over great swathes of Sub-Saharan Africa thus contributing to the wealth of the continent.

South Asia

The countries of South Asia, present-day India, Bangladesh, Bhutan, Pakistan, the Maldives, Nepal, and Sri Lanka, separated from the rest of Asia by the Himalayas, developed cultures quite distinct from those of the Near East, the Far East, and Southeast Asia. Much of we know about disease in the past comes from the sixth century BC Ayurvedic texts, the Caraka and Sushruta, which mix spiritual well-being with descriptions of diseases some of which are difficult to interpret. For the next 1,000 years or so, trade brought the region in contact with the Arab and European world and their diseases, but there are only sporadic references to infectious diseases which probably included cholera, leprosy, typhoid, smallpox, and malaria. The first detailed accounts of smallpox date from AD 1160. Epidemics of plague occurred in 1443, 1543, and 1573 after which the disease became endemic with occasional epidemics such as that in 1812 that killed half the population of Gujarat. Cholera, however, is the disease that is most associated with India and the epicenter seems to have been the Ganges delta. The first Indian epidemic occurred in 1503 and in 1817 it killed 4,000 in Calcutta from where it spread throughout the subcontinent to the Far East and to Cuba and Mexico in 1833, Europe in 1835–1837, and Africa in 1837. From the nineteenth century onward there have been periodic cholera pandemics nearly all of which originated from the Ganges region where the religious ritual of bathing in the river is thought to have contributed to the spread of the disease.

The European colonization of the subcontinent began in 1498 with the voyages of Vasco da Gama and later Portuguese traders whose accounts of recognizable diseases appear as more Europeans began to arrive. Because India had already experienced some of the diseases prevalent in Europe, it suffered none of the disastrous epidemics experienced in the Americas and Australasia. India effectively came under British rule from 1765 and inherited a sophisticated health system which it supplemented with the introduction of Western medicine.

Despite its long history of civilization and knowledge of infectious diseases, no particular event in South Asia can be said to have changed the course of world history although diseases that contributed to the outcome of wars that plagued the region throughout its history had significant local consequences and, as in Africa, slowed and curtailed the development of roads and railways.

East Asia

East Asia which encompasses China, Japan, and Korea, like South Asia, is a geographically distinct region with well-defined disease etiologies. The Chinese civilization emerged about 4000 BC and from 1765 to 1122 BC experienced a growth in both labor-intensive agriculture and the construction of walled cities. By 221 BC there was massive growth in the population and considerable expansion followed by a period during which great dynasties emerged and declined. In the first century BC China reached as far north as Bengal and by the time of the Tang Dynasty (AD 618–907) there were over 20 cities and a population of about 2 million. Population growth, the congregation of people in cities, and increasing trade with the outside world created conditions conducive to the spread of infectious diseases: smallpox arrived from the north in 250 BC and from the south in AD 48 and thereafter became endemic throughout the region. In 1206 Mongol nomads invaded China and established the Yuan Dynasty which in 1368 was replaced by the native Ming Dynasty characterized by trade with Southeast Asia, South Asia, Africa, and Europe. This period of trading brought new diseases to China and toward the end of the Ming period the pattern of diseases in China resembled that in South Asia and Europe. In 1633 the Ming Dynasty came under threat from the Manchu army, descended from non-Chinese Manchurian tribes. The Manchu were so aware of the dangers of smallpox that they used only soldiers who had recovered from the disease or had been "immunized" against it [42], a successful strategy that ended the Ming Dynasty in 1644 and began the Qing Dynasty which ruled until 1911. Increased trade and the arrival of Europeans in the seventeenth century did not have the devastating effects seen in the Americas as the local people had already experienced all the diseases likely to have been carried by foreigners.

From earliest times China was in conflict with its neighbor, Japan, and this came to a head with the "Sino-Japanese war" 1894–1895 when the two countries went of war over Korea. The Chinese were comprehensively defeated and this marked the beginning of Japan as a world power. The Japanese despised the Chinese and this led to the creation of the infamous "Unit 731" the objective of which was to manufacture biological weapons for use against the Chinese [43]. Between 1940 and 1942 the Japanese bombed over 12 Chinese cities with a variety of agents including plague-infested fleas and, in one attack on Quzhou, 50,000 died and in Ningbo 97% of the population were killed. Altogether 200,000–400,000 people perished. The Allied defeat of Japan in 1945 brought these activities to an end.

Humans have inhabited Japan for over 10,000 years, but our knowledge of diseases during the early history of Japan is very limited because of the country's self-imposed isolation which, coupled with the fact that the population was widely distributed in small groups, also rendered it relatively free from infectious diseases. Early chronicles dating from about 710 to 720 BC refer to diseases which might have been malaria, tuberculosis, and leprosy, but the whole period 200 BC–AD 495 seems to have been free of any significant impact of any diseases despite the growth in population over this period. However, in AD 495 smallpox arrived from Korea but did not spread very far because population movements were limited largely due to the nature of the terrain. Between AD 700 and 1050 Japan suffered from a series of 10 devastating "plagues." These included smallpox in 735–737 ("the great smallpox epidemic"), 790, 812–814, 833, and 853, bubonic plague in 808, influenza between 862 and 1015, and measles in 998 and 1025. The 735–737 "great smallpox" epidemic alone killed between 30% and 40% of those infected. These plagues had effects similar to those of the Black Death in Europe including economic stagnation. In addition, Chinese influence declined and Buddhism was adopted. These plagues also allowed the population to build up their herd immunity and between 1050 and 1260 infectious disease had ceased to dominate people's lives and smallpox had become a disease of childhood. With the expansion of trade routes and the arrival of Europeans in 1543, the only disease passed on to the naive population was syphilis.

The Japanese economy continued to thrive and with one exception (apart from the venture into biological warfare discussed earlier) disease played little part in the development of the country or its economy. The exception was in the early twentieth century when the Japanese used their knowledge of malaria to persuade the population of Taiwan to abandon their way life and to become more Japanese [44].

Korea was established in the late third millennium BC by people from northern China and was conquered by the Chinese in 108 BC, by the Mongols in 1231, and became a Japanese Protectorate in 1904–1905. The first records of smallpox epidemics, via India and China, are from the third century BC and there were epidemics in AD 552, 585–587, 735–737, and 765 from whence the disease passed to Japan. There were further epidemics in 1418, between 1424 and 1675 and 1680, all with devastating effects, during which kings, princes, and other important leaders died. The population of Korea had not been exposed to European diseases in the same way as the Japanese and in 1707 and between 1752 and 1775 there were epidemics of measles, called "dot eruption disease." By 1883 smallpox had become a childhood disease and virtually everyone had scars from the disease or inoculation. By the end of the century smallpox had been virtually eradicated and the pattern of infectious diseases in Korea closely resembled that in the Americas. Infectious diseases in Korea, although they had important effects locally and in the neighboring countries, made negligible impact on world history.

Conclusions

Infectious diseases have played a significant role in determining the political maps of the world that have evolved over millennia. Cholera, leprosy, typhoid, typhus, plague, tuberculosis, measles, smallpox, yellow fever, and malaria have all contributed to important historical events such as the decline of the powers of Athens and Rome, the rise of Islam, the end of the feudal system in Europe, the colonization of the Americas, Africa, and Australasia, the end of French colonialism in the Americas, and numerous examples of disruption of economic development and subsequent political consequences. In addition, there must have been thousands, if not millions, of minor recorded and unrecorded events, the effects of which have not been evaluated, that might have turned out differently had disease not intervened.

Acknowledgment

I would like to thank Prof. Sir Roderick Floud for his careful reading of the penultimate draft of this chapter and for his helpful suggestions. Any errors, however, are my own.

References

1. Kjellén R. Der Staat als Lebenstraum. Leipzig: S. Hirzel, 1917.
2. Jackson WAD. Politics and Geographic Relationships. Englewood Cliff: Prentice Hall, 1964.
3. Kohn GC. Dictionary of Wars. New York: Checkmark, 1999.
4. Smallman-Raynor MR, Cliff AD. Impact of infectious diseases on war. Infect Dis Clin North Am 2004;18:341–68.
5. Zinsser H. Rats, Lice and History. London: Routledge, 1935. Reprinted London: Penguin Books, 2000.
6. Stringer C, McKie R. African Exodus. The Origins of Modern Humanity. London: Jonathan Cape, 1997.
7. Fernádex-Armesto F. 1492 The Year Our World Began. London: Bloomsbury, 2010.
8. Anderson R, May R. Infectious Diseases of Humans: Dynamics and Control. Oxford: Oxford University Press, 1991.
9. McKeown T. The Modern Rise of Population. London: Edward Arnold, 1976.
10. American Academy of Pediatrics. Red Book 2009. Report on the Committee on Infectious Diseases 2009. Washington, DC: American Academy of Pediatrics, 2009.
11. Ackernecht EH. History and Geography of the Most Important Diseases. New York and London: Hafner, 1965.
12. Creighton C. A History of Epidemics in Britain, 2 vols. Cambridge: Cambridge University Press, 1965.
13. Cliff A, Haggett P, Smallman-Raynor M. Deciphering Global Epidemics. Cambridge: Cambridge University Press, 1989.
14. Diamond J. Guns, Germs and Steel. London: Jonathan Cape, 1997.
15. Hays JN. The Burdens of Disease. Epidemics and Human Response in Western History. New Brunswick, NJ: Rutgers University Press, 1998.

16. Kipple KF (ed). The Cambridge World History of Human Disease. Cambridge: Cambridge University Press, 1993.
17. Lockwood JA. Six-Legged Soldiers. Oxford: Oxford University Press, 2009.
18. McKeown T. The Origins of Human Disease. Oxford: Blackwell, 1988.
19. McNeill WH. Plagues and People. New York: Bantam Doubleday, 1976.
20. Major RH. Classic Descriptions of Disease, 3rd edn. Springfield, IL: CT Thompson, 1945.
21. Oldstone MBA. Viruses, Plagues, and History. New York: Oxford University Press, 1998.
22. Sherman IW. Twelve Diseases That Changed Our World. Washington: ASM Press, 2007.
23. Kinder H, Hilgeman W. The Penguin Atlas of World History, 2 vols. New York: Penguin Books, 1978.
24. Overy R (ed). The Times Complete History of the World, 6th edn. London: Harper Collins, 2004.
25. Parker P. World History. London: Dorling Kindersley, 2010.
26. Ingram A. The new geopolitics of disease: between global health and global security. Geopolitics 2005;10:522–45.
27. Cunha BA. The death of Alexander the Great: malaria or typhoid fever? Infect Dis Clin North Am 2004;18(1):53–63.
28. Stobart JC. The fourth century. In: Hopper RJ (ed). The Glory That Was Greece, 4th edn. London: Sidgewick and Jackson, 1964:182–217.
29. Longrigg J. The great plague of Athens. Hist Sci 1980;18:209–25.
30. Stobart JC. The growth of the Empire. In: Maguinness WS, Scullard HH (eds). The Grandeur That Was Rome, 4th edn. London: Sidgewick and Jackson, 1961:201–75.
31. Horrox R. The Black Death. Manchester, UK: Manchester University Press, 1994.
32. Hirst LH. The Conquest of Plague. Oxford: Clarendon Press, 1953.
33. Phillips H, Killingray D. The Spanish Influenza Pandemic of 1918–1919: New Perspectives. London and New York: Routledge, 2003.
34. Verano JW, Ubelaker DH. Disease and Demography in the Americas. Washington: Smithsonian Institute, 1992.
35. Augustin G. History of Yellow Fever. New Orleans: Searcy and Pfaff, 1909.
36. Crosby MC. The American Plague. New York: Berkley Books, 2006.
37. Pierce JR. Yellow Jack: How Yellow Fever Ravaged America and Walter Reed Discovered Its Deadly Secrets. Hoboken, NJ: John Wiley & Sons, 2005.
38. Campbell J. Invisible Enemies: Smallpox and Other Diseases in Aboriginal Australia. Melbourne: Melbourne University Press, 2002.
39. Curston P, McCracken K. Plague in Sydney. Kensington, NSW: Sydney University Press, 1980.
40. Vincent W. The Periplus of the Erythrean Sea. London: T Cadell and W Davies, 1800.
41. Cox FEG. History of sleeping sickness (African trypanosomiasis). Infect Dis Clin North Am 2004;18(2):231–45.
42. Serruys H. Smallpox in Mongolia during the Ming and Ching dynasties. Zentralasiat Stud 1980;14:41–68.
43. Harris SH. Factories of Death: Japanese Biological Warfare 1932–45 and the American Cover-Up, Revised edn. New York and London: Routledge, 2002.
44. Ku Ya Wen. Anti-malarial policy and its consequences in colonial Taiwan. In: Ka-che Yip (ed). Disease, Colonisation and the State: Malaria in Modern East Asian History. Hong Kong: Hong Kong University Press, 2009:31–48.

Chapter 2
Detection of infectious diseases using unofficial sources

Lawrence C. Madoff[1] and David O. Freedman[2]

[1]Division of Infectious Diseases, Beth Israel Deaconess Medical Center, Harvard Medical School and Brigham and Women's Hospital, Boston, MA, USA
[2]Division of Infectious Diseases, University of Alabama at Birmingham, Birmingham, AL, USA

Infectious disease surveillance systems have embraced the Internet. ProMED-mail is a rapid reporting system of emerging infectious diseases in humans, animals, and plants. ProMED-mail relies on local news sources like newspapers and their web sites and local rapporteurs submitting reports of unusual events such as the first English language report of SARS. Each report on ProMED-mail is placed into perspective by an expert in the field and whether the report is credible or not is discussed. Provider-based surveillance of travelers has also become increasingly sophisticated. Monitoring disease trends geolocation of acquired diseases among travelers can inform both pretravel advice and posttravel management. Data from sentinel travelers upon their return to medically sophisticated environments can also benefit local populations in resource-limited countries. Networks such as GeoSentinel have provided cumulative trends in travel-related illness to assess pretravel risk for mass gathering events such as the Beijing Olympic Games or the FIFA World Cup in South Africa. Data provided by the GeoSentinel also helped in determining the seasonality of dengue by region of travel and risk of acquiring schistosomiasis by destination. Global surveillance of travel-related disease represents a powerful tool for the detection of infectious diseases. Such data should encourage clinicians to take a detailed travel history during every patient encounter.

Introduction

Informal source surveillance

Traditional public health surveillance depends on a hierarchy of reporting systems. Practitioners, field personnel, laboratories, hospitals, and other health-care facilities report on selected diseases and outbreaks first through local, state, or provincial agencies, who in turn report these events, often in aggregated numerical form, to higher governmental and then regional or international groups. Such reporting is often regulated and mandated by governmental authorities and is the basis of publicly available health statistics, and often forms the basis for governmental responses to outbreaks. International agencies such as the World Health Organization (WHO) or the Office International des Épizooties (OIE; World Organisation for

Infectious Diseases: A Geographic Guide, First Edition.
Edited by Eskild Petersen, Lin H. Chen & Patricia Schlagenhauf.
© 2011 John Wiley & Sons, Ltd. Published 2011 by John Wiley & Sons, Ltd.

Animal Health) may then communicate news of significant outbreaks to health agencies in other countries or to the public and often forms the basis for international responses. Such reporting systems have many advantages. Particularly in parts of the world where the public health infrastructure is well funded and robust, these systems can effectively capture important infectious disease events and do so in a thorough and sensitive manner.

However, formal public health reporting systems are not without disadvantages. Delays at any level (or at several levels) can result in unacceptable lags as reports must traverse numerous officials prior to reaching national and international attention. Likewise, failure at any level to collect or transmit the information to the next level can result in information never reaching those with the capacity to respond—a break in any link in the chain resulting in failure of the system. Moreover, there is often incentive not to report on the presence of diseases or to delay reporting as long as possible. Disease outbreaks can disrupt commerce, discourage tourism, or damage the reputation of a locality, region, or country. For example, the discovery of Bovine Spongiform Ecephalopathy (BSE) in a single cow in the United States led to a ban on importation of US beef into Japan that persisted for years [1].

In addition, many official surveillance systems focus on specified "reportable" diseases. As such, they may fail to detect or report newly emerged, undiagnosed, or undefined illnesses even if they threaten public health.

A convergence of trends

In the 1970s and 1980s, some authorities believed that infectious diseases were, or were soon to be, "conquered." Adherents to this notion believed that antimicrobials, improved public health measures, vaccines and general improvements in the human condition would virtually eliminate infectious diseases. Indeed, it was argued that the medical specialty of infectious diseases might become unnecessary, at least in developed countries. This thought was soon challenged, however, by the evidence of a multitude of diseases that appeared during this era, not the least of which was HIV infection. By the 1990s, the concept of disease emergence and reemergence had become prominent and the 1992 publication by the Institute of Medicine report entitled "Emerging Infections: Microbial Threats to Human Health in the United States" brought these ideas to the forefront.

At the same time, the Internet was moving from an exclusive tool of the military and academia into the mainstream. With advent of commercial Internet service providers such as America Online, the use of e-mail became common even outside of academic institutions. The birth of the World Wide Web meant that individuals around the world without specific technical skills were exchanging more and more information. Moreover, the dissolution of the Soviet Union had revealed the existence of a massive biological warfare program, raising awareness of the threat of the intentional or accidental release of agents that could cause biological harm.

Indeed, it was at a WHO-sponsored meeting on the threat of biological weapons, that the use of the Internet for exchanging information on biological threats was pioneered. Attendees at this meeting, held in 1993, began to exchange e-mails regarding outbreaks of diseases potentially related to biological weapons in August of 1994. The members began a "listserv" that allowed anyone to send an e-mail to all members of the group. Soon, others heard of this list and requested to join. The originators dubbed this service "ProMED-mail" for the e-mail service of the Program for Monitoring Emerging Diseases.

As ProMED-mail rapidly grew, its founders realized it needed to better regulate the flow of information, and the service began to moderate posts to the lists. A report would flow through a central moderator who would select posts that would be sent to all members of the list and provide commentary on the contents of the reports. Reports included firsthand information from clinicians or laboratories on disease outbreaks as well as media reports of outbreaks. These reports from "informal" sources often preceded official reports of the same outbreaks, and often encouraged official sources to hasten the release of confirmatory reports, leading to an overall improvement in the reporting of outbreaks.

By 1999, ProMED outgrew its unstructured roots and became a part of the International Society for Infectious Diseases. This membership organization for infectious disease clinicians around the world provided financial backing for the fledgling organization and created a more formal organizational structure with an advisory board, an Editor, Associate Editors, and Subject Area Moderators. Infrastructure was reinforced with support provided by the Oracle Corporation and the Bill and Melinda Gates Foundation.

ProMED-mail today (www.promedmail.org)

ProMED is open to all sources of information. Much of the information comes from readers, who may send firsthand information such as a clinician witnessing an unusual syndrome or cluster. They may send local news media reports, not just those visible on the web, but also local radio or television broadcast reports. Laboratorians may report unusual emerging disease findings from public health, private, or academic laboratories. They may also report "rumors"—unverified often secondhand or thirdhand information. One notable example occurred when a ProMED reader, Steve Cunnion, sent ProMED a message relating to what a friend had told him regarding a teacher's chat room in China. This report of widespread pneumonia in Guangdong formed the basis of ProMED's report on severe acute respiratory syndrome (SARS), which occurred well in advance of most formal and informal reports. Currently ProMED has over 45 staff in 17 countries who communicate via the Internet (with face-to-face meetings held every year or two). ProMED's staff includes specialists in many aspects of emerging infectious diseases: virology, parasitology, bacteriology, epidemiology, toxicology, veterinary health, and medical infectious disease. ProMED staff and volunteers scour official and unofficial sites daily for news regarding outbreaks of emerging diseases. These include the sites of well-known international organizations like OIE, FAO, and WHO, but also many local and regional official health department sites, as well as blogs and specialized disease-focused web sites, and mailing lists [2–4].

As of this writing (November 2010) ProMED counts over 53,000 subscribers to its e-mail subscription service to the global list. A number of subscription options are available, including digest forms, animal- and plant-only, and a daily and weekly update that provides only the titles of reports with links to the full text. The web site attracts approximately 2 million to 20 million hits in a given month, with considerable variation apparently related to headline-generating outbreaks (e.g., the H1N1 pandemic). The web site also provides the ability to search using free text and by date range through the entire ProMED-mail archive of over 60,000 reports going back to 1994.

HealthMap (www.healthmap.org)

In the past 3 years, ProMED has begun an exciting collaboration with HealthMap.org based at Children's Hospital Boston and Harvard Medical School. This global service includes multilingual web-crawling capacity that automatically finds information on disease outbreaks in publicly available web sites, processes the information, and places it on a detailed Google map of the world. Since its beginning, HealthMap incorporated ProMED reports into its system. The collaboration began through the development of a specialized map of ProMED reports. Fostered in part by a grant from Google.org, this collaboration has now expanded and includes:

1 The provision of automated e-mail alerts of disease information mined by the HealthMap web crawler. These alerts can be tailored by disease, geography, and other features that allow ProMED specialty moderators to keep tabs on areas of their particular interest.

2 The capacity for ProMED staff to "curate" HealthMap reports: refining the disease name and adding accuracy and precision to the mapping process.

3 The inclusion of HealthMap detailed maps corresponding to areas of disease activity within ProMED reports.

4 The organization of ProMED's vast repository of disease reports (over 60,000 reports going back 16 years) into a structured database; this allows research activities concerning the timing, quality, and accuracy of both informal and official disease reports. This research in turn, will allow improvements to be made in the detection of disease outbreaks.

Provider-based surveillance in travelers

In recent years, clinicians have been faced with the emergence and rapid worldwide spread of novel influenza strains, SARS, Chikungunya virus, drug-resistant tuberculosis, and other conditions and pathogens. Modern transportation and increased tourism, business travel, and immigration contributed to dissemination of these high-impact pathogens. Human movement has occurred for centuries and will continue, despite the threats posed by infectious agents.

As a result a closer look at globally mobile populations that move pathogens across international borders is necessary. Travelers can spread new and reemerging infectious diseases that initially appear in developing countries, and they act as ideal sentinels for the early detection of these diseases. Specialized travel/tropical medicine clinics are ideally situated to effectively detect emerging infections and to track ongoing trends in travel-related illness. Returning travelers seen at a few sentinel sites by such collaborative provider networks as GeoSentinel (www.geosentinel.org) [5,6] provide a sample of disease agents in more than 230 different countries. Real-time data are captured at the clinical point of service.

Sharing locally acquired disease information on Internet discussion forums and news groups such as ProMED-mail facilitates responses to rapidly evolving situations. More recently, automated news scanning software that aggregates and prioritizes potential sentinel disease events has allowed platforms such as HealthMap to publicly display on a Google Maps background all key travel-related infectious disease concerns. These resources may all be used in concert with existing public health system responses to inform infectious disease practitioners and improve diagnosis of ill-returned travelers.

Structure of the GeoSentinel Surveillance Network

GeoSentinel established in 1995, is the major provider-based surveillance network for travel-related illness. The GeoSentinel communications and data collection network currently comprises 53 travel/tropical medicine International Society of Travel Medicine (ISTM) member clinics. The 53 GeoSentinel sites participate in full sentinel surveillance and are located in 25 countries on all 6 continents (Figures 2.1 and 2.2). These clinics contribute clinic-based sentinel surveillance data on ill-returned travelers using direct Internet data entry at the point of care. GeoSentinel surveillance data enable patient diagnoses, country of exposure, chronology of travel, and standardized exposure details to be collected for detailed analysis of travel-related morbidity. In addition, such networks can detect disease outbreaks, enhance surveillance, and facilitate rapid communication, response, and dissemination of information among providers and public health partners. The GeoSentinel dataset (to March 1, 2011) contains 143,614 patient records and these records cover traveler exposures in over 237 countries and territories. In 2010 the database grew by 22,347 records.

An additional 199 ISTM clinics have joined the GeoSentinel Network Members program from 39 countries on 6 continents. They communicate unusual or alarming cases to GeoSentinel and as well as participate in enhanced surveillance and response. Alerts and advisories covering important disease risks and outbreaks in collaboration with CDC and other international organizations are channeled through GeoSentinel clinics as well as through the remaining 2,500 ISTM members in 75 countries.

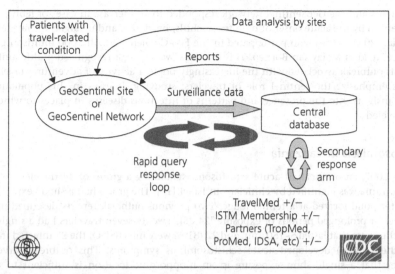

Fig. 2.1 How does GeoSentinel work?

What is GeoSentinel?

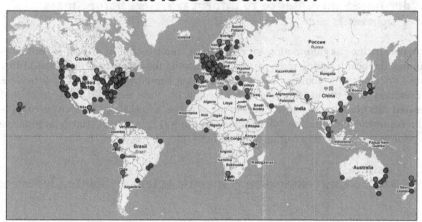

 • <u>Provider-based Surveillance</u> of international travelers and migrants.
Does not cover endemic diseases in local populations
● 53 travel/tropical medicine clinics globally (since 1996)
● 199 Network Members on all 6 continents (since 2002)

Fig. 2.2 The 53 travel/tropical medicine clinics and 199 network members from 6 continents, all members of ISTM, participate in provider-based surveillance of international travelers and migrants. Surveillance does not cover endemic diseases in local populations.

Examples of provider-based surveillance response capabilities

Leptospirosis in Borneo

A good example of effective detection of outbreaks among travelers was the outbreak report of leptospirosis among "Eco-Challenge" athletes [7–9]. In September 2000, two US health departments and the GeoSentinel network responded to an increase in cases of febrile illness, characterized by the acute onset of high fever, chills, headache, and myalgias in travelers from more than 20 countries who participated in the Eco-Challenge-Sabah 2000 multisport endurance race, held in Malaysian Borneo. This outbreak was the first recognized multicountry leptospirosis outbreak associated with the increasingly popular activity of adventure travel. These findings emphasize the sentinel role of travelers; studying illnesses in this population can provide insights into the presence and patterns of infectious diseases in places to which they have traveled.

Schistosomiasis in Tanzania

In April 2007, an outbreak of acute schistosomiasis among a group of 34 travelers returning from Tanzania was identified by clinicians in Israel [10]. The group had a single exposure to a freshwater pond located at a tented lodge. Two previous outbreak reports described multiple exposures or prolonged periods of exposure [24,25]. Twenty-seven travelers had a single exposure to the water that lasted 5–150 min, and 22 (81%) were infected. Of the 22 infected travelers, 19 of them (86%) developed acute schistosomiasis symptoms. This outbreak serves as a reminder that a single short exposure in an inopportune location is sufficient to acquire schistosomiasis. Thus, clinicians should be aware that screening tests for schistosomiasis should be performed on returned travelers with freshwater exposure in Africa.

Provider-based surveillance to inform travelers before mass gathering events

Identifying specific risk information for destination countries can be critical to protect public and individual health during mass gatherings. Ongoing data collection by global health surveillance systems allows country-specific analyses that can provide travelers and their healthcare providers with useful information to prepare for their trips. An early 2008 study of aggregated data from ill travelers to China in the previous decade allowed provision of evidence-based recommendations for the 2008 Beijing Olympics [11]. A similar study was published in 2010 prior to the FIFA World Cup in South Africa [12].

Provider-based surveillance and specific travel-associated infections

Dengue

A recent GeoSentinel study from 1997 through 2006 defined, for the first time, seasonality of dengue in 522 returned travelers [13]. Most (68%) of the travelers went to Asia, 15% to Latin America, 9% to the Caribbean, 5% to Africa, and 2% to Oceania. Thailand, India, Indonesia, and Brazil reported the most cases among returned travelers. Data showed peaks of infections in south-east Asia in June and September, south-central Asia (i.e., India and Bangladesh) in October, South America in March and August, and the Caribbean in October. These data provide information on relative risk according to season. Also, detecting dengue cases at atypical times in sentinel travelers can inform the international community of epidemic activity in specific areas. In April 2002, GeoSentinel alerted the international community when it posted a notice of the increase in travel-related dengue from Thailand on ProMED-mail [14]. Official surveillance data from local populations were not immediately available. Data reported later by Thai authorities to the WHO confirmed the observation.

Geolocalization and visualization on the HealthMap platform

The GeoSentinel HealthMap (Figure 2.3) collaboration displays a subset of key GeoSentinel diagnoses from individual patients on a worldwide Google map in real time as soon as patient records are entered into the system. Event icons display links to relevant web pages in seven languages from HealthMap's (www.healthmap.org) proprietary news-crawling software allowing for detection of diagnosis clusters or of suspicious syndromes (e.g., unknown fever) that arise in close proximity [15,16]. Patient icons also contain real-time generation of time-series visualizations of that event in the context of all previous occurrences of that diagnosis in the GeoSentinel database. This is a customized GeoSentinel version of the public HealthMap in collaboration with the HealthMap team at Harvard. HealthMap has also provided contextualized outbreak information integration with GeoSentinel data, such as HealthMap news stories and ProMED alerts visible on the GeoSentinel HealthMap.

Analysis of morbidity and estimating risk by destination

GeoSentinel provides a rich database of travel-related morbidity which has allowed for considerable analysis of destination-specific infectious disease profiles and risk factors [17]. When

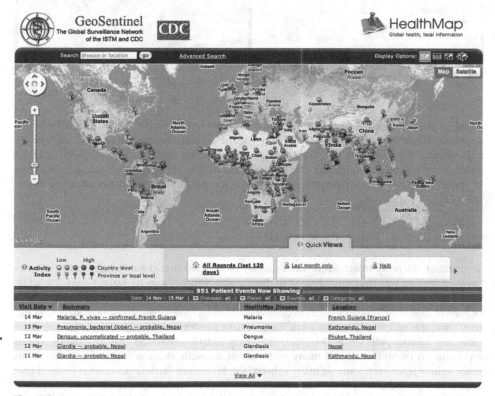

Fig. 2.3 Output of significant events is visually geolocated using a Google Maps platform. HealthMap heralds a generation of surveillance technology that complements existing travelers' health surveillance systems [12,13].

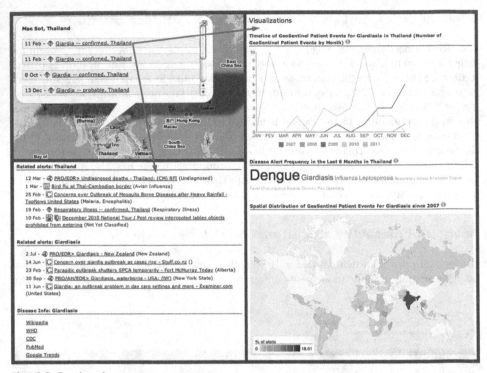

Fig. 2.3 Continued

patients present to clinicians after travel to the developing world, travel destinations are associated with the probability of the diagnosis of certain diseases. Diagnostic approaches and empiric therapies can be guided by these destination-specific differences. In addition advice for the prospective traveler can be prioritized and tailored. A large number of analyses of specific diseases, specific destinations, and specific patient characteristics are cited below [18–44].

One medicine: animal and plant health

Students of emerging infectious diseases quickly recognized that the movement of pathogens between species was frequently linked to disease emergence. From its earliest days, ProMED-mail espoused a "one medicine" or "one health" philosophy that recognized the commonality of human and animal diseases. Just as disease outbreaks crossed geographic boundaries, so did they cross species boundaries. Zoonotic diseases have proven to be the most frequent source of emerging human pathogens. Therefore, veterinary health has always played a major role in reporting on ProMED-mail and many outbreaks of zoonotic diseases (plague, anthrax, tularemia, yellow fever, rabies among many others) [45]. Moreover, ProMED's founders realized that animal and plant diseases, even if they did not cross over to humans, could affect human health by impacting food supplies. Therefore foot and mouth disease, bluetongue (diseases exclusively of animals), and wheat rust could cause natural disasters and be used as agents of biological warfare.

Regional networks

Some regions of the world are underserved by communications technology and Internet access. These areas often include the very areas that are recognized as emerging disease hotspots, such as the Amazon region of South America, Southeast Asia, and sub-Saharan Africa. To help address these inequities, to improve cross-border communication within these regions and to improve the flow of emerging disease reports into and out of these regions, ProMED-mail has launched several regional networks. These networks have a degree of independence from the global ProMED list, although ProMED provides the infrastructure, funding and training for them, they are administered by a regional top moderator who makes decisions on which posts to carry, based on local interests. ProMED's first regional network was ProMED-ESP, a Spanish-language network based in Latin America and ProMED-Port similarly covers Portuguese-speaking Latin America. Other networks include ProMED-MBDS (Mekong Basin Diseases Surveillance) based in Southeast Asia and providing posts in English with limited translation capacity for other regional languages such as Vietnamese, Thai, and Chinese. ProMED-RUS provides Russian-language reports for the newly independent states of the former Soviet Union. The two most recent additions, ProMED-EAFR and ProMED-FRA provide reports in English and French respectively covering the African region.

Each service has a separately available e-mail list as well as its own web site for those interested in those particular areas of the world. As expected, these regional networks have provided enormously rich content that is rebroadcast on the global ProMED-mail service.

Effectiveness of informal source surveillance

Numerous other programs have begun to use informal source surveillance including automated systems like HealthMap and Canada's Global Public Health Information Network (GPHIN), Biocaster, Medisys, and others as well as more human-driven systems such as Georgetown's Argus project [46]. Moreover, the use of informal sources and the Internet for outbreak detection has been widely accepted by the global public health community and codified in the revisions to the International Health Regulations ratified by the World Health Assembly in 2005 and taking effect in 2007. Recent work has demonstrated that the time from the beginning of an outbreak until its detection has been reduced as informal source surveillance has blossomed [47].

Conclusion

Surveillance of imported infectious diseases facilitates the detection of outbreaks of international public health concern. Surveillance data can inform guidelines to protect the health of future travelers. Collection of population-based data from 230 countries is difficult and, therefore provider-based sentinel systems in returned travelers are an innovative way to sample disease trends and emerging infections globally. Automated news scanning and data fusion technologies show promise in generation of early warning systems for disease emergence.

References

1. ProMED-mail. BSE, bovine–USA (WA)(16): new regulations. ProMED-mail 2004. 18-MAR-2004. Archive Number: 20040318.0747. Accessed November 1, 2010 at http://www.promedmail.org.

2. Cowen P, Garland T, Hugh-Jones ME, et al. Evaluation of ProMED-mail as an electronic early warning system for emerging animal diseases: 1996 to 2004. JAMA 2006;229(7):1090–99.

3. Madoff LC, Woodall JP. The Internet and the global monitoring of emerging diseases: lessons from the first 10 years of ProMED-mail. Arch Med Res 2005;36(6):724–30.

4. Madoff LC. ProMED-mail: an early warning system for emerging diseases. Clin Infect Dis 2004;39:227–32.

5. Freedman DO, Kozarsky PE, Weld LH, Cetron MS, for the GeoSentinel Study Group. Special report: GeoSentinel: the Global Emerging Infections Sentinel Network of the International Society of Travel Medicine. J Travel Med 1999;6(2):94–8.

6. Freedman DO, Weld LH, Kozarsky PE, et al., for the GeoSentinel Surveillance Network. Spectrum of disease and relation to place of exposure among ill returned travelers. N Engl J Med 2006;354(2):119–30.

7. Freedman DO. Leptospirosis—UK, USA, Canada ex Malaysia (Borneo). ProMED-mail. 12-SEP-2000. Archive Number: 20000912.1553.

8. Update: Outbreak of acute febrile illness among athletes participating in Eco-Challenge-Sabah 2000—Borneo, Malaysia, 2000. MMWR Morb Mortal Wkly Rep 2001;50;21–4.

9. Sejvar J, Bancroft E, Winthrop K, et al. and the Eco-Challenge Investigation Team. Leptospirosis in "Eco-Challenge" athletes, Malaysian Borneo, 2000. Emerg Infect Dis 2003;9(6):702–7.

10. Freedman DO, Schwartz E, von Sonnenburg F. Schistosomiasis—Tanzania (Lake Eyasi). ProMED-mail. 04-SEP-2007. Archive Number: 20070904.2912.

11. Davis XM, MacDonald S, Borwein S, et al., for the GeoSentinel Surveillance Network. Health risks in travelers to China: the GeoSentinel experience and implications for the 2008 Beijing Olympics. Am J Trop Med Hyg 2008;79(1):4–8.

12. Mendelson M, Davis X, Jensenius M, et al. Short report: health risks in travelers to South Africa: the GeoSentinel experience and implications for the 2010 FIFA World Cup. Am J Trop Med Hyg 2010;82(6):991–5.

13. Schwartz E, Weld LH, Wilder-Smith A, et al., for the GeoSentinel Surveillance Network. Seasonality, annual trends, and characteristics of dengue among ill returned travelers, 1997–2006. Emerg Infect Dis 2008;14(7):1081–8.

14. Freedman DO, Kozarsky PE. Dengue/DHF updates (16): April 26, 2002 (2) Thailand: out of season dengue outbreak in travellers to Koh Phangan. ProMED-mail. 26-APR-2002. Archive Number: 20020426.4039.

15. Brownstein JS, Freifeld CC, Madoff LC. Digital disease detection – harnessing the Web for public health surveillance. N Engl J Med 2009;360(21):2153–5, 2157.

16. Brownstein JS, Freifeld CC, Reis BY, Mandl KD. Surveillance sans frontières: Internet-based emerging infectious disease intelligence and the HealthMap project. PLoS Med 2008;5(7): e151.

17. Leder K, Wilson ME, Freedman DO, Torresi J. A comparative analysis of methodological approaches used for estimating risk in travel medicine. J Travel Med 2008;15(4):263–72.

18. Hagmann S, Neugebauer R, Schwartz E, et al. Illness in children after international travel: analysis from the GeoSentinel Surveillance Network. Pediatrics 2010;126(5):e1072–80. Published online April 5, 2010.

19. Schlagenhauf P, Chen LH, Wilson ME, et al. Sex and gender differences in travel-associated disease. Clin Infect Dis 2010;50(6):826–32.

20. Torresi J, Leder K. Defining infections in international travellers through the GeoSentinel Surveillance Network. Nat Rev Microbiol 2009;7(12):895–901.

21. Chen LH, Wilson ME, Davis X, et al., for the GeoSentinel Surveillance Network. Illness in long-term travelers visiting GeoSentinel clinics. Emerg Infect Dis 2009;15(11):1773–82.

22. Gautret P, Schlagenhauf P, Gaudart J, et al., for the GeoSentinel Surveillance Network. Multicenter EuroTravNet/GeoSentinel study of travel-related infectious diseases in Europe. Emerg Infect Dis 2009;15(11):1783–90.

23. Jensenius M, Davis X, von Sonnenburg F, et al., for the GeoSentinel Surveillance Network. Multicenter GeoSentinel analysis of rickettsial diseases in international travelers, 1996–2008. Emerg Infect Dis 2009;15(11):1791–8.

24. Swaminathan A, Torresi J, Schlagenhauf P, et al., for the GeoSentinel Network. A global study of pathogens and host risk factors associated with infectious gastrointestinal disease in returned travellers. J Infect 2009;59 (1):19–27.

25. Nicolls DJ, Weld LH, Schwartz E, et al., for the GeoSentinel Surveillance Network. Characteristics of schistosomiasis in travelers reported to the GeoSentinel Surveillance Network 1997–2008. Am J Trop Med Hyg 2008;79(5):729–34.

26. Lederman E, Weld LH, Elyazar IRF, et al., for the GeoSentinel Surveillance Network. Dermatologic conditions of the ill returned traveler: an analysis from the GeoSentinel Surveillance Network. Int J Infect Dis 2008;12 (6):593–602.

27. Greenwood Z, Black J, Weld L, et al., for the GeoSentinel Surveillance Network. Gastrointestinal infection among international travelers globally. J Travel Med 2008;15(4): 221–8.

28. Lipner EM, Law MA, Barnett E, et al., for the GeoSentinel Surveillance Network. Filariasis in travelers presenting to the GeoSentinel Surveillance Network. PLoS Negl Trop Dis 2007;1 (3):e88.

29. Wilson ME, Weld LH, Boggild A, et al., for the GeoSentinel Surveillance Network. Fever in returned travelers: results from the GeoSentinel Surveillance Network. Clin Infect Dis 2007;44:1560–68.

30. Gautret P, Schwartz E, Shaw M, et al., for the GeoSentinel Surveillance Network. Animal-associated injuries and related diseases among returned travellers: a review of the GeoSentinel Surveillance Network. Vaccine 2007;25(14): 2656–63.

31. Fenner L, Weber R, Steffen R, Schlagenhauf P. Imported infectious disease and purpose of travel, Switzerland. Emerg Infect Dis 2007;13 (2):217–22.

32. Leder K, Tong S, Weld L, et al., for the GeoSentinel Surveillance Network. Illness in travelers visiting friends and relatives: a review of the GeoSentinel Network. Clin Infect Dis 2006;43(9):1185–93.

33. Boggild AK, Yohanna S, Keystone JS, Kain KC. Prospective analysis of parasitic infections in Canadian travelers and immigrants. J Travel Med 2006;13(3):138–44.

34. CDC. Reported by Kay C, Patrick D, Keystone J, et al. Transmission of malaria in resort areas—Dominican Republic, 2004. MMWR Morb Mortal Wkly Rep 2005;53(51–52):1195–8.

35. Leder K, Black J, O'Brien D, et al., for the GeoSentinel Surveillance Network. Malaria in travelers: a review of the GeoSentinel Surveillance Network. Clin Infect Dis 2004;39(8):1104–12.

36. Elliott JH, O'Brien D, Leder K, et al., for the GeoSentinel Surveillance Network. Imported *Plasmodium vivax* malaria: demographic and clinical features in nonimmune travelers. J Travel Med 2004;11(4):213–17.

37. Leder K, Sundararajan V, Weld L, Pandey P, Brown G, Torresi J, for the GeoSentinel Surveillance Group. Respiratory tract infections in travelers: a review of the GeoSentinel Surveillance Network. Clin Infect Dis 2003;36(4): 399–406.

38. Shaw MT, Leggat PA, Weld LH, Williams ML, Cetron MS. Illness in returned travellers presenting at GeoSentinel sites in New Zealand. Aust N Z J Public Health 2003;27(1):82–6.

39. Simon F, Freedman DO. Chikungunya (08)—France ex Singapore. ProMED-mail. 23-APR-2009. Archive Number: 20090423.1524.

40. Freedman DO, Gkrania-Klotsas E, Jensenius M, Hagmann S. Malaria—Europe, USA, ex Gambia. ProMED-mail. 01-DEC-2008. Archive Number: 20081201.3775.

41. Parola P, Gautret P, Freedman DO. Dengue/DHF update (32): France ex Cote d'Ivoire. ProMED-mail. 08-AUG-2008. Archive Number: 20080808.2446.

42. Freedman DO, Burchard G. Malaria—Germany ex Bahamas: (Great Exuma). ProMED-mail. 16-APR-2008. Archive Number: 20080416.1369.

43. Nutman T. Trypanosomiasis—USA ex Tanzania (Serengeti): RFI. ProMED-mail. 13-JUL-2005. Archive Number: 20050713.1989.

44. Freedman DO. Wound infections, tsunami-related—Asia. ProMED-mail. 10-JAN-2005. Archive Number: 20050110.0079.

45. Madoff L. Cooperation between animal and human health sectors is key to the detection, surveillance, and control of emerging disease. Euro Surveill 2006;11(12):E061221.4.

46. Hartley D, Nelson N, Walters R, et al. The landscape of international event-based biosurveillance. Emerg Health Threats 2010;3:e3. doi:10.3134/ehtj.10.003.

47. Chan E, Brewer TF, Madoff LC, et al. Global capacity for emerging infectious disease detection. Proc Natl Acad Sci USA 2010; 107:21701–6.

Chapter 3
Microbes on the move: prevention, curtailment, outbreak

Patricia Schlagenhauf,[1] Giles Poumerol[2] and Francisco Santos-O'Connor[3]

[1]Center for Travel Medicine, University of Zürich and WHO Collaborating Centre for Travellers' Health, Zürich, Switzerland
[2]International Health Regulations Department, World Health Organization, Geneva, Switzerland
[3]European Centre for Disease Control (ECDC), Stockholm, Sweden

Infectious diseases are mobile and global. This chapter provides a brief overview of the prevention of infection during international travel, the revised International Health Regulations (IHR) with respect to curtailment of infection, and the European Centre for Disease Prevention and Control (ECDC) approach to outbreak investigation. Travel is an important factor in the spread of infection. Many disease risks can be mitigated by effective preventive measures such as the use of vaccines and chemoprophylaxis but there are no consensus guidelines worldwide on the global prevention of infectious disease in travelers. Individual travelers are ultimately responsible for their health and well being while traveling and on their return as well as for the prevention of the transmission of communicable disease to others. Yellow fever is the single disease for which proof of vaccination may be required as a condition of entry. It is difficult to curtail infectious disease as it can rapidly cross borders. The revised IHR (2005) were unanimously agreed upon by the World Health Assembly on May 23, 2005 as a global legal framework on the use of international law for public health purposes. Compared with the previous regulations, IHR 2005 expands the scope of internationally reportable diseases and events from three diseases (cholera, plaque, and yellow fever) to "all events which may constitute public health emergencies of international concern," thus providing criteria for identifying novel epidemic events, and specifying conditions for involvement of the international community in outbreak responses. The investigation and response to disease outbreaks requires a coordination of national and international organizations as well as multidisciplinary partnerships. Outbreak investigation, as practiced by the ECDC, extends beyond detection, assessment, and response support and includes a large range of activities and proactive work to strengthen public health capacity.

Prevention of disease in travelers

"Viruses and bacteria don't ask for a green card" a fact astutely observed in 1993 by the Surgeon General Antonia C. Novello. Human travel is subject to some degree of regulation but who

Infectious Diseases: A Geographic Guide, First Edition.
Edited by Eskild Petersen, Lin H. Chen & Patricia Schlagenhauf.
© 2011 John Wiley & Sons, Ltd. Published 2011 by John Wiley & Sons, Ltd.

MODEL INTERNATIONAL CERTIFICATE OF VACCINATION OR PROPHYLAXIS

This is to certify that [name].............................., date of birth.............., sex........................,

nationality..........................., national identification document, if applicable......................

whose signature follows...

has on the date indicated been vaccinated or received prophylaxis against:

(name of disease or condition)..

in accordance with the International Health Regulations.

Vaccine or prophylaxis	Date	Signature and professional status of supervising clinician	Manufacturer and batch No. of vaccine or prophylaxis	Certificate valid from... until.........	Official stamp of administering centre
1.					
2.					

Fig. 3.1 International Certificate of Vaccination and Prophylaxis. (Reproduced with permission from WHO [4].)

checks the microbial baggage? Most countries have no requirements regarding disease avoidance or vaccination coverage for visitors or travelers.

Protection of travelers and destination populations

Modern travel is swift and easy; it takes 36 h to travel around the world, much faster than the fanciful 80 days of Jules Verne's 1873 era. Today, international tourist arrivals exceed 900 million annually and are expected to top 1.5 billion by the year 2020. Who protects the traveler from the global onslaught of microbes encountered during travel that differ so markedly from those of his own home terrain? The destination country may also be impacted by the traveler who can introduce a pathogen into a new geographic or ecological niche such as the introduction of measles into the New World by Europeans or the transmission of the Chikungunya virus in Italy introduced by a traveler from India to local *Aedes albopictus*. Apart from some "obligatory entry requirements" such as yellow fever vaccination (Figure 3.1), general disease preventive measures are largely voluntary. Ultimately the traveler is responsible for his or her own health. He or she should seek pretravel advice on the risks of infectious disease at the destination, should use precautions to avoid transmitting any infectious disease to others during or after travel, should report any illness on return including information on recent travel. Who provides the traveler with all this information? In Europe, individual countries have national guidelines [1]. The US guidelines are formulated by the US Centers of Disease Control. The World Health Organization (WHO) publishes an annual volume entitled "International Travel and Health" which aims to meet the needs of national health administrations, practising travel health advisors, tourist agencies, shipping companies, airline operators, and all who are called on to give health advice to travelers (http://www.who.int/ith). A number of travel medicine web sites suggest global measures based on country of destination (Box 3.1) and these web sites are updated frequently. Concise, up-to-date information is key in the provision of advice on the prevention of disease in travelers.

Box 3.1 A selection of travel medicine web sites

WHO International Travel and Health   www.who.int/ith
CDC Centers for Disease Control   www.cdc.gov/travel/default.aspx
NaTHNaC National Travel Health Network and Centres   www.nathnac.org
For a broader listing see http://www.who.int/ith/links/national_links/en/index.html.

Travel health is an increasingly complex specialty and encompasses travel health advice and recommendations that should be evidence based and rooted in the epidemiology of travel-associated infections and diseases and their global, geographic distribution. Practitioners of preventive travel medicine include general practice health professionals such as general practice doctors and nurses, tropical medicine specialists, specialist "travel clinics," pharmacists, and occupational medicine professionals [1]. Those seeking pretravel health advice need indivi-dualized information on the disease profile at the destination and preventive measures such as vaccinations (routine and travel specific), malaria chemoprophylaxis or standby treatment as appropriate, vector bite protection, and also competent advice on a myriad of "minor to major" infectious conditions including travelers' diarrhea, waterborne and food-borne infections, droplet or contact infections, sexually transmitted diseases, and rabies. Recent analyses have shown that vaccine-preventable diseases are significant contributors to morbidity and potential mortality in travelers. More research is needed on the uptake, cost-effectiveness, and efficacy of travel medicine preventive measures. Increasingly, the Internet is becoming an important source of information for those seeking travel medicine advice and the importance of this source is likely to increase dramatically in the coming years and is recognized by the travel medicine community as a major player. Ideally, the travel industry should also play a role in informing potential travelers about possible health risks but this is a gray area and advice is usually confined to information about "obligatory vaccines." Currently, in terms of international regulations, yellow fever is the single disease with international require-ments with the exception of an obligatory quadrivalent meningococcal vaccination for Hajj pilgrims.

Yellow fever

The documented international certificate of vaccination is required by various countries as a condition of entry particularly if travelers are arriving from infected or potentially infected areas (see http://www.who.int/ith for this listing). An international certificate is for one individual only and is valid for 10 years provided that the yellow fever vaccine used has been approved by the WHO. The former "International Certificate of Vaccination or Revaccination Against Yellow Fever" has been revised to "International Certificate of Vaccination or Prophylaxis" and includes documentation, not just on yellow fever, but on any vaccine or prophylaxis (Figure 3.1). Currently, no European or North American country requires a yellow fever vaccination certificate as a condition of entry. An historical anecdote explains why the inter-national vaccination book is yellow; apparently in earlier times, ships entering a port could raise a yellow flag to indicate that the crew was free of infectious disease.

Imported disease

Infectious disease is mobile and global. Often, infection in the returned traveler develops only after a certain incubation period. In fourteenth century Europe, this led to the invention of the practice of "quarantine" (Italian *quaranta giorne* 40 days), a precaution which was adapted widely in Mediterranean ports (1348 Venice; 1377 Ragusa; and 1383 Marseille). In recent years, surveillance networks such as GeoSentinel [2] have made great progress in elucidating the epidemiology of travel-associated illness and have shown how the profile of acquired infections vary according to the geographic areas visited by the traveler (Figure 3.2). This knowledge can be used as an evidence base for the formulation of geography-cum-pathogen recommendations.

Curtailment of disease

The revised International Health Regulations (IHR) have a role in the curtailment of infectious disease. In the wake of the 2003 outbreak of severe acute respiratory syndrome (SARS), pre-paredness for public health emergencies was propelled into worldwide consciousness. The appearance and rapid international spread of SARS demonstrated to all—including global leaders, ministers of health, prime ministers, and heads of state—how an infectious disease can rapidly cross borders and deliver health threats and economic blows on an unimaginable scale [3] and the IHR 2005 were unanimously agreed upon by the World Health Assembly on May 23, 2005 [4].

This global legal framework constitutes a "major development in the use of international law for public health purposes."

New times, new requirements

The revised regulations reflect a growing understanding that the best way to prevent the global spread of diseases is to detect and contain them while they are still local. WHO member states have obligations to rapidly assess and alert the global community about potential disease threats as well as to prevent and control the spread of disease inside and beyond their borders. Compared with the previous regulations, adopted in 1969, IHR 2005 expands the scope of internationally reportable diseases and events, provides criteria for identifying novel epidemic events, and specifies conditions for involvement of the international community in outbreak responses. The revision includes the following five substantive changes.

Expanded scope

The previous regulations applied to only three infectious diseases: cholera, plague, and yellow fever. IHR 2005 reflect shifting concepts about disease control, shaped by recent and impending disease threats and the experiences of the past two decades in detecting and responding to disease outbreaks. The revised regulations replace the previous disease-specific framework with one built on timely notification of all events that might constitute a public health emergency of international concern, taking into account the context in which an event occurs. The advantage of this approach is its applicability to existing threats as well as to those that are new and unforeseen.

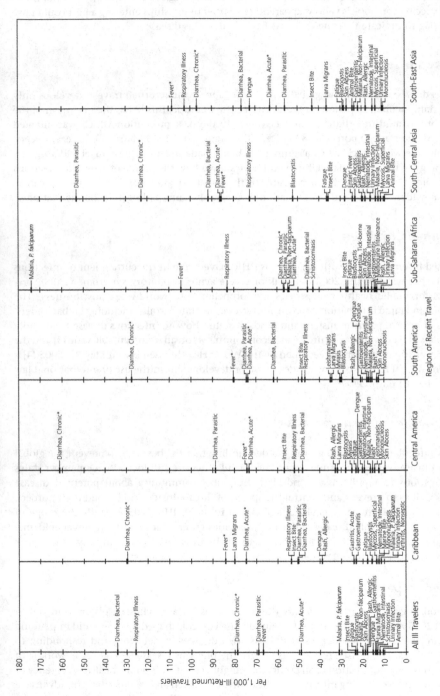

Fig. 3.2 Proportionate morbidity of disease according to region of travel. (Reproduced from Freedman et al. [2], with permission from Massachusetts Medical Society.)

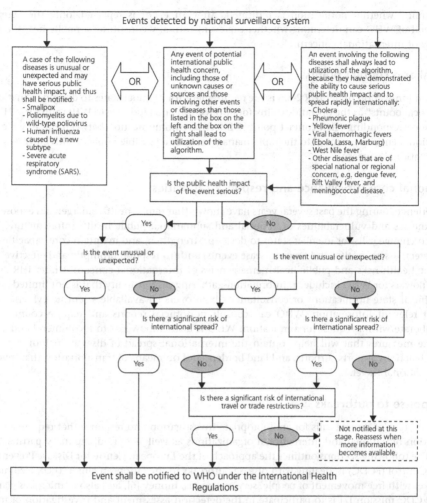

Fig. 3.3 Decision instrument for the assessment and notification of events that may constitute a public health emergency of international concern. Annex 2—International Health Regulations (IHR).

Decision instrument and notification

Expanding the scope of the IHR beyond reporting of three diseases to reporting of any public health emergency of international concern required an algorithm to assist in identification of such events. The resulting decision instrument (Figure 3.3) identifies a limited set of criteria for use by member states for fulfilling the obligation to determine whether an event occurring within their territory might constitute a public health emergency of international concern and therefore require formal notification to WHO within 24 h of assessment.

IHR 2005 include a list of diseases for which a single case must be reported to WHO immediately, regardless of the context in which the disease occurs. This list includes smallpox, poliomyelitis due to wild-type poliovirus, human influenza caused by a new subtype, or SARS. In addition, an event involving certain other diseases (e.g., cholera, pneumonic plague, yellow fever, viral hemorrhagic fevers) calls for a careful evaluation using the decision instrument to determine whether notification is indicated. After an event is reported, only the Director General of WHO can determine whether the event formally constitutes a public health emergency of international concern.

Focal and contact points

A third innovation under IHR 2005 is the requirement for member states to designate "national IHR focal points" as the operational link for notification and reporting to WHO and for WHO to name corresponding "IHR contact points." Effective communication between these two organizational entities is central to the rapid management of a possible public health emergency of international concern.

National core surveillance and response capacities

Experiences during the past several years have shown that public health emergencies expose the weaknesses and vulnerabilities of national and subnational public health infrastructure. The fourth change calls for member states to develop, strengthen, and maintain core capacities to: (i) detect, assess, notify, and report disease events; and (ii) respond promptly and effectively to public health risks and public health emergencies of international concern. Under IHR 2005, new powers for WHO include an information-gathering responsibility that is not limited solely to official state notifications or consultations but covers all available scientific evidence and other relevant information. WHO can consult nonofficial reports and require countries to collaborate with a request for verification. WHO is also empowered to recommend and coordinate measures that will help contain the international spread of disease, including public health actions at ports, airports, and land borders, and on means of transportation that involve international travel.

Response to outbreaks

An outbreak of disease calls for an appropriate investigation and response that require a coordination of national and international organizations as well as multidisciplinary partnerships [5]. The following sections outlines the approach of the European Centre for Disease Prevention and Control (ECDC) in dealing with disease outbreaks in the European Union (EU), a common market with free movement of people, services, goods, money [6], and also of microbes. Part of the ECDC mission [7] is to participate in the detection assessment and investigation of international outbreaks according to the following steps.

Identification of communicable disease public health alerts   The process starts by searching for information signals heralding potential EU concern outbreaks. Surveillance systems should be sensitive enough to detect signals indicating outbreaks with epidemic potential efficiently to implement control measures as soon as possible. ECDC achieves this by analyzing data from indicator-based surveillance systems (at EU level, The European Surveillance System [TESSy, see http://www.ecdc.europa.eu/en/activities/surveillance/Pages/Surveillance_Tessy.aspx] provides a one-stop-shop for case-based reporting from the Member States (MS) for the routine surveillance of the 46 diseases listed in the Decisions 2002/253/EC and 2003/534/EC plus SARS, West Nile Fever, and Avian Influenza [8, 9]) and filtering information from event-based surveillance systems (which gather unstructured data from sources of any nature [10], e.g., MedISys [see http://medusa.jrc.it]). Unofficial sources (e.g., media) require validation (i.e., confirmation of authenticity) by cross-checking the information against independent sources. In this context, the newly developed Epidemic Intelligence Information System (EPIS, see http://ecdc.europa.eu/en/activities/epidemicintelligence/Pages/EpidemicIntelligence_Tools.aspx), a real-time European web-based communication platform, offers a valuable tool for MS experts to exchange information on outbreak identification, validation, and assessment. Some sources always report validated events, such as the EU Early Warning and Response System (EWRS) [11], the WHO through the IHR, and institutional web sites. Moreover, MS communicate validated events having a potential to affect other countries through the EWRS assessed by their public health authorities against established notification criteria [11, 12]. The ECDC then gathers all available information to characterize the reported outbreaks by time, place, and persons affected to assess the risk for EU spread. Signals of potential or definite outbreaks with potential public health and EU relevance in terms of severity, spread, and need for further actions, generate public health alerts which are evaluated to decide the need for a European level coordinated response.

Outbreak response and rapid risk assessment Response activities include risk assessment, risk management, and risk communication. In the EU, the MS are responsible for risk management, supported by the coordination of the European Commission (EC) that is also engaged in risk communication. The ECDC mandate [7] covers risk assessment and communication but it can also provide scientific support to the risk management activities. Other stakeholders such as European and international networks, other European agencies, and international organizations (i.e., the WHO) can be involved.

EU response action plan The EC may then coordinate a plan of action as was the case with the 2009 influenza A (H1N1) pandemic, creating an ad hoc response team with representatives from the affected MS, the ECDC, the EC and, if relevant, other stakeholders. It includes the coordination of an EU wide outbreak investigation, complementing the investigation being carried out in the affected Member States. This usually includes the following stages, several of which may have begun before and can occur simultaneously:

1 Confirm outbreak and diagnosis.
2 Case definition: to facilitate common dataset collection and comparable analysis when several EU countries are involved a common case definition is used (EU case definition where relevant [13]).
3 Case finding: efforts are made to search for additional cases and for further descriptive and analytical epidemiology in all MS and outside the EU, through indicator and event-based surveillance.
4 Data collection: a common line listing for cases and key variables at an EU level allows uncovering previously unsuspected associations between cases.
5 Descriptive epidemiology: cases are described by time, place, and person.
6 Generating a hypothesis: the epidemiological description can provide a hypothesis regarding the infection source.
7 Testing the hypothesis: Different types of analytical studies can be considered (e.g., case–control or cohort studies, seroprevalence studies, spatial mapping) to reveal an association between a risk factor and disease. Additional epidemiological, environmental, and microbiological investigations may be required.
8 Control measures (coordinated by the EC): these involve controlling the infection source (if needed liaising with other stakeholders, e.g., Rapid Alert System for Food and Feed, RASFF [http://ec.europa.eu/food/food/rapidalert/index_en.htm]), interrupting transmission or protecting those at risk.

The outbreak team meets regularly to review the investigation and control status, focusing on the protocols and tests in place for patient management, diagnostics and contact tracing, the identification of the population at risk, and the measures to prevent new cases in the different MS. The team communicates regularly, exchanging information on the investigation and control measures and sharing updated situation reports and risk assessments. After considering public opinion risks and preparing media messages the team decides how information about the event will be made public. Confirmed outbreaks require an active follow-up of all relevant information until fully contained. The documentation of all related activities facilitates information sharing and allows for auditing and evaluation. When considered useful, the lessons learnt at national and EU level can be documented and shared with all involved actors.

References

1. Schlagenhauf P, Santos-O'Connor F, Parola P, The practice of travel medicine in Europe. Clin Microbiol Infect 2010;16:203–8.

2. Freedman DO, Weld LH, Kozarsky PE, et al. Spectrum of disease and relation to place of exposure among ill-returned travellers. N Engl J Med 2006;354:119–30.

3. Heymann DL. The international response to the outbreak of SARS in 2003. Philos Trans R Soc Lond B Biol Sci 2004;359:1127–9.

4. World Health Organization. Revision of the International Health Regulations, WHA 58.3. Available from http://www.who.int/gb/ebwha/pdf_files/wha58/wha58_3-en.pdf.

5. MacLehose L, Brand H, Camaroni I, et al. Communicable disease outbreaks involving more than one country: systems approach to evaluating the response. BMJ 2001;323(7317):861–863.

6. Consolidated Version of the Treaty on the Functioning of the European Union in Article 26.2. Official Journal of the European Union 9.5.2008. Page C 115/59. Available online at: http://eur-lex.europa.eu/LexUriServ/LexUriServ.do?uri=OJ:C:2008:115:0047:0199:EN:PDF.

7. Regulation (EC) No 851/2004 of the European Parliament and of the Council of 21 April 2004 establishing a European Centre for Disease Prevention and Control, T.E.P.a.t.C.o.t.E. Union, Editor. OJEU 2004;L:142/1–11.

8. 2002/253/EC: Commission Decision of 19 March 2002 laying down case definitions for reporting communicable diseases to the Community network under Decision No. 2119/98/EC of the European Parliament and of the Council T.C.o.t.E. Communities, Editor. OJEU 2002;L:86/44–62.

9. 2003/534/EC: Commission Decision of 17 July 2003 amending Decision No. 2119/98/EC of the European Parliament and of the Council and Decision 2000/96/EC as regards communicable diseases listed in those decisions and amending Decision 2002/253/EC as regards the case definitions for communicable diseases, T.C.o.t.E. Communities, Editor. OJEU 2003;L:184/35–9.

10. Bohigas PA, Santos-O'Connor F, Coulombier D, Epidemic intelligence and travel-related diseases: ECDC experience and further developments. Clin Microbiol Infect 2009;15(8):734–9.

11. Commission Decision of 22 December 1999 on the early warning and response system for the prevention and control of communicable diseases under Decision No. 2119/98/EC of the European Parliament and of the Council T.C.o.t.E. Communities, Editor. OJEU 2000; L:21/32–5.

12. Commission Decision of 28/IV/2008 amending Decision 2000/57/EC as regards events to be reported within the early warning and response system for the prevention and control of communicable diseases. The Commission of the European Communities. 2008. Available online at: http://ec.europa.eu/health/ph_threats/com/docs/1574_2008_en.pdf.

13. 2008/426/EC: Commission Decision of 28 April 2008 amending Decision 2002/253/EC laying down case definitions for reporting communicable diseases to the Community network under Decision No 2119/98/EC of the European Parliament and of the Council (notified under document number C(2008) 1589), T.C.o.t.E. Communities, Editor. OJEU 2008;L:159/46–90.

Chapter 4
Diagnostic tests and procedures

Larry I. Lutwick,[1,2] Marc Mendelson[3] and Eskild Petersen[4]

[1]Infectious Diseases, VA New York Harbor Health Care System, Brooklyn, NY, USA
[2]State University of New York Downstate Medical School, NY, USA
[3]Division of Infectious Diseases and HIV Medicine, Department of Medicine, Groote Schuur Hospital, University of Cape Town, Cape Town, South Africa
[4]Department of Infectious Diseases, Aarhus University Hospital, Skejby, Aarhus, Denmark

This chapter provides guidelines for diagnostic procedures to be performed on admission and the following period until a diagnosis is clear. It is divided according to the focal symptoms from an infection including the central nervous system (CNS); ear, nose, and throat; cardiopulmonary; gastrointestinal; hepatobiliary; genitourinary including those that are sexually transmitted; joint and muscle; and cutaneous as well as fever of unknown origin without focal symptoms and patients with eosinophilia. It will also include a section regarding interpreting positive and negative test results.

Understanding diagnostic tests

What are you testing for?

Other than microscopy and culture, most diagnostic tests for microorganisms are aimed at detecting a subunit part of the pathogen in the patient's blood, tissue, or body fluid. These subunits include the capsule of the organism (such as the polysaccharide capsule of *Cryptococcus neoformans*), the surface coat protein (such as hepatitis B surface antigen, HBsAg), and nucleic acid, either DNA or RNA (such as the genome of HIV or a specific DNA insertion sequence of *Mycobacterium tuberculosis*).

In certain situations, directly detecting a pathogen subunit antigen is the most common way of identifying it because specific culture techniques are not available or are hazardous. Hepatitis B virus is the classic example of a pathogen detected in this way. Likewise, detection of *C. neoformans* capsule in blood or cerebrospinal fluid (CSF) in the untreated patient reflects ongoing cryptococcal illness, especially in the CSF, where capsule antigen is cleared quite slowly and its persistence per se does not necessarily mean treatment failure unless the culture is positive. The detection of parts of a pathogen's genome in blood or body fluid is generally a reflection of replication at some time but not necessarily at that time. As an extreme example, scientists have detected the DNA of the prehistoric wooly mammoth in archived material, although the wooly mammoth is not currently living.

Infectious Diseases: A Geographic Guide, First Edition.
Edited by Eskild Petersen, Lin H. Chen & Patricia Schlagenhauf.
© 2011 John Wiley & Sons, Ltd. Published 2011 by John Wiley & Sons, Ltd.

In addition to the above tests, many pathogens are identified by finding antibodies directed against the organism in the patient's serum. Such an antibody can be a surrogate screening marker for infection such as antibody tests for HIV and hepatitis C. Every pathogen consists of multiple antigenic sites, called epitopes, and the immune system will develop antibodies and cellular immune recognition directly against these epitopes. In most circumstances, some of these antibodies produced will be neutralizing, binding to a vital part of the pathogen to "neutralize" it. Other antibodies can be readily produced while infection is occurring but have no role in clearing the infection. In some cases, the antibody test is a polyclonal one, directed at the organism as a whole. In others, antibodies against specific parts of the pathogen can be detected and are helpful in defining the state of the disease process just as early antibody (IgM) production can be measured along with the IgG response. As an example, antibodies directed against the Epstein–Barr virus (EBV) early antigens and IgM antibody against EBV viral capsid antigen (VCA) occur early in EBV infection, followed by prominent IgG anti-VCA and antibodies against EBV nuclear antigens (EBNAs) generally develop only in convalescence from acute EBV infection.

Antibody detection can also be used as a presumptive measure for immunity against a particular pathogen usually to decide whether vaccination is required or if an exposure has occurred. Disease immunity measured this way includes measles, mumps, varicella, and parvovirus B19. The absence of detectable antibody following vaccination can reflect primary vaccine failure or waning immunity requiring booster immunization but not necessarily. As an example, the "protective" antibody for HBV, anti-HBs, wanes over time following vaccination, but immunity lasts substantially longer than detectable antibody either because of an amnestic immune response or because of the persistence of a protective cellular immune response.

Is a result positive or not?

Laboratory tests are meant to make a definitive diagnosis but, in almost every situation including culture, the clinician must consider the results in perspective. As an example, the growth of M. tuberculosis in a sputum culture could reflect a true positive result, a mislabeled specimen or cross-contamination in the laboratory. Likewise, specific organism stains can be contaminated or could be staining in response to a related, nonpathogenic strain. A result can be negative simply because the density of the pathogen is below the detection limit of the assay. This is particularly important in PCR, microscopy and rapid tests.

Most importantly, and seen daily by every Infectious Disease physician, the growth of a new gram-negative bacillus such as Klebsiella or Pseudomonas in the respiratory secretions of an endotracheally intubated ICU patient does not necessarily require specific antimicrobial therapy as the organism may be just colonizing the airway of the ill person.

The terms sensitivity and specificity are often used in the interpretation of laboratory data [1]. Sensitivity is the proportion of positives that are actually positive, hence its expression as %. Similarly, specificity is the proportion of negatives which are correctly identified.

Tests can also be analyzed by their predictive value; that is, a positive predictive value (PPV) is the proportion of patients with a positive test who are correctly diagnosed. It differs from sensitivity, in taking into account the number of false positives, that is, PPV = Number of true positives/(number of true positives + number of false positives). In short, it actually predicts the probability that a positive test reflects the underlying condition that you are testing for. PPV is also directly proportional to the prevalence of an infection or condition in the population. Hence in high prevalence tuberculosis settings for example, as the number of false positive tests is usually low, the PPV will be much higher than in a low prevalence setting.

The negative predictive value (NPV) reflects the proportion of patients with a negative test who are correctly diagnosed, and also takes into account the number of true and false negatives.

NPV is indirectly proportional to prevalence and thus in contrast to PPV, when an infection or condition is highly prevalent in the population, the NPV will be lower than in areas of low prevalence.

Setting the limits

How sensitive one might want a test to be may be related to wanting to find all of those with the condition so that therapeutic interventions can be put in place early to avoid complications or spread of the condition. Using the PPD tuberculin skin test (TST), in HIV-infected individuals or household contacts of a case of infectious tuberculosis, a low degree of induration (5 mm) giving a higher sensitivity is used despite the fact that a 5-mm set point may misdiagnose individuals as having tuberculosis when they do not (false positive). On the other hand, for individuals without any risk factors for reactivation of tuberculosis and no epidemiologic risk factors increasing their risk of exposure, a 15-mm set point is used. In this case, the specificity is more important so that if chemopreventative therapy is used, it will be more appropriate.

CNS infections—meningitis and encephalitis

The classic symptoms of bacterial meningitis are fever, neck stiffness, altered mental status, and headache. Certain patient populations, such as the young and the immunocompromised, may have an atypical presentation and, for these patients, clinicians must have a particularly low threshold for obtaining diagnostic studies including lumbar puncture.

The key diagnostic tests are lumbar puncture to obtain CSF, serologic assays, and computerized tomography (CT) and/or magnetic resonance imaging (MRI) scanning of the head and neuroaxis.

Biochemistry/cytology

CSF leukocyte count and concentration of protein and glucose lack specificity and sensitivity for the diagnosis of meningitis. A normal cell count is less than 5 cells/μl, protein less than 45–50 mg/l, and a glucose ratio above 0.5 between blood and CSF. Because of time for the blood glucose to be equal to CSF glucose, the blood glucose should ideally be obtained 30 min prior to the lumbar puncture.

Cells are differentiated into polymorphs (neutrophils) and mononuclear cells. An elevated polymorph cell count is typical of bacterial infection, whereas mononuclear cells dominate in viral, mycobacterial (or certain other intracellular growing bacteria), and fungal infections. Note that lymphoma cells in the CSF will be counted as mononuclear cells.

Microbiology

The Gram stain of CSF reveals bacteria in about 50–80% of cases and culture is positive in 80% of cases at best. Antimicrobial therapy prior to lumbar puncture decreases the sensitivity; however, culture can identify common pathogens like *Streptococcus pneumoniae*, *Haemophilus influenzae*, *Neisseria meningitidis*, and *Listeria monocytogenes*. The sensitivity of stains for acid-fast bacteria in *Mycobacterium tuberculosis* meningitis (TBM) is low as are stains for most fungal meningitides. Direct antigen detection of *C. neoformans* and culture for *M. tuberculosis* play an important role. PCR for *M. tuberculosis* is a good "rule in" test, but lacks sensitivity. Viruses can be identified by PCR, serum antibodies, or intrathecal antibody synthesis expressed as a serum/CSF ratio.

Microbiological diagnosis of CNS infections

Microorganism	Culture	16-S-PCR	PCR for specific agent	IgG index for intrathecal antibody synthesis	Agent-specific antibodies (IgM, IgG)
Bacteria	+	+	–	–	–
M. tuberculosis	+	–	+	–	Interferon-gamma release assays in blood positive[a]
Herpes simplex, enterovirus, herpes zoster, EBV	–	–	+	+	Herpes simplex meningitis is usually due to HSV-2, whereas HSV encephalitis is usually due to HSV-1
HIV	–	–	+	–	–
West Nile virus	–	–	+	–	+
Japanese encephalitis	–	–	+	–	+
St. Louis encephalitis, tick-borne encephalitis (TBE), and other arboviruses	–	–	+	–	+
Nipah and Hendra viruses	–	–	+	–	Serum neutralization assay
Chandipura virus	–	–	+	–	+
Rabies	–	–	(+)[b]	(+)[b]	+
Borrelia spp.[c]	–	–	–	+	–
Syphilis	–	–	+	–	+[d]
Eosinophilic meningoencephalitis[e]	–	–	–	–	+
Cryptococcus	+	–	Pan-fungal PCR	–	The methods used are direct microscopy in tusch stained wet mount, antigen detection by enzyme immunoassay (ELISA), culture, and PCR

[a]The interferon-gamma release assays do not differentiate between latent and acute tuberculosis. The result is very dependent on the patient's origin in the developed world. It should not be used in areas highly endemic for tuberculosis, many of which will be positive without active tuberculosis disease.

[b]Postexposure immunization should be started as soon as possible after exposure. PCR and intrathecal antibody synthesis can only be helpful after CNS symptoms develop.

[c]In Europe, lyme borreliosis is caused by Borrelia burgdorferi sensu stricto, Borrelia afzelii, Borrelia garinii, and the recently described species Borrelia spielmanii, whereas B. burgdorferi dominates in North America. Diagnosis can be difficult and the role of immunoblot using recombinant antigens has not been studied in population-based studies. The methods available were recently reviewed [2].

[d]VDRL (Venereal Disease Research Laboratory) or equivalent specific antibody tests.

[e]Suspected in patients with CNS symptoms and eosinophilia in peripheral blood often with elevated total IgE. Organisms associated with this entity include the parasites Angiostrongylus cantonensis, Baylisascaris procyonis, and Gnathostoma spinigerum, and the dimorphic fungus Coccidioides immitis. IgG detection to A. cantonensis L3 larvae is available.

Imaging

MRI is generally more sensitive compared to CT scans in patients with encephalitis [3]. The results are generally nonspecific but can be very suggestive in patients with herpes simplex encephalitis and the immunosuppressed host with *Toxoplasma gondii* brain infection. Because of a small but finite risk of cerebral herniation when a lumbar puncture is done and when high intracerebral pressure is present (from intracerebral hemorrhage, tumor, or cerebral abscess), a brain imaging study is often performed before lumbar puncture.

Ear, nose, and throat

The majority of infections are related to respiratory viruses, and EBV is of particular importance. Streptococcal infection, notably *Streptococcus pyogenes* (Group A *Streptococcus*), is important to diagnose as treatment can prevent rheumatic fever.

Basic diagnostics for ear, nose, and throat infections

Microorganims	Diagnostic procedure
Streptococcal infections	Throat swab culture, rapid tests for group A *Streptococcus* [4]
Tuberculosis	Culture and microcopy of biopsy. 16S rRNA PCR Peripheral blood ELISpot and Mantoux test
Peritonsillar abscess[a]	MR or CT scan of the neck
Necrotizing fasciitis[b]	MR or CT scan of the neck
Influenza	Viral culture, serology, rapid antigen testing, reverse transcriptase PCR, and immunofluorescence assays
EBV	Specific antibody profiling, rapid test of EBV antibodies (monospot, heterophile agglutination test)
HSV I and II	PCR of vesicular fluid. Serology (type-specific)
HIV	Serology, PCR, and antigen/antibody rapid tests

[a]Requires acute ENT evaluation.
[b]Requires acute surgical evaluation.

Biochemistry/cytology

In viral infections, the C-reactive protein (CRP) is only moderately elevated and the differential white blood cell (WBC) count is normal or, especially in the case of EBV (mononucleosis), dominated by a lymphocytosis. Influenza, however, can cause a polymorph leukocytosis. In streptococcal and other bacterial infections, the WBC is usually elevated with a polymorph predominance, and the CRP more elevated. The CRP response has a lag time of 18–24 h which means that in the setting of an acute presentation, the CRP may still be normal or low despite the bacterial etiology. It should be remembered that pertussis (whooping cough) is a bacterial upper respiratory infection due to *Bordetella pertussis* that can cause a peripheral lymphocytosis.

Rapid tests

There are several rapid tests on the market detecting group A *Streptococcus* and EBV (the most common cause of infectious mononucleosis). The sensitivity varies considerably between kits from 62% to 95%, but show good specificity [4]. Rapid detection tests of the mononucleosis heterophile antibody are often insensitive in the first week of illness.

Microbiology

Group A *Streptococcus* is readily grown from the oropharynx; however, other classical upper respiratory pathogens such as *B. pertussis* and diphtheria-causing *Corynebacterium diphtheriae* have a much lower yield from culture. Vincent's angina is an acute necrotizing infection of the pharynx caused by a combination of fusiform bacilli (*Fusiformis fusiformis*—a gram-negative bacillus) and spirochetes.

Imaging

A number of focal, potentially life-threatening bacterial infections of the head and neck can be suspected clinically but are usually confirmed with MRI or CT scan. These infections, for which the microbiological causes (usually aerobic and anaerobic normal mouth flora) are identified by culture of the pus and/or blood, include peritonsillar abscess, pharyngeal abscess, retropharyngeal abscess/fasciitis, and jugular vein septic thrombophlebitis.

Cardiopulmonary

Pulmonary infections

Biochemistry/cytology   The CRP is only a rough guideline to differentiate between viral infections or atypical bacteria like *Mycoplasma* and *Chlamydia* and bacterial infections such as *S. pneumoniae* [5–7]. The CRP response has a lag time of 18–24 h which means that with a short history the CRP will still be normal or low despite a bacterial infection. An elevated peripheral WBC count with increased polymorphs is characteristic of pyogenic bacterial infections.

Microbiology and rapid tests

Microorganism	Culture[a]	16-S-PCR	PCR for specific agent	Agent-specific antibodies (IgM, IgG) obtained with at least 2 weeks interval	Microscopy	Other tests
Viruses	−	−	+	+	−	
Mycoplasma and chlamydiae	−	−	+	+	−	
Chlamydophila psittaci	−	−	+	+	−	
S. pneumoniae and other bacterial infections	+	+	+	−	−	
Fungal infections[b]	+	−	−	−	−	
Pneumocystis jirovecii[c]	−	−	+		+	
M. tuberculosis	+	−	+	−	+	TST or an interferon-gamma release assays[d]
Melioidosis [8]	+	+	−	−	Specific direct immuno-fluorescence	Hemagglutination assay

[a]Culture of expectorate or, if negative, after BAL.

[b]Detection of galactomannan for *Aspergillus*. *Candida* mannan is being introduced and in under evaluation, but seems promising with invasive candidiasis.

[c]Gomori-methenamine silver stain or direct fluorescent stain of BAL or expectorate.

[d]Interferon-gamma release assays and TSTs will be negative in immunocompromised patients for instance HIV infected with a low CD4 T-cell count. In severe tuberculosis these tests can also be negative despite disseminated tuberculosis so-called anergy.

For details regarding eosinophilia and pneumonia see "Eosinophilia and elevated IgE" section.

Imaging A plain chest X-ray will show an infiltrate in most cases of pneumonia if symptoms have persisted for more than 2 days. CT or MRI is usually not needed in uncomplicated pneumonia, but if symptoms persist despite treatment, CT or MRI is helpful to diagnose empyema and/or lung abscess. CT or MRI can be more sensitive than chest X-ray to differentiate between inflammation and malignancy.

Cardiac infections

Endocarditis is usually a clinical diagnosis and is most often associated with bacteremia or fungemia. Continuously positive blood cultures is the most sensitive finding to distinguish the intravascular location of an infection (usually endocarditis) as compared to the intermittent or transient positive blood culture in most infections [9]. A normal procalcitonin and CRP do not exclude endocarditis [10].

Microbiological diagnosis of infections causing endocarditis, myocarditis, and pericarditis

Microorganism	Culture[a]	16-S-PCR	PCR for specific agents	Agent-specific antibodies (IgM, IgG) obtained with at least 2 weeks interval	Microscopy	Other tests
Bacterial infections	+	+	+	−	−	
Virus	−	−	+	+	−	
Mycoplasma and chlamydiae	−	−	+	+	−	
Q fever (*Coxiella burnetii*)	−	+	+	+	−	
Fungal infections[b]	+	−	−	−	−	
M. tuberculosis	+	−	+	−	+	TST or an interferon-gamma release assays
Chagas' disease, *Trypanosoma cruzi*	−	−	+[c]	+	−	

[a]Culture of blood or pericardial aspirates.
[b]Detection of galactomannan in *Aspergillus* infections.
[c]Chagas disease is a cause of cardiomyopathy in South and Central America. PCR can be performed on blood or biopsy material [11].

Imaging Transthoracic echocardiography (TTE) and/or transesophageal echocardiography (TEE) should always be performed in suspected endocarditis, myocarditis, and pericarditis.

Positron emission tomography (PET) may provide additional information on extracardial foci of infection, but do not replace TTE and TEE in the acute phase.

Gastrointestinal infections

Biochemistry/cytology

Elevated WBC count is generally found in bacterial infections of the gastrointestinal tract especially when there is invasive disease. The toxin-associated *Clostridium difficile*-associated colitis can also be associated with an elevated WBC.

Microbiology

Microscopy for cysts from protozoa like *Giardia*, helminth eggs like *Ascaris*, and routine culture will identify common bacterial pathogens such as *Salmonella* spp., *Campylobacter*, *Yersinia*, and *Shigella*. *Vibrio cholerae* and pathogenic *E. coli* like enterotoxin-producing *Escherichia coli* (ETEC) and verotoxin-producing *Escherichia coli* (VTEC) require more specific media. In outbreak situations a rapid dipstick test for *V. cholerae* can be useful [12]. In the immunocompromised host, special stains for coccidian parasites such as *Cryptosporidium* are important.

Microbiological diagnosis of gastrointestinal infections

Microorganism	Culture	Agent-specific culture	PCR for specific agent	Microscopy	Other specific diagnostic tests
Salmonella, Shigella spp., *Campylobacter, Yersinia*	+	−	−	−	−
V. cholerae	−	+	+	−	Rapid dipstick tests [9]
C. difficile (Cd)	+	+	−	−	Toxin detection in feces PCR for 027 and other Cd
ETEC, VTEC	−	+	−	−	Toxin detection in culture supernatants
Viruses	+	−	+	−	Rapid tests for rotavirus
Giardia intestinalis	−	−	+	+	Immunofluorescence of fecal smear with labeled specific antibodies
Cryptosporidium spp., *Cyclospora cayetanensis*[a]	−	−	+	+	Immunofluorescence of fecal smear with labeled *Cryptosporidium*-specific antibodies
Entamoeba histolytica and *Entamoeba dispar*	−	−	+	+	Staining of feces preserved in formalin, SAF, or polyvinyl alcohol
Presumed nonpathogenic intestinal protozoan parasites like *Blastocystis hominis* and *Dientamoeba fragilis*	−	−	+	(+)	Staining of feces preserved in formalin, SAF, or polyvinyl alcohol
Microsporidia spp.	−	−	+[b]	+[c]	Electron microscopy has been used, PCR
Schistosoma mansoni	−	−	−	+[d]	*Schistosoma* antibodies are more sensitive than microscopy in patients with a low worm load Egg detection in feces and urine
Other intestinal helminths	−	−	−	+	See section 11

Microorganism	Culture	Agent-specific culture	PCR for specific agent	Microscopy	Other specific diagnostic tests
Helicobacter pylori	−	−	+[e]	−	Urea breath test, rapid antigen detection tests under evaluation [13]. *Helicobacter*-specific antibodies cannot be used to confirm eradication [14]
Tropheryma whipplei	−	−	+[e]	−	
M. tuberculosis	−	+	+	−	TST or an interferon-gamma release assays may be false negative

[a]Modified Ziehl–Neelsen staining.
[b]PCR on corneal scrapings and intestinal biopsies.
[c]Polychrome staining.
[d]Microscopy of feces concentrated a.m. Kato or microscopy of biopsies from the rectal mucosa.
[e]PCR on biopsy material.

Imaging

Imaging is not specific for most intestinal infections, but is helpful if the diagnosis is not clear or inflammatory bowel diseases such as Crohn's disease and ulcerative colitis or diverticulitis are considered. CT or MRI may show inflammation in the intestinal wall and a capsule endoscopy and biopsy will be able to show inflammation in the small intestine [15]. Imaging can confuse ileocecal tuberculosis with Crohn's disease and amebiasis with ulcerative colitis. Pancolitis with colon wall thickening is common in *C. difficile* toxin disease.

Direct visualization via fiber-optic endoscopy may be employed and allows biopsy of relevant areas. In the immunosuppressed patient, duodenal biopsy may play an important role in determining the etiology of chronic diarrhea due to, for example, *Isospora belli*.

Hepatobiliary infections

Biochemistry/cytology

The liver enzymes, alanine aminotransferase (ALT) or aspartate aminotransferase (AST) (the latter being less specific for the liver), will be elevated in viral hepatitis and reflects a parenchymal destruction of hepatocytes. The elevation is not pathognomonic of a particular etiology, as the serum enzymes rise in any cause of liver cell damage such as alcohol, adverse reactions to drugs, or hypotension. In certain hepatic infections such as cytomegalovirus (CMV), EBV, and Q fever (*C. burnetii*), the biochemical response can be more cholestatic with more prominently elevated alkaline phosphatase and total bilirubin. Abnormalities in liver function during leptospirosis infection are characterized by elevated bilirubin with a proportionately modest elevation in transaminases. This is due to the abnormality of bilirubin transport.

Parasitic infections like liver flukes and echinococcosis may sometimes result in elevated eosinophil count and elevated total IgE, but not always.

Microbiological diagnosis of hepatobiliary infections

Microorganism	Culture	16-S-PCR	PCR for specific agent	Agent-specific antibodies (IgM, IgG) obtained with at least 2 weeks interval	Microscopy	Other tests
Hepatitis A	−	−	+	+	−	
Hepatitis B	−	−	+	+	−	
Hepatitis C, D, E	−	−	+	+	−	
CMV, EBV	−	−	+	+	−	
Bacterial liver abscess	+	+	+	−	−	Imaging with CT or MRI will show a hypodense lesion without a wall
Leptospirosis	−	−	+	+	−	
M. tuberculosis	+	−	+	−	+	TST or an interferon-gamma release assays may be false negative
Amebic liver abscess (E. histolytica)	−	−	+	+	−	Imaging with CT or MRI will show a hypodense lesion without a wall
Fasciola hepatica, Fasciola gigantum, Opisthorchis spp., Clonorchis sinensis	−	−	−	+[a]	+[b]	Imaging with CT or MRI will show hypodense lesions often multiple, some of which may be subcapsular
Echinococcus granulosus	−	−	−	+	+	Imaging with CT or MRI will show hypodense lesions often with smaller cysts inside and a dense, fibrous capsule often with calcifications [16]
Echinococcus multilocularis	−	−	−	+[c]	+	Imaging with CT or MRI will show hypodense lesions often with smaller cysts inside and a dense, fibrous capsule often with calcifications [16]
Leishmania spp.	−	−	+[d]	+	+[d]	

[a]Antibody assays are available for fascioliasis.
[b]Eggs can be detected in feces.
[c]Serology is cross-reactive between E. granulosus and E. multilocularis and the diagnosis rest on a combination of serology and imaging, and has recently been reviewed.
[d]PCR and microscopy of bone marrow aspirate.

Imaging

CT or MRI is generally not of any value in acute hepatitis although the granular pattern in acute Q fever is suggestive of this disease. Ultrasound, CT, or MRI is essential in the diagnosis and staging of echinococcosis and diagnosis of the liver flukes, liver abscess, and cholecystitis.

Genitourinary tract infections including STI

Upper and lower urinary tract infections

Biochemistry/cytology CRP and WBC will usually be elevated in upper urinary tract infections (pyelonephritis) but may be normal in uncomplicated cystitis. A rapid urine dipstick test for leukocytes, blood, protein, nitrite, and leukocyte esterase will often be positive in both lower and upper urinary tract infections. Dipstick tests, urine culture for bacteria, and clinical symptoms should all be considered together for a diagnosis of lower or upper urinary tract infection [17].

Microbiology and rapid tests A urinary sample for culture is essential before antibiotic treatment is started.

Microbiological diagnosis of genitourinary tract infections

Microorganism	Culture	16-S-PCR	PCR for specific agent	Agent-specific antibodies (IgM, IgG) obtained with at least 2 weeks interval	Microscopy	Other tests
Bacterial infections	+ [a]	–	–	–	+	
M. tuberculosis	+	–	+	–	+	TST or an interferon-gamma release assays
Schistosoma haematobium	–	–	–	+	+	Biopsy of bladder wall and urine sediment may show *Schistosoma* eggs with a terminal spine

[a]In patients with fever and a suspected urinary tract infection, blood samples for culture should be obtained before antibiotic treatment is started.

Imaging Ultrasound, CT, or MRI is usually not needed in lower urinary tract infection, but if symptoms persist despite treatment, imaging is helpful to diagnose a renal stone, hydrone-phrosis, perirenal abscess, and strictures seen in long-standing schistosomiasis, brucellosis, and tuberculosis.

Sexually transmitted diseases and other genital infections

Acute venereal diseases are usually a clinical diagnosis based on the history, physical examination, and tests for specific agents.

Biochemistry Biochemistry will seldom be of great help.

Microbiological diagnosis of sexually transmitted diseases and other genital infections

Microorganism	Culture	16-S-PCR	PCR for specific agent	Agent-specific antibodies (IgM, IgG) obtained with at least 2 weeks interval	Microscopy	Other tests
Neisseria gonorrhoeae	+	?	+	−	+[a]	
Chlamydia trachomatis[b] including lymphogranuloma venereum (LGV)[c]	+	−	+	−	−	−
Mycoplasma genitalium[b]	−	−	+[d]	−	−	
Syphilis [18,19]	−	?	+	+	+	Serial tests often necessary
Chancroid (Haemophilus ducreyi)	+	?	+	−	−	
Granuloma inguinale (Calymmatobacterium granulomatis)	(+)[e]	?	+	−	+	Painful chancre
Herpes genitalis	−	−	+	(+)[f]	−	
Gardnerella vaginalis	+	?	−	−	−	−
Scabies	−	−	−	−	+	
M. tuberculosis	+	−	+	−	+	TST or an interferon-gamma release assays

[a]Less sensitive than culture and PCR.
[b]Sample by urinary tract scrapings.
[c]LGV is caused by C. trachomatis serovars L1, L2, and L3 and can be differentiated from other Chlamydia by PCR [20,21].
[d]PCR only increase diagnostic sensitivity in primary syphilis, not in the secondary or tertiary syphilis.
[e]Not routinely available.
[f]Many people will have antibodies against herpes from a previous infection, and the diagnosis rely on clinical findings and PCR.

Joint, muscle, skin, and soft tissue infections

Some infections like streptococcal skin infections, erysipelas, are a clinical diagnosis but the deeper joint, muscles, and soft tissue infections need biopsies or aspirates for culture and or 16-S-PCR for diagnosis. Necrotizing fasciitis is an acute, surgical emergency necessitating surgical debridement.

Biochemistry/cytology

CRP or PCT and WBC will usually be elevated in bacterial infections like septic arthritis, streptococcal skin infections, and necrotizing fasciitis. Long-standing osteomyelitis will often be followed by a normocytic normochromic anemia.

Microbiology

Culture should be obtained from blood before treatment is started. Culture from wounds will usually often show bacteria which contaminate the wound which in most cases are not representative of bacteria causing invasive infection.

Culture should be obtained from relevant samples by taking biopsies (osteomyelitis), aspirating abscesses and joint fluid for culture, and/or PCR (16-S-PCR).

Microbiological diagnosis of joint, muscle, skin, and soft tissue infections

Microorganism	Culture	16-S-PCR	PCR for specific agent	Microscopy	Other tests
Bacterial infections (septic arthritis, osteomyelitis, myositis)	+	+	–	–	
Necrotizing fasciitis[a]	+	+	–	–	
M. tuberculosis	+	–	+	+	TST or an interferon-gamma release assays
Trichinella spp.	–	–	+[b]	+	Serology available

[a]Necrotizing fasciitis is most commonly caused by invasive group A *Streptococcus* (iGAS), but almost all bacteria has been reported to cause necrotizing fasciitis including *E. coli*, and *Vibrio vulnificus* is especially seen after wounds in maritime environments.
[b]From muscle biopsy.

Imaging

X-ray or CT imaging is needed if necrotizing fasciitis is suspected and air in soft tissues is an important indicator of this condition.

MRI is needed to diagnose soft tissue infections and osteomyelitis. CT is less sensitive. Osteomyelitis may show on plain X-rays, but rarely before 4 weeks after the infection started. PET scans are helpful to identify multiple foci.

Rash

A rash is a nonspecific symptom that can be seen in many viral, fungal, and some bacterial infections, and noninfection-related conditions like autoimmune disorders and hypersensitivity reactions to drugs.

A rash is a diffuse reddening (erythema) of the skin and can be divided into macular (non-elevation of the affected areas), papular (elevation of the involved skin areas), vesicular (small clear vesicles), or pustular (vesicles containing pus). A rash with bleeding in the skin is a purpura or ecchymosis. If the manifestation of bleeding is pinpoint, it is referred to as a petechia. Acute febrile illnesses with petechiae and purpurae include meningococcemia and spotted fever group rickettsioses such as African tick bite fever and Rocky Mountain spotted fever.

Biochemistry

CRP and WBC will usually be only slightly elevated or normal in uncomplicated viral infections. Total IgE and eosinophil count are elevated in invasive helminth infections like filariasis and onchocerciasis.

Microbiological diagnosis of patients with a rash

Microorganism	Culture	16-S-PCR	PCR for specific agent	Microscopy	Specific antibodies either IgM or paired samples for increase in IgG titer	Other tests
Streptococcal group A infections (scarlet fever)	+[a]	+	–	–	+	
Bacterial infections with an erythematous rash[b]	(+)	(+)	–	–	+	
Viral infections with an erythematous rash[c]	–	–	(–)	–	+	
Viral infections with a vesicular rash[d]	–	–	+	–	(+)	
Viral infections with a hemorrhagic rash (purpura)[e]	–	–	+	–	+	
Rickettsial infections with a hemorrhagic rash (purpura)[f]	–	+	+	–	+	
Mycobacterium leprae	–	+	+[g]	+[h]	–	
Fungal infections with rash[i]	–	–	+	+	–	

[a]Throat swab.

[b]Bartonella quintana, B. henselae, B. bacilliformis, Borrelia recurrentis, Borrelia burgdorferi, Chlamydia psittaci, Francisella tularensis, Mycoplasma pneumoniae, Leptospira spp., L. monocytogenes, Salmonella typhi, Spirillum minus.

[c]Adenovirus, EBV, CMV, enterovirus (coxsackie, echo), dengue fever, HIV, human herpes virus 6, measles, parvovirus B19, rubella.

[d]Herpes simplex, monkey pox, varicella zoster, vaccinia.

[e]Ebola, Marburg, yellow fever, Crimean–Congo hemorrhagic fever.

[f]Rickettsial spotted fever (SF) group (Rocky Mountain SF, Mediterranean SF, rickettsial pox, endemic typhus, murine typhus, scrub typhus).

[g]Not routinely available.

[h]Microscopy of biopsies from peripheral nerves or nasal scrapings.

[i]Candida spp., Cryptococcus spp., Histoplasma capsulatum, Blastomyces dermatitidis, C. immitis, mucormycosis.

Imaging

Imaging is only indicated if systemic, deep infections are suspected.

Fever without focal symptoms

The classical definition of fever of unknown origin (FUO) requires, among other things, that the fever has persisted for 3 weeks or more and that the patient has undergone basic investigations which will have ruled out common infections. However, a common scenario is the patient presenting with undifferentiated fever, that is, one with few or no focal symptoms, in whom it is important to establish a diagnosis as soon as possible. This section proposes an approach to such patients.

Always consider underlying HIV infection in patients with unexplained symptoms.

Initial tests on admission

The approach to a patient with an undifferentiated febrile illness starts with a thorough history including travel and exposure risks. It depends on a number of factors including the perceived degree of illness of the individual, the length of time that the person has been ill relative to the likely risk exposure, the geographic location and, in prolonged illness, whether the patient has lost weight.

Other factors of relevance may be exposure to household pets, livestock, or other animals, the occupation of the patient, and specific dietary habits.

Fever unrelated to infection, such as from autoimmune disorders, malignancies, endocrinology disorders, and drug reactions, should be considered when planning diagnostic investigations.

Biochemistry/cytology

Hemoglobin, WBC plus differential count, liver parameters, serum electrolytes, BUN, creatinine, CRP, ESR.

However, ESR should not be performed in patients with HIV as it is very difficult to interpret in the setting of hyperimmune activation which increases the ESR.

Screening for autoimmune diseases by antinuclear antibodies, ANA, ANCA, and rheumatoid factor.

Microbiology

Microscopy and culture from blood, urine, throat, sputum, wounds, sores, pustules, or vesicles.

HIV testing.

Imaging

Chest X-ray as a minimum, ultrasound, ±CT or MRI of thorax and abdomen to rule out intra-abdominal abscess, pleural effusions enlarged glands in the mediastinum or abdomen.

PET scan may be useful to visualize inflammatory foci and small malignancies.

Other

Electrocardiogram (ECG).

Consider TTE or TEE.

Further tests

Biochemistry should be repeated on a daily basis and blood cultures should be taken at 1 or 2 days interval or if there is a rigor or rapid rise in temperature.

Specific cultures and serologic studies are indicated based on particular aspects of the clinical circumstances in patients with undifferentiated febrile illnesses. For example, see the next section.

Specific cultures and serologic studies in particular clinical circumstances

Exposure to cats, especially kittens with fleas	*Bartonella* (Cat scratch disease)
Exposure to freshwater (river rafting)	Leptospirosis
Exposure to rodents	Lymphocytic choriomeningitis virus infection, leptospirosis
Exposure to rabbits	Tularemia
Ingestion of unpasteurized dairy products	Brucellosis, Salmonellosis
Ingestion of uncooked bivalve molluscs	Typhoid fever
Exposure to ticks	Spotted Fever Group (SFG) rickettsiosis, e.g., African Tick Bite Fever (ATBF), RMSF (Rocky Mountain spotted fever), MSF (Mediterranean spotted fever), babesiosis, Colorado tick fever, and other rickettsial fevers. See the chapter(s) on the parts of the world where the patient traveled
Travel to central valley of California, Mexico, or parts of Central America	Coccidioidomycosis

Travel to malaria-endemic area: Malaria (remember that *Plasmodium vivax* and *Plasmodium ovale* can relapse later, usually within 12 months after return) can be transmitted by *Anopheles* mosquitoes carried on an airplane or via blood transfusion.

Rapid tests do not pick up *Plasmodium malariae*, *Plasmodium knowlesi*, or variant *P. ovale*.

Travel to USA, Ohio and/or Upper Mississippi River valleys or parts of Central and South America or the Caribbean; Entry into bat-infested caves worldwide: Histoplasmosis.

A bone marrow aspirate and/or biopsy with culture can be useful for infections including typhoid fever, brucellosis, histoplasmosis, mycobacteriosis (tuberculosis and atypical mycobacteria), leishmaniasis, and Q fever as well as diagnostic for lymphoproliferative diseases such as leukemia and lymphoma.

Biochemistry   Total IgE elevated in active helminth infections.

Other   TST or IFN-γ release assay (Quantiferon) for tuberculosis, depending on the clinical setting. Consider TTE and TEE if not done previously.

Eosinophilia and elevated IgE

Eosinophilia and/or increased total IgE is a common finding in systemic, helminth infections, that is, infections with roundworms (nematodes), tapeworms (cestodes), and flukes (trematodes). Eosinophilia and IgE can be normal in chronic infections with low activity.

Biochemistry   CRP may or may not be slightly to moderately elevated, depending on the particular microorganism.

Microbiology   Diagnosis rests on a history of exposure in a relevant geographical area, symptoms and detection by microscopy, PCR, or specific antibodies as shown in the following table.

Imaging   MRI and CT scan are of value in infections with the liver flukes and echinococcosis.

Key symptoms and method of diagnosis for helminths

Name	Key symptoms	Diagnosis
Cestodes (tapeworms)		
Diphyllobothrium latum	Diarrhea, anemia	*Microscopy:* eggs in feces
E. granulosus	Cysts in liver or other organs	*Antibodies:* in blood
		Microscopy: cyst material Eosinophilia and elevated *total IgE* may be seen in active, expanding cysts
		Imaging: cysts in affected organs
E. multilocularis	Expanding, semisolid liver tumor without fibrous capsule	*Antibodies:* in blood. Cross-reactivity with *E. granulosus*
		Microscopy: cyst material Eosinophilia and elevated *total IgE* may be seen in active, expanding cysts
		Imaging: expanding mass often in the liver
Hymenolepis nana	Diarrhea, often asymptomatic	*Microscopy:* eggs in feces
Taenia saginata	Diarrhea, often asymptomatic	*Microscopy:* eggs in feces
Taenia solium Cysticercosis	Can cause cysticercosis with multiple small cysts in muscles and brain by ingestion of eggs. Common course of epilepsy in poor countries. Subcutaneous nodules	*Microscopy:* eggs in feces but cannot be distinguished from *T. saginata*
		Antibodies: used in cysticercosis, cross-reactivity with other helminthes
		Eosinophilia and elevated *total IgE* may be seen but not always
		Imaging: cysts in the brain and other organs
Trematodes (flukes)		
C. sinensis	Biliary cirrhosis, often asymptomatic	*Microscopy:* eggs in feces
		Imaging: hypodense lesions in the liver
F. hepatica	Biliary cirrhosis	*Microscopy:* eggs in feces
		Antibodies: tests have been developed
		Eosinophilia and elevated *total IgE* may be seen but not always
		Imaging: hypodense lesions in the liver
Fasciolopsis buski	Diarrhea, intestinal wall abscess, intestinal hemorrhaging	*Microscopy:* eggs in feces
		Eggs are very similar to *F. hepatica*
		Imaging: hypodense lesions in the liver

(Continued)

Name	Key symptoms	Diagnosis
Opisthorchis felineus	Biliary cirrhosis, often asymptomatic	*Microscopy:* eggs in feces *Antibodies:* tests have been developed *Imaging:* hypodense lesions in the liver
Paragonimus westermani, Paragonimus africanus	Lung lesions with fibrosis and hemoptysis. May be located in other organs including the brain	*Microscopy:* eggs in sputum *Antibodies:* tests have been developed *Imaging:* lesions in the lungs which may resemble tuberculosis
S. haematobium, S. japonicum, S. mansoni, S. intercalatum, S. mekongi	Liver cirrhosis can be seen in all *Schistosoma* infections *S. haematobium* causes hematuria, scarring of the bladder and urinary tract, abdominal cramps *S. mansoni* causes diarrhea, abdominal cramps, and rectal cancer *S. japonicum* more likely leads to liver fibrosis	*Microscopy:* eggs seen in urine, bladder, and rectal biopsy. *S. mansoni* eggs found in feces in heavy infections. (Urine collected at midday for *S. haematobium* and *S. japonicum* consider filter enrichment.) Advanced cases might require biopsies (rectal for all species and bladder for *S. japonicum* and *S. haematobium*) *Antibodies:* more sensitive compared to microscopy *Eosinophilia* and elevated *total IgE* may be seen but not always *Imaging:* fibrotic scarring in the bladder and upper urinary tract
Nematodes (roundworms) *Ascaris lumbricoides*	Often nonpathogenic. May cause eosinophilic pneumonia in heavy infections. Intestinal obstruction	*Microscopy:* eggs in feces *Eosinophilia* and elevated *total IgE* may be seen often but not always *Imaging:*
Enterobius vermicularis *Strongyloides stercoralis*	Pruritus ani Often nonpathogenic. May cause diarrhea, rash, urticaria, pruritus, and overwhelming infection in immunocompromised. Can remain silent for years	*Microscopy:* Scotch tape test *Microscopy:* larvae found in feces *Antibodies:* blood
Trichuris trichiura *Trichinella spiralis* native a.o.	Diarrhea, rectal prolapse, malabsorption Fever, muscle pain, myocarditis, rash Diarrhea in the acute stage	*Microscopy:* eggs in feces *Microscopy:* muscle biopsy *Antibodies:* blood, preferred method in humans *Eosinophilia* and elevated *total IgE* may be seen often but not always and depend on the time after infection

Ancylostoma duodenale, Necator americanus	Hookworms	Penetrate skin and may give a rash at the site of invasion. Diarrhea, anemia, malabsorption	*Microscopy:* eggs in feces
Wuchereria bancrofti, Brugia malayi, and Brugia timori	Filariasis Elephantiasis	Fever, lymphadenopathy, after many years of repeated infections elephantiasis may develop	*Microscopy:* microfilaria, thick blood film Giemsa stained. ICT for rapid and early antigen detection, direct detection (Giemsa) of microfilariae in blood. Caveat daytime/nocturnal patterns, concentration technique, skin snips PCR *Antibodies:* extensive cross-reactivity between filarial species *Eosinophilia* and *total IgE* almost always elevated to very high levels
Loa loa		Rash, anterior and posterior uveitis Moving edema "Calabar swellings"	*Microscopy:* microfilaria, thick blood film Giemsa stained *Antibodies:* extensive cross-reactivity between filarial species *Eosinophilia* and *total IgE* almost always elevated to very high levels
Onchocerca volvulus	African river blindness Onchocerciasis	Anterior uveitis, subcutaneous, painless nodules Fever, lymphangitis	*Microscopy:* Microfilaria found in skin snips Antibodies: extensive cross-reactivity between filarial species *Eosinophilia* and *total IgE* almost always elevated
Dracunculus medinensis	Guinea worm	Long worm protruding from wound often at the lower extremities Superinfection	Long worm protruding from wound often at the lower extremities *Eosinophilia* and *total IgE* almost always elevated
Toxocara canis, Toxocara cati	Cutaneous and visceral larva migrans Creeping eruption	Moving eruption, intense itching, sometimes multiorgan, systemic infection	*Antibodies:* extensive cross-reactivity between filarial species *Eosinophilia* and *total IgE* almost always elevated to very high levels in visceral larva migrans but not in cutaneous larva migrans
Baylisascaris		Itching rash, cough, loss of eye sight, variable CNS symptoms due to larvae migration in the brain, seizures, and coma	Usually eosinophilia (peripheral and in CNS), elevated total IgE, and elevated ALAT. Changes in the CNS on MR and CT scans [22]. PCR and specific-antibody assays have been described in the litterature but are not available as a routine

Diagnostics in areas with limited resources

More emphasis is commonly put on accruing clinical evidence to help diagnose infections in resource-limited countries where access to expensive tests is often unavailable outside of central hospitals or reference centers. One such example is specialist imaging such as CT scan and MRI which is often unavailable outside of tertiary academic teaching hospitals. When available, they may be employed in the diagnostic workup of infection and are particularly useful in assessment of occult infection in the immunocompromised host with HIV.

Ultrasound is cheaper and more commonly available outside of specialist centers. Specialist etiological investigations are similarly hard to access, such as PCR or serology. In rural areas the diagnostic armamentarium may be limited to basic microscopy ± basic biochemistry such as for tests on CSF.

Some diagnostic tests are not applicable in countries where an infection is highly prevalent due to their almost universal positivity in the general population. This is particularly relevant with respect to tuberculosis investigations. Interferon-gamma release assays such as Quantiferon-in-tube are rarely used to diagnose active tuberculosis due to high background prevalence of latent tuberculosis infection. The same is true for the TST in adults, although the TST is employed in the assessment of children who are contacts of tuberculosis patients.

The result of a paucity of diagnostic tests in resource-limited settings is an increase in the use of syndromic management and empiric antimicrobial regimens for clinically diagnosed infections. Switches in treatment are commonly dictated not by new information from sensitivity results, but rather by lack of improvement in the clinical condition.

Basic diagnostics of pulmonary infections

Fiber-optic bronchoscopy, bronchiolar lavage, and transbronchial biopsy are only available in specialist centers and CT is not routinely used for diagnosis of pneumonia. Chest X-ray is the standard.

Basic diagnostics of endocarditis

High index of suspicion in any patient with fever, murmur ± extracardiac embolic phenomena such as Roth's spots, Osler's nodes, etc. Echocardiography is limited to specialist centers; hence more reliance is made on clinical diagnosis and use of criteria such as the Duke criteria.

Basic diagnostics of gastrointestinal symptoms

Empiric/syndromic treatment of diarrhea with antibiotics is common in resource-limited countries, which may eliminate the chance of making an etiologic diagnosis. Endoscopy and intestinal biopsy is restricted to specialist centers, yet when available, such direct imaging and biopsy plays a vital role in management of HIV patients with complicated or nonresolving infections after empiric treatment.

Basic diagnostics of sexually transmitted infections

The majority of countries with limited resources employ a syndromic approach to management of sexually transmitted infection and therefore do not use diagnostic tests, but rather treat individual syndromes.

Basic diagnostics of patients with adenopathy

Fine needle aspiration or biopsy should be performed on all suspicious lymph nodes, particularly those that are asymmetric and >1.5 cm. Specimens should be sent for tuberculosis microscopy, culture (±histology), and cytology. If a diagnosis is not forthcoming, the node should be excised whenever possible and sent for the above tests.

References

1. Spitalnic S. Test properties I: sensitivity, specificity, and predictive values. Hosp Physician 2004;September:27–31.
2. Aguero-Rosenfeld ME, Wang G, Schwartz I, Wormser GP. Diagnosis of lyme borreliosis. Clin Microbiol Rev 2005;18:484–509.
3. Noguchi T, Yoshiura T, Hiwatashi A, et al. CT and MRI findings of human herpesvirus 6-associated encephalopathy: comparison with findings of herpes simplex virus encephalitis. AJR Am J Roentgenol 2010;194:754–60.
4. Lasseter GM, McNulty CA, Richard Hobbs FD, Mant D, Little P; PRISM Investigators. In vitro evaluation of five rapid antigen detection tests for group A beta-haemolytic streptococcal sore throat infections. Fam Pract 2009;26:437–44.
5. Heiskanen-Kosma T, Paldanius M, Korppi M. Serum procalcitonin concentrations in bacterial pneumonia in children: a negative result in primary healthcare settings. Pediatr Pulmonol 2003;35:56–61.
6. Avni T, Mansur N, Leibovici L, Paul M. PCR using blood for diagnosis of invasive pneumococcal disease: systematic review and meta-analysis. J Clin Microbiol 2010;48:489–96.
7. Bewick T, Lim WS. Diagnosis of community-acquired pneumonia in adults. Expert Rev Respir Med 2009;3:153–64.
8. Ekpo P, Rungpanich U, Pongsunk S, Naigowit P, Petkanchanapong V. Use of protein-specific monoclonal antibody-based latex agglutination for rapid diagnosis of Burkholderia pseudomallei infection in patients with community-acquired septicemia. Clin Vaccine Immunol 2007;14: 811–2.
9. Rodriguez R, Alter H, Romero KL, et al. A pilot study to develop a prediction instrument for endocarditis in injection drug users admitted with fever. Am J Emerg Med 2010 (in press).
10. Knudsen JB, Fuursted K, Petersen E, et al. Procalcitonin in 759 patients clinically suspected of infective endocarditis. Am J Med 2010 (in press).
11. Shah DO, Chang CD, Cheng KY, et al. Comparison of the analytic sensitivities of a recombinant immunoblot assay and the radio-immune precipitation assay for the detection of antibodies to Trypanosoma cruzi in patients with Chagas disease. Diagn Microbiol Infect Dis 2010;67:402–5.
12. Mukherjee P, Ghosh S, Ramamurthy T, et al. Evaluation of a rapid immunochromatographic dipstick kit for diagnosis of cholera emphasizes its outbreak utility. Jpn J Infect Dis 2010; 63:234–8.
13. Kesli R, Gokturk HS, Erbayarak M, Karabagl P, Terzi Y. Comparison of the diagnostic value of 3 different stool antigen tests for noninvasive diagnosis of Helicobacter pylori infection. J Investig Med 2010 (in press).
14. Loy CT, Irwing LM, Katelaris PH, Talley NJ. Do commercial serological kits for Helicobacter pylori infection differ in accuracy? A meta-analysis. Am J Gastroenterol 1996;91:1138–44.
15. Lee NM, Eisen GM. 10 years of capsule endoscopy: an update. Expert Rev Gastroenterol Hepatol 2010;4:503–12.
16. Brunetti E, Kern P, Vuitton DA; Writing Panel for the WHO-IWGE. Expert consensus for the diagnosis and treatment of cystic and alveolar echinococcosis in humans. Acta Trop 2010; 114:1–16.
17. Schmiemann G, Kniehl E, Gebhardt K, Matejczyk MM, Hummers-Pradier E. The diagnosis of urinary tract infection: a systematic review. Dtsch Arztebl Int 2010;107:361–7.
18. Heymans R, van der Helm JJ, de Vries HJ, Fennema HS, Coutinho RA, Bruisten SM. Clinical value of Treponema pallidum real-time PCR for diagnosis of syphilis. J Clin Microbiol 2010; 48:497–502.
19. Herremans T, Kortbeek L, Notermans DW. A review of diagnostic tests for congenital syphilis in newborns. Eur J Clin Microbiol Infect Dis 2010;29:495–501.

20. Cai L, Kong F, Toi C, van Hal S, Gilbert GL. Differentiation of *Chlamydia trachomatis* lymphogranuloma venereum-related serovars from other serovars using multiplex allele-specific polymerase chain reaction and high-resolution melting analysis. Int J STD AIDS 2010;21:101–4.

21. Velho PE, Souza EM, Belda Junior W. Donovanosis. Braz J Infect Dis 2008;12:521–5.

22. Walker MD, Zunt JR. Neuroparasitic infections: nematodes. Semin Neurol 2005;25(3):252–61.

Chapter 5
East Africa: Madagascar and Indian Ocean islands

Philippe Gautret and Philippe Parola

Infectious Diseases and Tropical Medicine Unit, Hopital Nord, Marseille, France

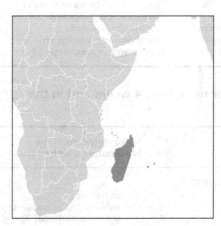

Comoros
Madagascar
Maldives
Mauritius
Réunion (Fr.)
Seychelles

In Reunion, Mauritius, Maldives and Seychelles, improved socio-sanitation conditions over the past years have dramatically decreased the incidence of tropical disease levels comparable with those observed in developed countries. Malaria, schistosomiasis, and lymphatic filariasis have been eradicated, as well as cysticercosis with the exception of Reunion. Amebiasis, typhoid fever, and leprosy have become rare. However, because of the geographical proximity of Madagascar and Comoros where the diseases are endemic, there is a risk of reintroduction of vector-borne infections. Epidemics of dengue and chikungunya were recently observed over all the islands. Tuberculosis remains a public health concern in the whole area.

Infectious Diseases: A Geographic Guide, First Edition.
Edited by Eskild Petersen, Lin H. Chen & Patricia Schlagenhauf.
© 2011 John Wiley & Sons, Ltd. Published 2011 by John Wiley & Sons, Ltd.

Central Nervous System (CNS) infections: meningitis and encephalitis

Acute infections with less than 4 weeks of symptoms

Besides cosmopolitan infections, local infections like Toscana virus infection, West Nile encephalitis, rabies, and typhus should be considered.

Frequently found microorganisms	Rare microorganisms	Very rare microorganisms
Enteroviruses, herpes virus, varicella zoster virus *Streptococcus pneumoniae, Haemophilus influenzae* [1,2], *Neisseria meningitidis*	Rabies virus (Madagascar only), West Nile virus (Madagascar) Neurosyphilis, *Listeria, Mycobacterium tuberculosis Angiostrongylus cantonensis* [3,4]	Influenza *Klebsiella pneumoniae*

Infection with symptoms for more than 4 weeks and in the immunocompromised host

Microorganisms with symptoms for more than 4 weeks	Microorganisms in the immunocompromised host
Human Immunodeficiency Virus (HIV) *M. tuberculosis*	*M. tuberculosis* *Cryptococcus* spp., *Candida* spp., *Aspergillus* spp., *Rhodotorula, Nocardia, Toxoplasma*
Consider noninfectious causes like lymphoma.	

Ear, nose, and throat infections

Ear, nose, and throat infections with less than 4 weeks of symptoms

Frequently found microorganisms	Rare microorganisms and conditions	Very rare microorganisms
Rhinovirus, coronavirus, Respiratory Syncytial Virus (RSV), myxovirus, herpes virus, adenovirus, enterovirus (tonsillitis, rhinitis, otitis), Epstein–Barr virus (EBV) (tonsillitis) *Streptococcus* (tonsillitis, otitis), *Haemophilus,* *B. catarrhalis* (otitis)	*M. tuberculosis* (tonsillitis, otitis)	Diphtheria (tonsillitis)

Ear, nose, and throat infections with symptoms for more than 4 weeks and in the immunocompromised host

Microorganisms with symptoms for more than 4 weeks	Microorganisms in the immunocompromised host
Tuberculosis, syphilis (tonsillitis)	*Candida* spp.
Consider noninfectious causes like cancer.	

Cardiopulmonary infections

Pneumonia with less than 4 weeks of symptoms

Frequently found microorganisms	Rare microorganisms and conditions	Very rare microorganisms
Influenza *Streptococcus pneumoniae, Mycoplasma pneumoniae, H. influenzae, Staphylococcus aureus, Chlamydia pneumoniae* [5–8]	*Legionella pneumophila*	Diphtheria, *K. pneumoniae*

Endocarditis with less than 4 weeks of symptoms

Frequently found microorganisms	Rare microorganisms and conditions
Staphylococcus and *Streptococcus* spp.	*Neisseria gonorrhoeae*

Pulmonary symptoms for more than 4 weeks and in the immunocompromised host

Microorganisms and diseases with symptoms for more than 4 weeks	Microorganisms in the immunocompromised host
Tuberculosis [9] *Aspergillus*	Cytomegalovirus (CMV) *Aspergillus, Candida, Pneumocystis*
Consider noninfectious causes like lung cancer, autoimmune lung fibrosis, and Wegener's granulomatosis.	

Endocarditis for more than 4 weeks and in the immunocompromised host

Microorganisms and diseases with symptoms for more than 4 weeks	Microorganisms in the immunocompromised host
Staphylococcus and *Streptococcus* spp., *Enterococcus*	*Aspergillus, Candida*
Consider noninfectious causes like sarcoidosis.	

Gastrointestinal infections

Gastrointestinal infections with less than 4 weeks of symptoms

Frequently found microorganisms	Rare microorganisms and conditions	Very rare microorganisms
Adenovirus, norovirus and calicivirus, rotavirus, hepatitis A virus		
		Tuberculosis
Escherichia coli, Salmonella spp., *Campylobacter, Shigella*		
Giardia intestinalis, Trichomonas intestinalis	*Cryptosporidia* spp.	*Cyclospora cayetanensis*
Consider noninfectious causes like inflammatory bowel disease and intestinal malignancies like colon cancer.		

Diarrhea is often associated with infections with bacteria, virus, and parasites. Repeated negative bacterial cultures and microscopy for parasites should lead to the consideration that the symptoms may not be caused by an infection. Inflammatory bowel diseases like colitis and Crohn's disease are differential diagnosis and malabsorption and celiac disease must also be considered.

Gastrointestinal infections with symptoms for more than 4 weeks and in the immunocompromised host

Microorganisms with symptoms for more than 4 weeks	Microorganisms in the immunocompromised host
Hepatitis A	Herpes virus, CMV
Tuberculosis	*Isospora*, Microsporidium
G. intestinalis, Entamoeba histolytica, cryptosporidia, *T. intestinalis*, helminths [*Ascaris lumbricoides, Trichuris trichiura, Hymenolepis nana, Strongyloides stercoralis* (Madagascar, Comoros) [10,11], *Schistosoma mansoni* (Madagascar)]	*Candida*
Consider noninfectious causes like inflammatory bowel disease, intestinal malignancies like colon cancer, malabsorption, and celiac disease.	

Infections of liver, spleen, and peritoneum

Acute infections of liver, spleen, and peritoneum with less than 4 weeks of symptoms

	Frequently found diseases	Rare diseases
Jaundice	Hepatitis A	Hepatitis C
	Hepatitis B	Hepatitis E
	EBV, CMV infection	Rickettsiosis
		Leptospirosis
		Syphilis II
		Crimean–Congo Hemorrhagic Fever[a]
Space-occupying lesion in liver	Bacterial liver abscess	Amebic liver abscess
Splenomegaly	Typhoid fever	Visceral leishmaniasis
	Bacterial endocarditis	Relapsing fever
	Viral hepatitis	Brucellosis
	EBV, CMV	Tuberculosis

[a]Has not been described.

Chronic infections of liver, spleen, and peritoneum with more than 4 weeks of symptoms

	Frequently found diseases	Rare diseases
Jaundice	Chronic viral hepatitis	Toxocariasis
	Schistosomiasis[a]	Hepatic tuberculosis[b]
		Leprosy (Madagascar, Comoros)
		Histoplasmosis
Space-occupying lesion in liver		Tuberculosis
Ascites	Tuberculous peritonitis	Schistosomiasis[a]
Splenomegaly	Hepatosplenic schistosomiasis	Tuberculosis
		Brucellosis

[a]Hepatic schistosomiasis is most often due to *S. mansoni* and only present in Madagascar.
[b]Hepatic TB may occur as miliary, nodular, and solitary abscess form.

Infections of liver, spleen, and peritoneum in the immunocompromised host

Infections in the immunocompromised host are no different from the immunocompetent host.

Genitourinary infections

Cystitis, pyelonephritis, and nephritis with less than 4 weeks of symptoms

Frequently found microorganisms	Rare microorganisms and conditions	Very rare microorganisms
E. coli, K. pneumoniae, Staphylococcus saprophyticus, Proteus mirabilis	*Pseudomonas aeruginosa, Enterococcus faecalis*	Tuberculosis

Consider noninfectious causes, especially malignancies like renal cell carcinoma.

Sexually transmitted infections with less than 4 weeks of symptoms

Frequently found microorganisms	Rare microorganisms and conditions
Chlamydia spp., *N. gonorrhoeae, Gardnerella vaginalis*, syphilis *Trichomonas vaginalis*	Lymphogranuloma venereum, *Ducrey* *Entamoeba dispar* and *E. histolytica* (Madagascar, Comoros)

Cystitis, pyelonephritis, and nephritis with symptoms for more than 4 weeks and in the immunocompromised host

Microorganisms with symptoms for more than 4 weeks	Microorganisms in the immunocompromised host
Tuberculosis, *Schistosoma haematobium* (Madagascar) [12]	*Candida*

Consider noninfectious causes, especially malignancies like renal cell carcinoma.

Sexually transmitted infections with symptoms for more than 4 weeks and in the immunocompromised host

Microorganisms with symptoms for more than 4 weeks	Microorganisms in the immunocompromised host
HIV, herpes virus, papilloma virus, hepatitis B virus Syphilis, *N. gonorrhoeae*	Syphilis *Candida*

Joint, muscle, and soft tissue infections

Joint, muscle, and soft tissue infections with less than 4 weeks of symptoms

Frequently found microorganisms
S. aureus *S. pneumoniae*

Joint, muscle, and soft tissue infections with more than 4 weeks of symptoms and in the immunocompromised host

Microorganisms with symptoms for more than 4 weeks	Microorganisms in the immunocompromised host
Tuberculosis	*Candida*, dermatophytes

Skin infections

Skin infections with less than 4 weeks of symptoms

Frequently found microorganisms	Rare microorganisms and conditions
Erysipelas, *S. pneumoniae* *S. aureus* *Borrelia* spp. Dermatomycosis	Lice, scabies

We have not listed a rash due to viral infections as this is not considered an infection limited to the skin.

Skin infections with more than 4 weeks of symptoms and in the immunocompromised host

Microorganisms with symptoms for more than 4 weeks	Microorganisms in the immunocompromised host
Syphilis, tuberculosis, leprosy (Madagascar, Comoros) Scabies	*Candida* Dermatophytes

Adenopathy

Adenopathy of less than 4 weeks' duration

Frequently found microorganisms
EBV, CMV, parvovirus B19, HIV   *Toxoplasma gondii*

Adenopathy of more than 4 weeks' duration and in the immunocompromised host

Microorganisms with symptoms for more than 4 weeks	Microorganisms in the immunocompromised host
Rubella, T. gondii Tuberculosis	Adenovirus, HIV, CMV

If the diagnosis is not made within a few days, biopsies should be performed to exclude malignancies like lymphoma and carcinomas.

Fever without focal symptoms

Fever for less than 4 weeks without focal symptoms

Frequently found microorganisms	Rare microorganisms and conditions
Dengue, Chikungunya (La Reunion, Madagascar, Comoros, Mayotte, Seychelles) [13–18]	Rift Valley fever virus, Crimean–Congo fever (Madagascar), HIV, Influenza [19]
Salmonella typhi (Mauritius), leptospirosis (Seychelles, La Reunion, Mayotte, Maurice) [20,21]	Tuberculosis
Malaria (Madagascar, Comoros), *Plasmodium falciparum* predominant [22–24]	*S. mansoni* and *S. haematobium* (Madagascar only)

Fever for more than 4 weeks without focal symptoms and in the immunocompromised host

Microorganisms with symptoms for more than 4 weeks
Tuberculosis

Noninfectious causes should be considered from the beginning including malignancies like lymphoma and autoimmune diseases.

Noninfectious causes like lymphoma, other malignancies, and autoimmune diseases should be considered early.

Eosinophilia and elevated IgE

Eosinophilia and elevated IgE for less than 4 weeks

Frequently found microorganisms	Rare microorganisms and conditions
A. lumbricoides, T. trichiura, H. nana (Madagascar, Comoros)	Filaria (*Wuchereria bancrofti*)

Eosinophilia and elevated IgE for more than 4 weeks and in the immunocompromised host

Microorganisms with symptoms for more than 4 weeks
S. stercoralis (Comoros, Madagascar)
S. mansoni and *S. haematobium* (Madagascar)
Cysticercosis (Madagascar, Reunion, Comoros)
Visceral larva migrans
Angiostrongylus (La Reunion, Madagascar, Comoros)

Antibiotic resistance

Escherichia coli show high resistance rates against ampicillin, cotrimoxazol, nalidixic acid, and ciprofloxacin in Mauritius [25,26]. Methicillin-resistant *S. aureus* are still rare in the area. A low prevalence of multidrug-resistant tuberculosis was observed in Madagascar and Reunion [27,28]. In Madagascar and Comoros, *P. falciparum* exhibit a high level of resistance to antimalarials, including artemisinin derivatives and atovaquone–proguanil [29–32].

Vaccine-preventable diseases in children

According to World Health Organization (WHO) (http://www.who.int/immunization_ monitoring/data/en/), the childhood vaccination program includes vaccination against tuberculosis, diphtheria, tetanus, poliomyelitis (oral polio vaccine), pertussis, measles, and hepatitis B in all Islands. Vaccination against *H. influenzae* infection is provided in all Islands with the exception of Maldives. Vaccination against mumps and rubella is provided in Mauritius, Reunion, Seychelles, and Maldives. Of interest, rare cases of diphtheria are reported from Madagascar and Mauritius only. Cases of measles, rubella, and pertussis are reported from the entire region with local variations. Tetanus is mainly reported from Madagascar, Comoros, and Mauritius.

Background data

Basic economic and demographic data

Basic demographics[a]	GNI per capita (USD)	Life expectancy at birth (total, years)	School enrollment, primary (% net)
Comoros	750	65	55
Madagascar	410	61	98
Mauritius	6,400	72	95
Seychelles	10,290	73	99

GNI, gross national income.
[a]World Bank.

References

1. Razafindralambo M, Ravelomanana N, Randriamiharisoa FA, et al. [*Haemophilus influenzae*, the second cause of bacterial meningitis in children in Madagascar]. Bull Soc Pathol Exot 2004;97(2):100–3 (French).
2. Migliani R, Clouzeau J, Decousser JW, et al. [Non-tubercular bacterial meningitis in children in Antananarivo, Madagascar]. Arch Pediatr 2002; 9(9):892–7.
3. Graber D, Jaffar MC, Attali T, et al. [*Angiostrongylus* in the infant at Reunion and Mayotte. Apropos of 3 cases of eosinophilic meningitis including 1 fatal radiculomyeloencephalitis with hydrocephalus]. Bull Soc Pathol Exot 1997;90(5):331–2.
4. Picot H, Lavarde V, Donsimoni JM, Jay M. [Presence of *Angiostrongylus cantonensis* at la Réunion]. Acta Trop 1975;32(4):381–3.
5. Soares JL, Ratsitorahina M, Rakoto Andrianarivelo M, et al. [Epidemics of acute respiratory infections in Madagascar in 2002: from alert to confirmation]. Arch Inst Pasteur Madagascar 2003;69(1–2):12–19.

6. Michault A, Simac C. [Bacteriological and epidemiological data on *Streptococcus pneumoniae* in the hospital of southern Reunion Island]. Bull Soc Pathol Exot 2000;93(4):281–6.

7. Rakotoson JL, Rakotomizao JR, Andrianarisoa AC. [Acute community acquired pneumonia: 96 cases in Madagascar]. Med Trop (Mars) 2010;70(1):62–4.

8. Paganin F, Lilienthal F, Bourdin A, et al. Severe community-acquired pneumonia: assessment of microbial aetiology as mortality factor. Eur Respir J 2004;24(5):779–85.

9. Rasamoelisoa JM, Tovone XG, Razoeliarinoro HV, Rakotoarimanana DR. [Evaluation of the management of tuberculosis in children in Madagascar. Results of a multicentric study]. Arch Inst Pasteur Madagascar 1999;65(1–2): 82–5.

10. Buchy P. [Intestinal parasitoses in the Mahajanga region, west coast of Madagascar]. Bull Soc Pathol Exot 2003;96(1):41–5.

11. Brutus L, Watier L, Briand V, Hanitrasoamampionona V, Razanatsoarilala H, Cot M. Parasitic co-infections: Does *Ascaris lumbricoides* protect against *Plasmodium falciparum* infection? Am J Trop Med Hyg 2006;75(2):194–8.

12. Leutscher PD, Høst E, Reimert CM. Semen quality in *Schistosoma haematobium* infected men in Madagascar. Acta Trop 2009;109(1): 41–4.

13. Gautret P, Simon F, Hervius Askling H, et al.; EuroTravNet. Dengue type 3 virus infections in European travellers returning from the Comoros and Zanzibar, February–April 2010. Euro Surveill 2010;15(15):19541.

14. Receveur M, Ezzedine K, Pistone T, Malvy D. Chikungunya infection in a French traveller returning from the Maldives, October, 2009. Euro Surveill 2010;15(8):19494.

15. Pistone T, Ezzedine K, Schuffenecker I, Receveur MC, Malvy D. An imported case of chikungunya fever from Madagascar: use of the sentinel traveller for detecting emerging arboviral infections in tropical and European countries. Travel Med Infect Dis 2009;7(1):52–4.

16. Le Bomin A, Hebert JC, Marty P, Delaunay P. [Confirmed chikungunya in children in Mayotte. Description of 50 patients hospitalized from February to June 2006]. Med Trop (Mars) 2008;68(5):491–5.

17. Economopoulou A, Dominguez M, Helynck B, et al. Atypical chikungunya virus infections: clinical manifestations, mortality and risk factors for severe disease during the 2005–2006 outbreak on Réunion. Epidemiol Infect 2009; 137(4):534–41.

18. Sissoko D, Ezzedine K, Moendandzé A, Giry C, Renault P, Malvy D. Field evaluation of clinical features during chikungunya outbreak in Mayotte, 2005–2006. Trop Med Int Health 2010;15(5):600–7.

19. Staikowsky F, D'Andréa C, Filleul L, et al. [Outbreak of influenza pandemic virus A(H1N1) 2009 infections in Emergency Department, Saint-Pierre, Reunion Island. July–August 2009]. Presse Med 2010;39(7–8):e147–57.

20. Issack MI. Epidemiology of typhoid fever in Mauritius. J Travel Med 2005;12(5):270–4.

21. Agésilas F, Gey F, Monbrunt A, et al. [Acute leptospirosis in children in Reunion Island: a retrospective review of 16 cases]. Arch Pediatr 2005;12(9):1344–8.

22. Jambou R, Ranaivo L, Raharimalala L, et al. Malaria in the highlands of Madagascar after five years of indoor house spraying of DDT. Trans R Soc Trop Med Hyg 2001;95(1):14–18.

23. Parola P, Soula G, Gazin P, Foucault C, Delmont J, Brouqui P. Fever in travelers returning from tropical areas: prospective observational study of 613 cases hospitalised in Marseilles, France, 1999–2003. Travel Med Infect Dis 2006;4(2):61–70.

24. Parola P, Pradines B, Gazin P, Keundjian A, Silai R, Parzy D. [Chemosusceptibility analysis of *Plasmodium falciparum* imported from Comoros to Marseilles, France in 2001–2003]. Med Mal Infect 2005;35(10):489–91.

25. Randrianirina F, Soares JL, Carod JF, et al. Antimicrobial resistance among uropathogens that cause community-acquired urinary tract infections in Antananarivo, Madagascar. J Antimicrob Chemother 2007;59(2):309–12.

26. Issack MI, Yee Kin Tet HY, Morlat P. Antimicrobial resistance among Enterobacteriaceae causing uncomplicated urinary tract infections in Mauritius: consequences of past misuse of antibiotics. J Chemother 2007;19 (2):222–5.

27. Baroux N, D'Ortenzio E. [Tuberculosis in Reunion island: epidemiological characteristics of notified cases, 2000–2007]. Med Mal Infect 2010;40(1):12–17.

28. Ramarokoto H, Ratsirahonana O, Soares JL, et al. First national survey of *Mycobacterium tuberculosis* drug resistance, Madagascar, 2005–2006. Int J Tuberc Lung Dis 2010;14(6):745–50.

29. Andriantsoanirina V, Ratsimbasoa A, Bouchier C, et al. *Plasmodium falciparum* drug resistance in

Madagascar: facing the spread of unusual pfdhfr and pfmdr-1 haplotypes and the decrease of dihydroartemisinin susceptibility. Antimicrob Agents Chemother 2009;53(11):4588–97.

30. Savini H, Bogreau H, Bertaux L, et al. First case of emergence of atovaquone–proguanil resistance in *Plasmodium falciparum* during treatment in a traveler in Comoros. Antimicrob Agents Chemother 2008;52(6):2283–4.

31. Parola P, Pradines B, Simon F, et al. Antimalarial drug susceptibility and point mutations associated with drug resistance in 248 *Plasmodium falciparum* isolates imported from Comoros to Marseille, France in 2004–2006. Am J Trop Med Hyg 2007;77(3):431–7.

32. Andriantsoanirina V, Ménard D, Tuseo L, Durand R. History and current status of *Plasmodium falciparum* antimalarial drug resistance in Madagascar. Scand J Infect Dis 2010;42(1): 22–32.

Chapter 6
Eastern Africa

Andreas Neumayr and Christoph Hatz
Department of Medical and Diagnostic Services, Swiss Tropical and Public Health Institute, Basel, Switzerland

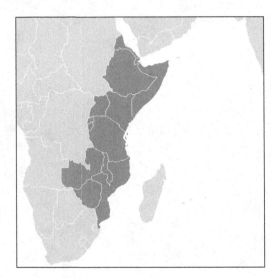

Eritrea
Djibouti
Somalia
Ethiopia
Kenya
Uganda
Rwanda
Burundi
Tanzania
Malawi
Mozambique
Zambia
Zimbabwe

Travelers in East Africa are potentially exposed to malaria, HIV, tuberculosis, and many other infectious diseases. Exposure determines the risk—from traveler's diarrhea and vector-borne diseases to extremely rare infections. Patients with a history of staying in or visiting Eastern Africa who present with an acute febrile illness may have acquired an infection specific for the region or one that is common worldwide (e.g. EBV, influenza).

Infectious Diseases: A Geographic Guide, First Edition.
Edited by Eskild Petersen, Lin H. Chen & Patricia Schlagenhauf.
© 2011 John Wiley & Sons, Ltd. Published 2011 by John Wiley & Sons, Ltd.

Parasites

Malaria occurs throughout the region—except for highland areas in Eritrea, Ethiopia, Kenya, and Tanzania—with varied transmission patterns. *Plasmodium falciparum* is the predominant species, with widespread chloroquine resistance. Emerging drug resistance of *Plasmodium vivax* to chloroquine exists in Ethiopia and Madagascar [1,2].

Malaria transmission in Eastern Africa

Country	Malaria-endemic areas	Malaria type
Burundi	All	*P. falciparum* >85%, *Plasmodium malariae*, *Plasmodium ovale*, and *P. vivax* <15%
Eritrea	All areas at altitudes <2,200 m, no malaria in Asmara	*P. falciparum* 85%, *P. vivax* 10–15%, *P. ovale* rare. *P. malariae* not described
Ethiopia	All areas at altitudes <2,500 m, no malaria in Addis Ababa	*P. falciparum* 85%, *P. vivax* 10–15%, *P. malariae* and *P. ovale* <5%
Kenya	All areas at altitudes <2,500 m, no malaria in Nairobi	*P. falciparum* 85%, *P. vivax* 5–10%, *P. ovale* up to 5%. *P. malariae* not described
Malawi	All	*P. falciparum* 90%, *P. malariae*, *P. ovale*, and *P. vivax* 10%
Mozambique	All	*P. falciparum* 95%, *P. malariae* and *P. ovale* 5%, *P. vivax* rare
Rwanda	All	*P. falciparum* <85%, *P. vivax* 5%, *P. ovale* 5%. *P. malariae* not described
Somalia	All	*P. falciparum* 95%, *P. vivax*, *P. malariae*, and *P. ovale* 5%
Tanzania	All areas at altitudes <1,800 m	*P. falciparum* >85%, *P. malariae* and *P. ovale* >10%, *P. vivax* rare
Uganda	All	*P. falciparum* 85%, *P. malariae*, *P. ovale*, and *P. vivax* <15%
Zambia	All	*P. falciparum* >90%, *P. vivax* up to 5%, *P. ovale* up to 5%. *P. malariae* not described
Zimbabwe	All	*P. falciparum* >90%, *P. vivax* up to 5%, *P. ovale* up to 5%. *P. malariae* not described

Adapted from information obtained from the CDC Malaria Map Application accessed at http://cdc-malaria.ncsa.uiuc.edu/index.php on September 16, 2010.

Viruses

Human Immunodeficiency Virus (HIV) shows a north–south distribution, with available figures ranging from 0.7% (rural)/5.5% (urban) in Ethiopia to 10.8% (rural)/23.1% (urban) in Zambia [3]. Dengue epidemics are infrequent in Eastern Africa, but all four serotypes have caused outbreaks in the region. Yellow fever may occur from Ethiopia to Tanzania, but the risk is low. Eritrea, Malawi, Mozambique, Zambia, and Zimbabwe are free of yellow fever.

Bacteria

Tuberculosis continues to be a major health issue in all countries in East Africa, especially as multidrug-resistant tuberculosis (MDR-TB) is on the rise and emergence of extensively drug-resistant tuberculosis (XDR-TB) has been reported from Mozambique and Kenya [4]. Among the 15 countries with the highest estimated TB incidence rates reported by the WHO are Zimbabwe (4th), Zambia (9th), and Mozambique (11th) [5]. Among the 27 high-burden MDR-TB countries the WHO lists are Ethiopia (16th), Kenya (20th), Mozambique (21st), and Zimbabwe (23rd) [6]. The classical sub-Saharan "Meningitis belt," with its infamous epidemics of meningococcal disease, ranges from Senegal to Eritrea and extends south through the Rift Valley to the Great Lakes region as far as Mozambique. Epidemic waves can last 2–3 years, typically occur in the dry season (December to June), and subside during the intervening rainy seasons.

CNS infections: meningitis, encephalitis, and other infections with neurological symptoms

Acute CNS infections with less than 4 weeks of symptoms

Frequently found microorganisms	Rare microorganisms	Very rare microorganisms
Adenoviruses	CMV	Chikungunya
Enteroviruses (Coxackie, Echo)	HHV 6 and 7	Trypanosomiasis
HSV 1 and 2	HIV	Filoviruses (Ebola, Marburg)
Varicella zoster	Influenza viruses	West Nile fever
Haemophilus influenzae	Measles	Polyomavirus (JC and SV-40)
Meningococci	Mumps	Polyomyelitis
Pneumococci	Parainfluenza viruses	Rabies
Staphylococci	EBV	LCMV
Streptococci	*Chlamydia pneumoniae*	Rift Valley fever
Malaria—*P. falciparum*	*Mycoplasma pneumoniae*	Sindbis
	Listeriosis	Angiostrongyloidiasis
		Primary amebic meningoencephalitis

CNS infections with more than 4 weeks of symptoms and in the immunocompromised host

Microorganisms with more than 4 weeks of symptoms	Microorganisms in the immunocompromised host
HIV	Tuberculosis
Brucellosis	Toxoplasmosis
Syphilis	Cryptococcosis
Tuberculosis	
Toxoplasmosis	
Trypanosomiasis[a]	
Angiostrongyloidiasis[a]	
Cysticercosis[a]	

[a]Rare infection.

Ear, nose, and throat infections

Ear, nose, and throat infections with less than 4 weeks of symptoms

Frequently found microorganisms	Rare microorganisms	Very rare microorganisms
Adenoviruses	Diphtheria	Filoviruses (Ebola,
EBV	*Neisseria gonorrhoeae* (initially pharyngitis)	Marburg)
Enteroviruses	Necrotizing fasciitis	
CMV	Peritonsillar abscess (*Fusobacterium*	
Coronaviruses	*necrophorum*)	
Human metapneumovirus	Vincent's angina (*Fusobacterium nucleatum,*	
HSV 1 and 2	*Treponema vincentii*)	
Measles		
Parainfluenza viruses		
Rhinoviruses		
Bordetella pertussis		
H. influenzae		
Moraxella catarrhalis		
M. pneumoniae		
Staphylococci		
Streptococci		

Ear, nose, and throat infections with more than 4 weeks of symptoms and in the immunocompromised host

Microorganisms with more than 4 weeks of symptoms	Microorganisms in the immunocompromised host
Syphilis	Tuberculosis
Tuberculosis	Candidiasis
Rhinoscleroma (*Klebsiella rhinoscleromatis*)[a]	Mucormycosis[a]
Lingulatosis[a]	Rhinosporidiosis[a] (*Rhinosporidium seeberi*)

[a]Rare infection.

Cardiopulmonary infections

Cardiopulmonary infections with less than 4 weeks of symptoms

Pulmonary infections with less than 4 weeks of symptoms

Frequently found microorganisms	Rare microorganisms	Very rare microorganisms
Adenoviruses	Q fever	Anthrax
Influenza viruses	Pulmonary symptoms due to	Melioidosis
Parainfluenza viruses	parasitic migration:	Plague
RSV	Ascariasis—Löffler's syndrome	Psittacosis
C. pneumoniae	Hookworm (*Necator americanus*)	Relapsing fever, borreliosis
	Strongyloidiasis	

(Continued)

Frequently found microorganisms	Rare microorganisms	Very rare microorganisms
Klebsiella pneumoniae *Legionella* *M. catarrhalis* *M. pneumoniae* *B. pertussis* *Staphylococcus aureus* Coagulase-negative staphylococci *Streptococcus pneumoniae*	Toxocariasis Tropical pulmonary eosinophilia (Filariasis) Schistosomiasis, Katayama fever	Rickettsiosis Acute bronchopulmonary aspergillosis (ABPA) *Aspergillus* spp. Blastomycosis Histoplasmosis (*H. capsulatum* var. *gati* and var. *duboisii*—African histoplasmosis)

Endocarditis with less than 4 weeks of symptoms

Frequently found microorganisms	Rare microorganisms	Very rare microorganisms
Streptococci *S. aureus* Coagulase-negative *Staphylococcus*	Q fever HACEK group bacteria *Bartonella* spp. Enterococci *N. gonorrhoeae* Salmonellosis *Pseudomonas aeruginosa* Rickettsiosis Tuberculosis	Rat-bite fever Histoplasmosis Propionebacterium

Myocarditis with less than 4 weeks of symptoms

Frequently found microorganisms	Rare microorganisms	Very rare microorganisms
Adenoviruses Enteroviruses (Coxsackie) Echoviruses	CMV Influenza viruses Mumps Parvovirus B19 Relapsing fever Rickettsiosis Staphylococci Streptococci Tuberculosis	Chikungunya Dengue EBV HSV Varicella zoster virus Brucellosis *Campylobacter* spp. Diphtheria Legionellosis *Neisseria meningitidis*

Frequently found microorganisms	Rare microorganisms	Very rare microorganisms
		Q fever
		Rickettsiosis
		Trichinellosis
		Trypanosomiasis

Pulmonary infections with more than 4 weeks of symptoms and in the immunocompromised host

Microorganisms with more than 4 weeks of symptoms	Microorganisms in the immunocompromised host
Atypical mycobacteria	Atypical mycobacteria
Melioidosis[a]	Melioidosis[a]
Pertussis	Nocardiosis
Tuberculosis	*Rhodococcus equi*
Paragonimiasis[a]	Tuberculosis
Pentastomiasis[a]	*Pneumocystis jirovecii*
Dirofilariasis[a]	*Aspergillus* spp.
	Blastomycosis
	Candida spp.
	Histoplasmosis (*H. capsulatum* var. *gati* and var. *duboisii*—African histoplasmosis)

[a]Rare infection.

Endocarditis with more than 4 weeks of symptoms and in the immunocompromised host

Microorganisms with more than 4 weeks of symptoms	Microorganisms in the immunocompromised host
Brucellosis	Bartonellosis
Q fever	Tuberculosis
	Aspergillosis
	Blastomycosis
	Candida spp.
	Cryptococcosis
	Histoplasmosis

Consider systemic lupus erythematodes (Libman–Sacks endocarditis).

Myocarditis with more than 4 weeks of symptoms and in the immunocompromised host   Brucellosis and tuberculosis should be considered. Aspergillosis, blastomycosis, candidiasis, cryptococcosis, and histoplasmosis are other rare possibilities.

Gastrointestinal infections

Gastrointestinal infections with less than 4 weeks

Frequently found microorganisms	Rare microorganisms	Very rare microorganisms
Adenoviruses	Cholera	Atypical mycobacteria
Astroviruses	*Vibrio parahaemolyticus*	Enteritis necroticans (pigbel,
Caliciviruses (Noroviruses)	*Yersinia* spp.	*Clostridium difficile* type C)
Rotaviruses	Cryptosporidiosis	*Isospora*
Sapoviruses	*Balantidium coli*	*Sarcocystis* spp.
Campylobacter spp.		*Trichinella*
Salmonella spp.		
Typhoid fever		
Shigellosis		
Enteropathogenic		
Escherichia coli		
Giardia intestinalis		
Entamoeba histolytica		

In gastroenteritis with a very short incubation period (hours) toxins should be considered (staphylococci, *Bacillus cereus*, and *Clostridium*).

Traveler's diarrhea: In a large prospective cohort study a 2-week incidence of traveler's diarrhea of 29.1% has been reported from the East Africa [7]. The spectrum of pathogens includes bacteria (pathogenic *E. coli*, *Salmonella*, *Shigella*, *Campylobacter*, etc.), viruses, and protozoa (*Amoeba*, *Giardia*, etc.).

Cholera: The risk for travelers to affected area is estimated to be less than 1 in 500,000 (0.001–0.01% per month of stay) [8].

Gastrointestinal infections with more than 4 weeks of symptoms and in the immunocompromised host

Microorganisms with more than 4 weeks of symptoms	Microorganisms in the immunocompromised host
Tuberculosis	Bartonellosis
E. histolytica	Tuberculosis
B. coli	Cryptosporidiosis
Ascariasis	Cyclosporiasis
Cyclosporiasis	Isosporiasis
Strongyloidiasis	*Microsporidia* spp.
Trichinellosis[a]	Strongyloidiasis
Trichuriasis	Candidiasis
Schistosomiasis	Blastomycosis
Taeniasis[a]	Histoplasmosis

Consider tropical enteropathy/sprue, postinfective irritable bowel syndrome, inflammatory bowel disease.
[a]Rare infection.

Infections of liver, spleen, and peritoneum

Acute infections of liver, spleen, and peritoneum with less than 4 weeks of symptoms

Frequently found microorganisms	Rare microorganisms	Very rare microorganisms
CMV	Coxsackieviruses	Yellow fever
EBV	HSV	Bartonellosis
Hepatitis A	Mumps	Blastomycosis
Hepatitis E	Leishmaniasis, visceral (*L. donovani, L. infantum*)	Histoplasmosis
Leptospirosis	Relapsing fever	
Q fever	Rickettsiosis	
Rickettsiosis	*Salmonella* spp.	
Typhoid fever	*Shigella*	
Amebic liver abscess	Syphilis	
	Yersinia spp.	

Hepatits A: Acute viral hepatitis A should be considered in any unvaccinated patient presenting with fever and jaundice.

Leptospirosis: Infections are caused by exposure to contaminated water. Symptoms include high fever, headache, chills, intense myalgia, conjunctival suffusion, jaundice, and gastro-intestinal symptoms. Liver failure, kidney failure, pulmonary hemorrhage as well as aseptic meningitis can manifest in severe cases. Leptospirosis should be suspected in adventure travelers (especially water sports).

Chronic infections of liver, spleen, and peritoneum with more than 4 weeks of symptoms and in the immunocompromised host

Microorganisms with more than 4 weeks of symptoms	Microorganisms in the immunocompromised host
Hepatitis B (±delta agent)	Atypical mycobacteriosis
Hepatitis C	Melioidosis[a]
Brucellosis	Tuberculosis
Tuberculosis	Strongyloidiasis
Amebic liver abscess	Candidiasis
Leishmaniasis, viceral[a]	Blastomycosis
Capillaria hepatica[a]	Histoplasmosis
Echinococcus granulosus[a]	Leishmaniasis, visceral
Fascioliasis[a]	(*L. donovani, L. infantum*)
Schistosomiasis	Cryptosporidiosis
Toxocariasis, visceral larva migrans	

[a]Rare infection, consider malignancy.

Genitourinary infections

Genitourinary infections with less than 4 weeks of symptoms

Cystitis, pyelonephritis, and nephritis with less than 4 weeks of symptoms

Frequently found microorganisms	Rare microorganisms	Very rare microorganisms
Enterococci	Hanta	Polyomaviruses (BK, JC)
Enterobacter spp.	Ascariasis (GN)	
E. coli	Strongyloidiasis (GN)	
K. pneumoniae	Lymphatic filariasis (GN)	
Leptospirosis	Onchocerciasis (GN)	
Mycoplasma—nongonococcal	Loiasis (GN)	
urethritis (NGU)		
Proteus spp.		
Relapsing fever, borreliosis		
Rickettsiosis		
Shigella (HUS)		
Staphylococci		
Ureaplasma urealyticum (NGU)		

GN, glomerulonephritis; HUS, hemolytic uremic syndrome.

Sexually transmitted infections with less than 4 weeks of symptoms

Frequently found microorganisms	Rare microorganisms	Very rare microorganisms
HSV 2	–	–
Gonorrhea—*N. gonorrhoeae*		

Cystitis, pyelonephritis, and nephritis with more than 4 weeks of symptoms and in the immunocompromised host

Microorganisms with more than 4 weeks of symptoms	Microorganisms in the immunocompromised host
Tuberculosis	Tuberculosis
Schistosomiasis—*Schistosoma haematobium*	Candidiasis

Consider para/postinfectious glomerulonephritis/nephrotic syndrome.

Sexually transmitted infections with more than 4 weeks of symptoms and in the immunocompromised host

Microorganisms with more than 4 weeks of symptoms	Microorganisms in the immunocompromised host
Papillomaviruses Chancroid—*Haemophilus ducreyi* Donovanosis (Granuloma inguinale)— *Calymmatobacterium granulomatis* Gonorrhea—*N. gonorrhoeae* Lymphogranuloma venereum—*Chlamydia trachomatis* serovar L1–L3 Syphilis veneral Trichomoniasis Ectoparasites (e.g., lice, scabies)	The same microorganisms are seen as in the immunocompetent host

Joint and muscle infections

Joint and muscle infections with less than 4 weeks of symptoms

Frequently found microorganisms	Rare microorganisms	Very rare microorganisms
Adenoviruses CMV Chikungunya Dengue EBV Enteroviruses (Coxackie, Echo) HIV Influenza viruses O'nyong nyong Parainfluenza viruses Sindbis	*Clostridium perfringens* (gas gangrene) Leptospirosis *N. gonorrhoeae* Nonclostridial myonecrosis: Anaerobic streptococcal myositis (e.g., GAS, peptostreptococci, streptococci) Synergistic nonclostridial myonecrosis (polymicrobial infection) Vascular gangrene (often polymicrobial infection) Relapsing fever, borreliosis Rickettsiosis *Salmonella* spp. Staphylococci (tropical pyomyositis) Streptococci	Hepatitis B and C HSV 2 Parvovirus B19 Varicella zoster West Nile virus Yellow fever Rat-bite fever (spirillosis, streptobacillosis) Trichinellosis *E. histolytica*

Consider reactive arthritis:
 Poststreptococcal reactive arthritis/rheumatic fever arthritis
 Reiter's syndrome (*C. trachomatis*)
 Shigella, Yersinia, Salmonella spp., etc.

Joint and muscle infections with more than 4 weeks of symptoms and in the immunocompromised host

Microorganisms with more than 4 weeks of symptoms	Microorganisms in the immunocompromised host
Chikungunya	Melioidosis[a]
Brucellosis	Tuberculosis
Tuberculosis	*Aspergillus* spp.
Melioidosis	*Candida* spp.
Syphilis endemic (Yaws)	Cryptococcosis
Cysticercosis[a]	Histoplasmosis
Dracunculiasis[a]	
Echinococcosis[a]	
Trichinellosis[a]	

[a]Rare infection, consider rheumatological diseases.

Skin infections

Skin infections with less than 4 weeks of symptoms

Frequently found microorganisms	Rare microorganisms	Very rare microorganisms
HSV 1 and 2	Hand, foot, and mouth disease (Coxackie A and Enterovirus 71)	Monkey pox
Varicella zoster		Orf virus
Staphylococci	Tungiasis	Tanapox
Streptococci		Anthrax
Cutaneous larva migrans		Diphtheria, cutaneous
Myiasis (*Cordylobia anthropophaga*)		*Erysipelothrix*
		N. gonorrhoeae, disseminated

Skin infections with more than 4 weeks of symptoms and in the immunocompromised host

Microorganisms with more than 4 weeks of symptoms	Microorganisms in the immunocompromised host
Molluscum contagiosum	Melioidosis[a]
Papillomaviruses	Tuberculosis, cutaneous
Leprosy[a]	Strongyloidiasis
Melioidosis[a]	Blastomycosis
Mycobacterium ulcerans (Buruli ulcer)[a]	Cryptococcosis
Necrotizing ulcer of skin (tropical ulcer)	Entomophtoromysosis (subcutaneous *Basidiobolus*)[a]
Noma[a]	Mycetoma—Madura foot[a]

Microorganisms with more than 4 weeks of symptoms	Microorganisms in the immunocompromised host
Syphilis endemic	Sporotrichosis
Syphilis veneral	Scabies
Tuberculosis, cutaneous	
Cutaneous amebiasis[a]	
Leishmaniasis, cutaneous[a]	
(*Leishmania tropica, Leishmania aethiopica, Leishmania Major*)	
Trypanosomiasis[a]	
Cysticercosis[a]	
Dracunculiasis[a]	
Gnathostomiasis[a]	
Loiasis[a]	
Lymphatic filariasis[a]	
Mansonelliasis (*Mansonella perstans*)[a]	
Onchocerciasis[a]	
Schistosomiasis (cercarial dermatitis)	
Strongyloidiasis	
Pityriasis versicolor	
Tinea/ringworm	
Mycetoma—Madura foot[a]	
Scabies	

[a]Rare infection.

Adenopathy

Adenopathy of less than 4 weeks duration

Frequently found microorganisms	Rare microorganisms	Very rare microorganisms
Adenoviruses	Diphtheria	Crimean–Congo hemorrhagic fever
CMV	Leptospirosis	Filoviruses (Ebola, Marburg)
Enteroviruses (Coxsackie)	Relapsing fever,	Rift Valley fever
Dengue	borreliosis	HTLV-1
EBV	Rickettsiosis	Anthrax
HHV 6 and 7	Syphilis	Bartonellosis
HIV	Typhoid fever	Brucellosis
HSV 1 and 2	Toxoplasmosis	Chancroid—*H. ducreyi*
Measles		Lymphogranuloma venereum
Mumps		Plague
Parvovirus B19		Rat-bite fever (spirillosis,
Rhinoviruses		streptobacillosis)
Rubella		
Varicella zoster		

Adenopathy of more than 4 weeks duration and in the immunocompromised host

Microorganisms with more than 4 weeks of symptoms	Microorganisms in the immunocompromised host
Atypical mycobacteria	Atypical mycobacteria
Bartonellosis	Bartonellosis
Brucellosis	Melioidosis[a]
Melioidosis[a]	Nocardiosis
Tuberculosis	R. equi
Toxoplasmosis	Tuberculosis
Trypanosomiasis[a]	Toxoplasmosis
Loiasis[a]	Blastomycosis
Lymphatic filariasis (Wuchereria bancrofti)[a]	Histoplasmosis
Mansonelliasis (M. perstans)[a]	Sporotrichosis
Sporotrichosis	

[a]Rare infection, consider malignancy.

African trypanosomiasis (African sleeping sickness) is transmitted by the tsetse fly and caused by the protozoa *Trypanosoma brucei*. East African trypanosomiasis is caused by *Trypanosoma brucei rhodesiense* and shows more acute and severe symptoms than the West African variant caused by *Trypanosoma brucei gambiense*. In the first stage (hemolymphatic stage) of the disease generalized swelling of lymph nodes (characteristically along the back of the neck: "Winterbottom's sign") and fever is seen. The second stage (meningoencephalitic stage), which coined the term "sleeping sickness," begins when the parasite invades the central nervous system (usually some weeks after infection). The presence of an inoculation chancre (a painful, circumscribed, indurated papule, 2–5 cm in diameter), which develops 5–15 days after the bite (and disappears after 2–3 weeks), facilitates the diagnosis. Trypanosomiasis in travelers has been reported from Tanzania, Botswana, Rwanda, Kenya, Malawi, Uganda, and Zambia.

Fever without focal symptoms

Fever less than 4 weeks without focal symptoms

Frequently found microorganisms	Rare microorganisms	Very rare microorganisms
Malaria	Hanta	Crimean–Congo hemorrhagic fever
CMV	Sindbis	Bunyamwera virus
Chikungunya	O'nyong nyong	Bwamba virus
Dengue	Rift Valley fever	Filoviruses (Ebola, Marburg)
EBV		Lujo hemorrhagic fever
Hepatitis A		Orungo virus
Hepatitis B		Wesselsbron virus
Hepatitis C		Yellow fever
HIV		Zika virus
Influenza		Anthrax
Measles		Bartonellosis, Trench fever— *Bartonella quintana*

Frequently found microorganisms	Rare microorganisms	Very rare microorganisms
Varicella zoster		Melioidosis
Adenoviruses		Plague
Relapsing fever, borreliosis		Psittacosis
Rickettsiosis		Rat-bite fever (spirillosis,
African tick bite fever		streptobacillosis)
Rickettsial pox		
Typhus epidemic/louse-borne		
Rickettsia prowazekii		
Typhus		
endemic/murine/		
tick-borne—*Rickettsia typhi*		
Typhoid fever		
Schistosomiasis, Katayama fever		

African tick bite fever (ATBF) caused by *Rickettsia africae* appears to be the most important "spotted fever" in East Africa [9]. Transmitted by Amblyomma ticks, safari tourists, backpackers, hunters, sports competitors, and foreign aid workers are particularly at risk. The average incubation period is 1 week. Eschars (often multiple) are observed in 95% of patients [10], and 4–9% of first-time Norwegian travelers to rural subequatorial Africa had specific antibodies to *R. africae* [11,12].

Louse-borne relapsing fever (LBRF) caused by *Borrelia recurrentis* is found in East African countries and is especially prevalent in Ethiopia [13]. The repeated episodes of fever, interrupted by periods of relative well-being, are often misdiagnosed as malaria.

Arthropod-borne virus infections Dengue fever, caused by a flavivirus, is transmitted by day-biting Aedes mosquitoes, and characterized by abrupt onset of fever, retro-orbital headache, myalgia ("breakbone" fever), a discrete uniform rash, and arthralgia. Eight percent of imported dengue fever cases in Europe are infected in Africa [14]. Among the arboviruses endemic in East Africa, the Togaviruses such as Chikungunya, O'nyong nyong, and Sindbis can cause fever with pronounced arthralgia. The characteristic polyarthralgic complaints of Chikungunya may persist for days, weeks, months, or in some cases even years. Zika virus and Wesselsbron virus are members of the Flaviviridae virus family. Common symptoms include mild headaches, maculopapular rash, fever, malaise, conjunctivitis, and arthralgia. Bunyamwera virus is an *Orthobunyavirus* belonging to the Bunyaviridae family that contains the La Crosse virus, the causative virus of La Crosse encephalitis. It causes a mild febrile illness sometime with conjunctivitis, rash, and mild CNS symptoms. Orungo virus belongs to the orbivirus family and has been described from Uganda, where it causes a mild febrile illness. Bwamba fever virus, transmitted by *Anopheles funestus*, is from the genus *Orthobunyavirus* and causes a mild febrile illness. Bwamba fever is believed to be endemic in East Africa, especially Kenya, Tanzania, and Uganda.

Viral hemorrhagic fevers The overall travel-related risk to contract a viral hemorrhagic fever is conservatively estimated at <1 in 1 million travel episodes to endemic African countries: Febrile patients returning from East Africa are at least 1,000 times more likely to have malaria [15].

Ebola and Marburg viruses: Cases and outbreak clusters of viral hemorrhagic fevers due to filoviruses are extremely rare events, but have occurred in Eastern Africa (Ebola: Uganda; Marburg: Kenya, Uganda). They are associated with very high case fatality rates. Current evidence suspects fruit bats to act as animal reservoir for Ebola and Marburg viruses. Index cases are often infected by handling corpses of primates. Nosocomial spread usually results from reuse of needles and syringes and direct contact to infected blood, body secretions, or tissues. Travelers should be informed that visits to bat-infested caves have a risk for infection, as documented by a fatal case of Marburg HF in a Dutch tourist 2008 [16]. Lujo virus and Ilesha virus are new hemorrhagic fever viruses. Only one outbreak of Lujo virus has occurred so far in Zambia with a case fatality rate of 80% [17]. *Rift Valley fever* (RVF) is a mosquito-borne viral zoonosis transmitted by mosquitoes or by contact with the blood or tissue of infected animals and possibly from the ingestion of raw milk. RVF is distributed throughout East Africa with single cases and epidemic outbreaks have been reported. Most human cases are relatively mild, but RVF-associated encephalitis, retinitis (leading to blindness), or the hemorrhagic form have been reported [18]. *Crimean–Congo hemorrhagic fever* (CCHF) is transmitted by ticks and occurs in Ethiopia, Kenya, Tanzania, Uganda, and Madagascar [19].

Fever for more than 4 weeks without focal symptoms and in the immunocompromised host

Microorganisms with more than 4 weeks of symptoms	Microorganisms in the immunocompromised host
Atypical mycobacteriosis	Atypical mycobacteriosis
Brucellosis	Bartonellosis
Infective endocarditis	Melioidosis[a]
Melioidosis[a]	Nocardiosis
Pyogenic intra-abdominal abscess	*R. equi*
Q fever	Tuberculosis
Relapsing fever, borreliosis	Leishmaniasis visceral (*L. donovani*,
Syphilis	*L. infantum*)
Tuberculosis	Toxoplasmosis
Amebic liver abscess	Strongyloidiasis
Leishmaniasis visceral (*L. donovani*,	*Strongyloides hyperinfection syndrome*
L. infantum)[a]	Blastomycosis
Strongyloidiasis	Cryptococcosis
Toxoplasmosis	Histoplasmosis
Trypanosomiasis[a]	
Toxocariasis, visceral larva migrans	

[a]Rare infection.

Eosinophilia and elevated IgE

Eosinophilia and elevated IgE less than 4 weeks

Frequently found microorganisms	Rare microorganisms	Very rare microorganisms
Acariasis	Hymenolepiasis	–
Cercarial dermatitis (Swimmer's itch, avian schistosoma spp.)		
Cutaneous larva migrans		
Strongyloidiasis		
Myiasis (*C. anthropophaga*)		

Eosinophilia and elevated IgE more than 4 weeks and in the immunocompromised host

Microorganisms with more than 4 weeks of symptoms	Microorganisms in the immunocompromised host
Angiostrongyloidiasis[a] Cysticercosis[a] Diphyllobotriasis[a] Dirofilariasis[a] *E. granulosus*[a] Gnathostomiasis[a] Hookworm (*N. americanus*) Loiasis[a] Lymphatic filariasis[a] *Mansonella*[a] *Onchocerca*[a] *Paragonimus* spp.[a] Schistosomiasis Strongyloidiasis Taeniasis (*Taenia saginata, Taenia solium*)[a] Toxocariasis, visceral larva migrans Trichinellosis[a] Trichostrongylus[a] Trichuriasis Scabies	Strongyloidiasis Scabies+the organisms listed under the immunocompetent host with symptoms both less and more than 4 weeks

[a]Rare infection.

Acute schistosomiasis (Katayama fever): Schistosomiasis is present throughout East Africa. The most prevalent species are *S. haematobium* and *S. mansoni*. *Schistosoma intercalatum* is only reported from Uganda [20]. In its second phase, fever, eosinophilia, urticaria, and possibly pulmonary symptoms appear as "Katayama fever." Parasite ova are absent from urine and stool during the prepatent period ($\sim$1–3 months). Serology is the diagnostic method of choice.

Antibiotic resistance

Uncontrolled over-the-counter sale and uncritical usage of antibiotics in humans as well as in livestock leads to antimicrobial resistance which is widespread in most African countries. Few appropriate laboratory facilities provide very scarce data on antibiotic resistance in East Africa.

Streptococcus pneumoniae: Isolates collected in Kenya, Uganda, and Tanzania remain susceptible to the most commonly used antibiotics with the exception of trimethoprim/sulfamethoxazole, and have exhibited no resistance to penicillin [21]. The prevalence of resistance to cefotaxime, erythromycin, and amoxicillin is low (0–1.5%). Worries about chloramphenicol resistance in meningitis cases appear to be unfounded as a decrease from 9% in 2004 to 2% in 2008 was observed [21].

Salmonella: Multidrug-resistant *Salmonella typhi* strains (ampicillin, trimethoprim, chloramphenicol, streptomycin, sulfonamides, and tetracyclines = MRSTY) have emerged in several East African countries (e.g., Kenya 1997–1998). This increasingly common resistance pattern prompted widespread use of fluoroquinolones, which was followed by the widespread emergence of reduced fluoroquinolone susceptibility of *S. typhi* in the early 1990s. Multidrug resistance is now an increasing problem as seen in Nairobi, where multidrug-resistant *S. typhi* isolates resistant to fluoroquinolones have increased from 5.6% in 2000 to 18.4% in 2008 [22]. Currently third-generation cephalosporins such as ceftriaxone or cefotaxime as well as the macrolide antibiotic azithromycin provide alternatives in fluoroquinolone-resistant *S. typhi*.

Shigella: Extensive outbreaks and epidemics of multidrug-resistant *Shigella dysenteriae* have been reported over the last four decades in the East Africa. The isolates have been resistant to ampicillin, chloramphenicol, tetracyclines, trimethoprim, and nalidixic acid. Third-generation cephalosporins such as ceftriaxone or cefotaxime as well as the newer fluoroquinolones and pivmecillinam provide alternatives.

Campylobacter: Multidrug resistance, including macrolides and fluoroquinolones, has increasingly been reported, but limited data are available from East Africa. Susceptibility testing, if available, should guide antimicrobial treatment.

Vaccine-preventable diseases in children

Immunization coverage among 1-year-olds in the Eastern African region

Immunization coverage among 1-year-olds (%)	Measles	Diphtheria Tetanus Polio (DTP3)	Hepatitis B (HepB3)
Burundi	75	74	83
Comoros	73	76	77
Djibouti	NS	NS	NS
Eritrea	84	83	83
Ethiopia	71	80	NS
Kenya	73	73	73
Madagascar	59	61	61
Malawi	80	89	89
Mauritius	98	98	98
Mozambique	77	72	72
Rwanda	84	89	89
Seychelles	99	99	99
Somalia	NS	NS	NS
Tanzania	94	95	95
Uganda	91	87	87
Zambia	84	80	NS
Zimbabwe	80	85	85
WHO-African region (total)	66	66	35

Adapted from WHO information obtained from http://www.afro.who.int/en/countries.html on September 16, 2010.
NS, not stated.

Basic economic and demographic data

	GNI per capita (USD)	Life expectancy at birth (total, years)	School enrollment, primary (% net)
Burundi	140	51	81
Djibouti	1,130	55	45
Eritrea	300	58	41
Ethiopia	280	55	71
Kenya	770	54	86
Madagascar	410	61	98
Malawi	290	48	87
Mozambique	370	42	76
Rwanda	410	50	94
Somalia	ND	48	ND
Tanzania	440	56	98
Uganda	420	53	95
Zambia	950	46	94
Zimbabwe	360	45	88

GNI, gross national income; ND, no data.
[a]World Bank.

Causes of death in children under 5 years expressed as % of the total number of deaths

Causes of death in children under 5 years (%)	Regional average—WHO African region	Burundi	Eritrea	Ethiopia	Kenya	Madagascar	Malawi	Mozambique	Rwanda	Tanzania	Uganda	Zambia	Zimbabwe
Neonatal causes	26.2	23.3	27.4	30.2	24.2	25.6	21.7	29.0	21.7	26.9	23.6	22.9	28.1
Pneumonia	21.1	22.8	18.6	22.3	19.9	20.7	22.6	21.2	23.2	21.1	21.1	21.8	14.7
Diarrheal diseases	16.6	18.2	15.6	17.3	16.5	16.9	18.1	16.5	18.5	16.8	17.2	17.5	12.1
Malaria	17.5	8.4	13.6	6.1	13.6	20.1	14.1	18.9	4.6	22.7	23.1	19.4	0.2
HIV/AIDS	6.8	8.0	6.2	3.8	14.6	1.3	14.0	12.9	5.0	9.3	7.7	16.1	40.6
Measles	4.3	3.0	2.5	4.2	3.2	5.0	0.3	0.3	1.6	1.3	3.0	1.2	2.9
Injuries	1.9	1.8	3.0	1.7	2.7	2.4	1.7	1.0	1.8	2.0	2.2	1.0	1.2
Others	5.6	14.6	13.0	14.3	5.3	8.0	7.6	0.1	23.7	0.0	2.1	0.1	0.3

Adapted from WHO information obtained from http://www.afro.who.int/en/countries.html on September 16, 2010.

Top 10 causes of death in all ages expressed as % of the total number of deaths

Top 10 causes of death in all ages (%)	Burundi	Eritrea	Ethiopia	Kenya	Madagascar	Malawi	Mozambique	Rwanda	Tanzania	Uganda	Zambia	Zimbabwe
Lower respiratory tract infections	12	16	12	10	14	12	7	13	12	11	12	4
Diarrheal diseases	8	6	6	7	9	8	8	10	6	8	7	2
HIV/AIDS	22	16	12	38	3	34	28	18	29	25	43	67
Perinatal conditions	6	6	8	4	7	3	5	7	4	4	4	2
Malaria	4	6	3	5	11	8	9	2	10	11	9	NS
Tuberculosis	3	5	4	5	4	2	3	4	18	4	3	3
Cerebrovascular diseases	3	4	3	4	5	3	2	3	3	3	2	2
Ischemic heart disease	3	3	3	4	4	3	2	3	3	3	2	2
Road traffic accidents	2	2	NS	2	3	1	ND	2	2	NS	1	NS
Measles	NS	3	4	NS	5	NS	3	2	NS	2	1	1

NS, not stated.

Adapted from WHO information obtained from http://www.afro.who.int/en/countries.html on September 16, 2010.

References

1. Teka H, Petros B, Yamuah L, et al. Chloroquine-resistant *Plasmodium vivax* malaria in Debre Zeit, Ethiopia. Malar J 2008;7:220.
2. Barnadas C, Ratsimbasoa A, Tichit M, et al. *Plasmodium vivax* resistance to chloroquine in Madagascar: clinical efficacy and polymorphisms in *pvmdr1* and *pvcrt-o* genes. Antimicrob Agents Chemother 2008;52:4233–40.
3. http://data.unaids.org/pub/FactSheet/2009/20 091124_FS_SSA_en.pdf. Accessed on September 16, 2010.
4. World Health Organization. Multidrug and extensively drug-resistant TB (M/XDR-TB): 2010 global report on surveillance and response. WHO/HTM/TB/2010. ISBN 978 92 4 159919 1.
5. World Health Organization. Global tuberculosis control: epidemiology, strategy, financing report. Geneva (Switzerland). WHO/HTM/TB/2009:411.
6. Schaaf HS, Moll AP, Dheda K. Multidrug- and extensively drug-resistant tuberculosis in Africa and South America: epidemiology, diagnosis and management in adults and children. Clin Chest Med 2009;30:667–83.
7. Pitzurra R, Steffen R, Tschopp A, Mutsch M. Diarrhoea in a large prospective cohort of European travellers to resource-limited destinations. BMC Infect Dis 2010;10:231.
8. Neilson AA, Mayer CA. Cholera—recommendations for prevention in travellers. Aust Fam Physician 2010;39:220–6.
9. Jensenius M, Fournier PE, Kelly P, Myrvang B, Raoult D. African tick bite fever. Lancet Infect Dis 2003;3:557–64.
10. Raoult D, Fournier PE, Fenollar F, et al. *Rickettsia africae*, a tick-borne pathogen in travelers to sub-Saharan Africa. N Engl J Med 2001;344:1504–10.
11. Jensenius M, Hoel T, Raoult D, et al. Seroepidemiology of *Rickettsia africae* infection in Norwegian travellers to rural Africa. Scand J Infect Dis 2002;34:93–6.
12. Jensenius M, Fournier PE, Vene S, et al. African tick bite fever in travelers to rural sub-Equatorial Africa. Clin Infect Dis 2003;36:1411–17.
13. Eguale T, Abate G, Balcha F. Relapsing fever in Hossana, Ethiopia: a clinical and epidemiological study. Ethiop J Health Sci 2002;12:103–8.
14. TropNetEurop: surveillance of imported dengue infections in Europe. Eurosurveill Weekly Arch 2003;7:32.
15. Beeching NJ, Fletcher TE, Hill DR, Thomson GL. Travellers and viral haemorrhagic fevers: what are the risks? Int J Antimicrob Agents 2010;36:26–35.
16. Timen A, Koopmans MP, Vossen AC, et al. Response to imported case of Marburg hemorrhagic fever, the Netherlands. Emerg Infect Dis 2009;15:1171–5.
17. Briese T, Paweska JT, McMullan LK, Hutchison SK, Street C, Palacios G. Genetic detection and characterization of Lujo virus, a new hemorrhagic fever-associated arenavirus from southern Africa. PLoS Pathog 2009;5(5):e1000455.
18. LaBeaud AD, Kazura JW, King CH. Advances in Rift Valley fever research: insights for disease prevention. Curr Opin Infect Dis 2010;23:403–8.
19. Mardani M, Keshtkar-Jahromi M. Crimean-Congo hemorrhagic fever. Arch Iran Med 2007;10(2):204.
20. http://www.who.int/wormcontrol/documents/maps/country/en/. Accessed on September 16, 2010.
21. Mudhune S, Wamae M; Network Surveillance for Pneumococcal Disease in the East African Region. Report on invasive disease and meningitis due to *Haemophilus influenzae* and *Streptococcus pneumonia* from the Network for Surveillance of Pneumococcal Disease in the East African Region. Clin Infect Dis 2009;48(Suppl. 2):S147–52.
22. Kariuki S, Revathi G, Kiiru J, Mengo DM, Mwituria J, Muyodi J. Typhoid in Kenya is associated with a dominant multidrug-resistant *Salmonella enterica* serovar Typhi haplotype that is also widespread in Southeast Asia. J Clin Microbiol 2010;48:2171–6.

Chapter 7
Central Africa

Gerd D. Burchard[1] and Stephan Ehrhardt[2]
[1]Department of Tropical Medicine and Infectious Diseases, University Medical Center Hamburg, Germany
[2]Clinical Research Unit, Bernhard Nocht Institute for Tropical Medicine, Hamburg, Germany

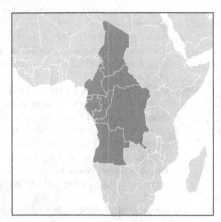

Angola
Cameroon
Central African Republic (CAR)
Chad
Congo
Democratic Republic of Congo (DRC)
Republic of Congo
Equatorial Guinea
Gabon
Sao Tomé and Principe

The pattern of infectious diseases in Central Africa is determined by geoclimatic conditions and socioeconomic factors. The climate in most parts is tropical hot and humid. The region is dominated by the Congo River and its tributaries; the area is covered mostly by savannah or tropical rain forest. Health care systems in some parts of Central Africa are disrupted. There are many diseases on which no data on prevalence and incidence are available. Prevalence data on these diseases can only be derived from single case reports or by analogy with other areas in Africa.

Sao Tomé and Principe is an island nation in the Gulf of Guinea with a different disease spectrum, however tropical disease like malaria, dengue, schistosomiasis, lymphatic filariasis by *Wuchereria bancrofti*, geohelminth infections do occur. No human cases of yellow fever have been reported. Ciguatera fish poisoning is endemic.

Infectious Diseases: A Geographic Guide, First Edition.
Edited by Eskild Petersen, Lin H. Chen & Patricia Schlagenhauf.
© 2011 John Wiley & Sons, Ltd. Published 2011 by John Wiley & Sons, Ltd.

CNS infections: meningitis and encephalitis

Acute CNS infections with less than 4 weeks of symptoms

	Frequently found diseases	Rare diseases
Meningitis	Meningococcal meningitis[a] Meningitis by gram-positive bacilli[c] Enterovirus meningitis Meningitis by other gram-negative bacilli	Tuberculous meningitis[b] Eosinophilic meningitis in schistosomiasis Neurosyphilis Listeriosis Leptospirosis
Encephalitis	Cerebral malaria[d] Herpes simplex and enterovirus encephalitis[f]	Trypanosomiasis[e] Rabies Ebola and Marburg fever West Nile virus[g] Loiasis[h] Cysticercal encephalitis
Myelitis	Spinal tuberculosis Tropical spastic paraparesis	HIV myelopathy Schistosomiasis Cerebral mycosis (cerebral phaeohyphomycosis)

[a]High incidence in countries of "Meningitis belt"—however, epidemics were also reported from a band of countries around the Rift Valley and Great Lakes regions extending as far south as Mozambique and from here west to Angola and Namibia in southern Africa.

[b]Tuberculous meningitis is more often chronic (often initially light symptoms and late diagnosis).

[c]Especially in children: *Haemophilus influenzae, Streptococcus pneumoniae.*

[d]Patient from malaria-endemic areas may have asymptomatic parasitemia plus meningitis by other microorganisms. In cerebral malaria, neck stiffness and photophobia are usually absent. When in doubt: perform lumbar puncture.

[e]West African trypanosomiasis (WAT) is a chronic disease with progression over months, even years to the final CNS stage of complete lethargy, coma, and death. East African trypanosomiasis (EAT) is an acute disease with involvement of the CNS within days to weeks after the infective tsetse fly bite. In most parts of Central Africa, *T. brucei gambiense* prevails in Democratic Republic of Congo (DRC), predominantly in the Plateaux Province.

[f]In malaria-endemic areas, the diagnosis of *Plasmodium falciparum* malaria is one of exclusion, because up to 70% of the children in the community may have parasitemia and yet be asymptomatic. However, in resource-poor countries, exclusion of viral encephalitis is problematic and practically no information is available on prevalence and manifestation of the neurotropic viruses in Central Africa.

[g]Serological evidence of human exposure to WNV has been reported in the CAR, Cameroon, Gabon, and the DRC.

[h]Antifilarial drugs can induce an encephalopathy in patients with very high *Loa loa* microfilaremias. Exceptionally, *L. loa* can provoke encephalitis in the absence of treatment.

Chronic CNS infections with more than 4 weeks of symptoms in immunocompetent and immunocompromised patients

The most common chronic CNS infection is tuberculous meningitis usually with gradual onset of fever, headache, altered consciousness, and cranial nerve palsies. Tuberculomas can give rise to focal neurological defects. Neurosyphilis should be considered in any patient with elevated spinal fluid WBC count.

WAT is a chronic disease with progression over months, even years to the final CNS stage of complete lethargy, coma, and death—see footnote e in the table under "Acute CNS infections with less than 4 weeks of symptoms." Neurocysticercosis is common and is an important cause of epilepsia in the region. Neurobrucellosis is to be expected in areas with livestock breeding only.

HIV-1 is another common neuroinfection in the region. Neurocognitive disorders are common in HIV patients. All HIV-related CNS infections can be seen, in particular cryptococcal meningitis, CMV, histoplasmosis. JC is a neurotropic virus and may cause progressive multifocal leukoencephalopathy (PML). Infections with *Nocardia, Candida,* and *Aspergillus* may be seen in immunocompromised patients, but data are not available from the region. Infection with *Toxoplasma gondii* is probably common in the region, and should be considered in HIV-positive patients with CNS symptoms especially if focal lesions are found on CNS scans. Encephalitis caused by the free-living ameba *Acanthamoeba* spp. and *Balamuthia mandrillaris* are probably found in immunocompromised patients, but has never been described from the region. Occasionally, immune reconstitution inflammatory syndrome (IRIS) may occur in the brain, when antiretroviral therapy is started.

Besides HIV-1, HIV-2 is also endemic in Central Africa. High prevalences have been reported in Equatorial Guinea. Longitudinal studies suggest that the rate of progression to advanced HIV-related disease and mortality are far lower for HIV-2 than for HIV-1. Dual infection with HIV-1 and HIV-2 is possible.

In patients with a gradually appearing symmetrical paraparesis of the lower limbs with signs of pyramidal tract involvement, sometimes also with bladder disorders, HTLV-1 infection has to be considered. In some parts of Central Africa up to 1–5% of the general population is infected [1]. Other subtypes have been described in that region, for example, HTLV-3 [2].

Ear, nose, throat, and upper respiratory tract infections

Acute and chronic infections

Acute and chronic suppurative otitis is highly prevalent in the area, affecting mainly children. Predominant bacterial agents in chronic discharging ears are gram-negative bacteria including *Pseudomonas aeruginosa*. Otomycosis is a differential diagnosis.

Streptococcal throat infection is common and patients may develop rheumatic fever. Other causes of pharyngitis: Vincent's angina and EBV. Diphtheria should be suspected in a patient if a creamy adherent membrane is present over part of the tonsil (no data from Central Africa).

Tuberculosis can affect nose, nasopharynx, oropharynx, middle ear, mastoid bone, larynx, deep neck spaces, and salivary glands—usually associated with pulmonary tuberculosis.

Rare diseases: Rhinoscleroma is a slowly developing granulomatous process in the nose caused by *Klebsiella rhinoscleromatis*. Rhinosporidiosis is another granulomatous disease caused by *Rhinosporidium seeberi* (Mesomycetozoea = unicellular parasites). Leprosy may affect the larynx, chronic nasal discharge, sometimes blood-stained, occurs in lepromatous leprosy. Nasal destruction is seen in yaws and leprosy (and in lupus vulgaris).

Ear, nose, and throat infections in immunocompromised host

ENT diseases in HIV patients include cervical lymphadenopathy, otitis media, oral candidiasis, and adenotonsillar diseases. The bacteriology of sinusitis in HIV infection often indicates opportunistic organisms not responsive to standard medical therapy, such as CMV, *Aspergillus*, and atypical mycobacteria. Tuberculosis must always be considered. In immunosuppressed patients, rare diseases have to be considered.

Sickle cell disease is a common inherited blood disorder in Central Africa. When bone is involved, infarction and osteomyelitis can be seen in the maxillofacial bone and skull base.

Children with protein-energy malnutrition may develop gangrenous stomatitis (cancum oris, noma).

Cardiopulmonary infections

Acute infections with less than 4 weeks of symptoms

Pulmonary infection with less than 4 weeks of symptoms

	Frequently found diseases	Rare diseases
Pneumonia	*S. pneumoniae*[a] *H. influenzae*[b] *Staphylococcus aureus*[c] Tuberculosis Viruses (rhino, adeno)	*Mycoplasma, Chlamydia, Legionella* Q fever Histoplasmosis, blastomycosis
Lung abscess	Gram-positive bacteria	Amebiasis[d]
Cough with eosinophilia	Schistosomiasis (Katayama syndrome) Ascariasis (Löffler's syndrome) Paragonimiasis	

[a]Most frequent; patients with hypogammaglobulinemia, asplenia, nephrotic syndrome, sickle cell anemia are at special risk.
[b]Responsible for 3–5% of episodes of pneumonia.
[c]Causing 1–2% of pneumonias.
[d]Liver abscess rupturing through diaphragm.

Endocarditis, myocarditis, and pericarditis with less than 4 weeks of symptoms

	Frequently found diseases	Rare diseases
Endocarditis	Subacute and acute bacterial endocarditis by *S. aureus* and *Streptococci* spp.	Q fever (*Coxiella burnetii*) *Bartonella quintana*—infection
Myocarditis	Acute virus myocarditis Malaria[a]	Trypanosomiasis
Pericarditis	Viral pericarditis[b] Pyogenic pericarditis[d] Tuberculosis	Amebic pericarditis[c]

[a]Mostly in addition to other organ complications.
[b]Fever, pericardial pain, but no evidence of systemic pyogenic infection.
[c]By rupture of left-sided liver abscess through diaphragm.
[d]Often in the course of bronchopneumonia or osteomyelitis, *S. pneumoniae, S. aureus.*

Chronic infections with more than 4 weeks of symptoms

Pneumonia with more than 4 weeks of symptoms   Tuberculosis should always be considered in patients with cough and fever for more than 4 weeks. *Nocardiosis* histoplasmosis, and blastomycosis are primarily infections in immunocompromised patients. Paragonimiasis is a differential diagnosis to tuberculosis and the main symptoms are cough and blood-flecked sputum. The radiological pictures show nodular infiltration and sometimes pleural fluid and/or cavities. Paragonimiasis is to be suspected in patients with pulmonary findings similar to tuberculosis but with negative tuberculosis diagnostics.

Endocarditis and pericarditis with more than 4 weeks of symptoms   Rheumatic heart disease (differential diagnosis: Libman–Sacks endocarditis in patients with SLE), tuberculosis, Q fever, and other rickettsial infection like *B. quintana* should be considered. Tuberculous pericarditis may be directly spread from the tracheobronchial tree or thoracic lymph nodes.

Infections in immunocompromised host

Pneumonia in immunocompromised host   Pneumonia in the immunocompetent host due to bacteria including tuberculosis is also found in the immunocompromised host. *Pneumocystis jirovecii* (previously *carinii*) should always be considered and seems to be frequent in Cameroon [3]. There are no data from other countries. CMV, adenovirus, and HSV are common viral causes and fungi such as *Candida* spp., *Aspergillus, Nocardia,* and *Actinomyces,* as well as gram-positive rod bacteria should be considered.

Endocarditis, myocarditis, and pericarditis in immunocompromised host   Myocarditis may be caused by HIV infection, *Cryptococcus, T. gondii,* and *Mycobacterium avium intracellulare* (MAI). Tuberculosis is a common cause of pericarditis.

Gastrointestinal infections

Gastrointestinal infections with less than 4 weeks of symptoms

	Frequently found diseases	Rare diseases
Diarrhea	Salmonellosis Shigellosis *Campylobacter* infection Giardiasis ETEC infection Norovirus and rotavirus infection *Clostridium difficile*	Amebic colitis[a] Cholera[b] *Escherichia coli* O157[c] Cryptosporidiosis Cyclosporiasis Strongyloidiasis Malaria[d] Pellagra[e]

[a]Typically with bloody diarrhea; diagnosis can be made when hematophagous trophozoites are found in stool.
[b]Cholera is endemic in Central Africa. Outbreaks as well as sporadic cases can be expected and notification is unreliable if existent at all. Notified outbreaks are published in the WHO Weekly Epidemiological Record (http://www.who.int/wer/en/index.html) and the data updated on the WHO website (http://www.who.int/topics/cholera/surveillance/en/index.html).
[c]Single cases have been reported [4].
[d]Falciparum malaria also can lead to febrile diarrhea.
[e]Main features of pellagra are the triad diarrhea, dermatitis and dementia.

Chronic gastrointestinal infections with more than 4 weeks of symptoms

Both infections with *Giardia intestinalis* and *Cryptosporidia* spp. may cause long-lasting, fluctuating gastrointestinal symptoms. Other intestinal parasites include hookworm infections, *Ascaris lumbricoides* and *Trichuris trichiura*. Infection with *Strongyloides stercoralis* is common but sometimes asymptomatic. It may, however, cause unspecific intestinal symptoms and in immunocompromised patients (e.g., in HTLV-1 infection) severe disease. Schistosomiasis by *Schistosoma mansoni* and rarely *Schistosoma intercalatum* is another common cause of chronic gastrointestinal symptoms. Enterocolitis caused by *Entamoeba histolytica* may present both as an acute dysenteria and as more prolonged infection in the colon mimicking inflammatory colitis.

Tuberculosis should always be considered in patients with long-lasting gastrointestinal symptoms. Morbus Whipple is found in Senegal, and it is assumed that Morbus Whipple is found in Central Africa, but reliable reports are lacking.

Diarrhea in immunocompromised host

Giardia lamblia, Cryptosporidia, Cyclospora cayetanensis, Isospora belli, and Microsporidia spp. should be considered. Other opportunistic infections include tuberculosis, intestinal cytomegaly, and *Mycobacterium avium intracellulare* infection.

Enteritis necroticans is a segmental necrotizing infection of the jejunum and ileum caused by *Clostridium perfringens* type C. It affects primarily children with severe protein malnutrition. There are, however, no data from Central Africa.

Infections of liver, spleen, and peritoneum

Acute infections of liver, spleen, and peritoneum with less than 4 weeks of symptoms

	Frequently found diseases	Rare diseases
Jaundice	Malaria[a] Hepatitis A Hepatitis B[b] EBV, CMV infection Hepatitis E[c]	Hepatitis C Hepatitis E Rickettsiosis Leptospirosis Syphilis II Relapsing fever Visceral leishmaniasis[d] Fitz-Hugh–Curtis syndrome[e] Ebola and Marburg fever Yellow fever CCHF[f] Trypanosomiasis
Space-occupying lesion in liver Splenomegaly	Bacterial liver abscess Malaria Typhoid fever Bacterial endocarditis Viral hepatitis EBV, CMV	Amebic liver abscess Trypanosomiasis Kala-azar Relapsing fever Dengue Brucellosis Tuberculosis

[a]Slight hemolytic jaundice is frequent. Elevation of liver enzymes >3× of the upper normal limit and marked jaundice may result from direct damage of hepatocytes and is indicative of severe malaria.
[b]Predominantly genotypes A and E.

(Continued)

[c]Has not been described, but is probably present.
[d]To be expected in the Northern part of Central Africa, e.g., Cameroon.
[e]Perihepatitis is seen in Fitz-Hugh–Curtis syndrome, which is a subgroup of pelvic inflammatory syndrome usually caused by gonorrhea (acute gonococcal perihepatitis) or *Chlamydia* infection.
[f]Virus was isolated in 1956 from a febrile patient in Belgian Congo. Outbreaks have been described in the DRC, otherwise there are only few data [5].

Chronic infections of liver, spleen, and peritoneum with more than 4 weeks of symptoms

	Frequently found diseases	Rare diseases
Jaundice	Chronic viral hepatitis	Brucellosis
	Schistosomiasis[a]	Q fever hepatitis
		Toxocariasis
		Hepatic tuberculosis[b]
		Leprosy[c]
		Histoplasmosis
		Porocephalosis[d]
Space-occupying lesion in liver		Tuberculosis
Ascites	Tuberculous peritonitis	*S. mansoni*
Splenomegaly	Hepatosplenic schistosomiasis	Tuberculosis
	Hyperreactive malarial syndrome[e]	Brucellosis

[a]Hepatic schistosomiasis is most often due to *S. mansoni*. The pathological effects of *S. intercalatum*—occurring in several foci in Central Africa—are mostly limited to mild intestinal disease.
[b]Hepatic tuberculosis may occur as miliary, nodular, and solitary abscess form.
[c]Granulomatous hepatitis may be seen in patients with lepromatous leprosy.
[d]Porocephalosis is a rare parasitic infection caused by the pentastomidae *Armillifer armillatus* and described primarily from Cameroon.
[e]Abnormal immunological reaction to plasmodium infection, huge splenomegaly >10 cm below costal margin, serum IgM more than 2 × standard deviation (2SD) above the local mean, high titer of malarial antibodies, and response to antimalarial drugs are the cornerstones of the diagnosis. Splenic lymphoma with villous lymphocytes coexists with this condition and it should always be considered in the differential diagnosis of unresponsive or poorly responsive cases of hyperreactive malarial splenomegaly.

Infections of liver, spleen, and peritoneum in immunocompromised host

Infections in the immunocompromised host are no different from the immunocompetent host.

Genitourinary infections

Acute genitourinary infections with less than 4 weeks of symptoms

Cystitis, pyelonephritis, and nephritis with less than 4 weeks of symptoms Uropathogenic *E. coli* are the most common cause of infection in patients with normal urinary tract anatomy.

Acute and chronic sexually transmitted diseases with less than 4 weeks of symptoms

	Frequent diseases	Rare diseases
Urethritis and discharge	Gonorrhea	Mycoplama urethritis
	Chlamydial urethritis	
	Trichomoniasis	
Genital ulcers	Syphilis	Lymphogranuloma inguinale
	Ulcus molle	Donovanosis[a]
	Genital herpes	

[a]The painless genital ulcers can easily be mistaken for syphilis.

Chronic genitourinary infections with more than 4 weeks of symptoms

Cystitis, pyelonephritis, and nephritis with more than 4 weeks of symptoms In patients from Central Africa with chronic genitourinary infections, tuberculosis and *Schistosoma haematobium* infection must be considered. *S. haematobium* may cause hematuria and hemospermia.

Hydrocele can occur in Bancroftian filariasis. Testicular enlargement may occur in mumps, filariasis, and during erythema nodosum leprosum. Chronic epididymo-orchitis is seen in tuberculosis and syphilis.

Cystitis, pyelonephritis, and nephritis infections in immunocompromised host

Infections in the immunocompromised host are similar to those in the immunocompetent host.

Patients with sickle cell disease are at increased risk for urinary tract infection.

Urinary tract infections in HIV-positive patients are more frequent than in uninfected patients. Necrotizing fasciitis of the genitalia (Fournier's gangrene) may develop. Impairment of kidney function is usually caused by HIV-associated nephropathy, direct infection of the renal cells with the HIV-1 virus, or changes in the release of cytokines during HIV infection.

Sexually transmitted diseases in immunocompromised host

Infections in the immunocompromised host are no different from the immunocompetent host.

Infections of joints, muscle, and soft tissue

Acute infections of bone, joints, and muscle with less than 4 weeks of symptoms

	Frequently found diseases	Rare diseases
Osteoarthritis	Septic arthritis	Chikungunya infection[a]
	Gonococcal arthritis	*Histoplasma duboisii* infection
	Rheumatic fever	Brucellosis[b]
		Leprosy

(Continued)

	Frequently found diseases	Rare diseases
Osteomyelitis	Acute hematogenous osteomyelitis[c]	
Myositis[d]	Pyomyositis[e]	Trichinosis
	Other bacterial myositis	Gas gangrene (clostridial myonecrosis)
	Group A streptococcal necrotizing myositis	
	Acute rhabdomyolysis[f]	

[a]Seen especially in Cameroon, Gabon, and Angola.

[b]*Brucella abortus* endemic from Sudan to Cameroon.

[c]Most often *S. aureus*, rarely streptococci and Enterobacteriaceae, and in sickle cell anemia very often *Salmonella*.

[d]Myositis is defined as inflammation of a muscle, especially a voluntary muscle, and characterized by pain, tenderness, swelling, and/or weakness.

[e]Pyomyositis is defined as an acute intramuscular bacterial infection which is neither secondary to a contiguous infection of the soft tissue or bone nor due to penetrating trauma. Infections result from hematogenous spread and are usually due to *S. aureus*.

[f]Seen in leptospirosis, pneumococcal sepsis, echovirus infections, and malaria (but also, e.g., in snake bite and other noninfectious conditions).

Chronic infections of bone, joints, and muscle with more than 4 weeks of symptoms and in the immunocompromised host

Tuberculosis should always be considered, additionally consider mycobacteria other than tuberculosis (MOTT) in the immunocompromised patient. Leprosy, brucellosis, and nocardiosis are rare causes of arthritis and osteomyelitis.

Patients with hemoglobinopathies like sickle cell disease and thalassemia have a high risk of osteomyelitis due to episodes of microthrombosis, osteonecrosis, and secondary infections.

In the immunocompromised host, HIV-associated arthritis should be considered. Rare causes—mainly in immunocompromised patients—are infections with *H. duboisii*, *Cryptococcus neoformans*, and microsporidia.

Infections of skin and soft tissues

Skin infections

	Frequently found diseases	Rare diseases
Maculopapular	Dengue, EBV, CMV, acute HIV infection, syphilis	Rickettsiosis[a]
		Relapsing fever
Papular, vesicular		Monkeypox[b]
		Tanapox[c]
Papular and petechia		Leptospirosis
Papillomatous		Yaws[d]
Chancre, erythematous		Trypanosomiasis
Hematoma	Meningococcal sepsis	Viral hemorrhagic fevers
Ulcer	Buruli ulcer	
	Tropical ulcer	
Subcutaneous nodules[e]	Onchocerciasis[f]	

	Frequently found diseases	Rare diseases
Migratory subcutaneous swellings, eye worm	Loiasis	
Itching	Filarial infection, including *Mansonella perstans*	
Multiple manifestations		Leprosy[g]

[a]Possibly reemerging, e.g., recently many cases in DRC.
[b]Recently reemerging in DRC [6].
[c]Sometimes with eschar.
[d]Still an issue in Central Africa, particularly in the pygmy population of south-western CAR and in DRC.
[e]Buruli ulcer may initially present as a subcutaneous nodule—rarely diagnosed in this stage.
[f]Uneven distribution in Central Africa: In Angola, onchocerciasis is distributed in discrete foci. In Cameroon and DRC, onchocerciasis is a countrywide public health problem. In Chad, the onchocerciasis focus is located in the southern part of the country. In the DRC, onchocerciasis is distributed in foci in the south of the country. Onchocerciasis is endemic on Bioko Island, which is situated off the coast of Cameroon and Gabon. In Gabon, there are only few villages where onchocerciasis remains a problem.
[g]For leprosy cases in Central Africa see: www.who.int/lep/situation/africa/en/index.html.

Soft tissue infections

Cellulitis and subcutaneous tissue infections including necrotizing fasciitis are frequently encountered.

Subcutaneous mycosis frequently seen: Chromoblastomycosis characterized by vegetative and verrucal lesions which occur predominantly on the lower limbs; mycetomas are chronic, inflammatory swellings with numerous sinuses, caused by molds or bacteria (in Africa predominantly eumycetomas, often caused by *Madurella mycetomatis*); entomophthoromycosis is slowly progressing infection of the subcutaneous tissue or paranasal sinuses caused by *Conidiobolus coronatus* leading to grotesque deformation of the face. The distribution of sporotrichosis in Central Africa is not well known, but single cases have been reported.

Skin infections in immunocompromised host

Skin infections that particularly affect HIV patients include herpes simplex, zoster, molluscum contagiosum, dermatophytosis, unusual forms of scabies, cryptococcosis, histoplasmosis, staphylococcal folliculitis (DD papular pruritic eruption). Bacillary angiomatosis is only rarely reported.

Adenopathy

Acute adenopathy with less than 4 weeks of symptoms

	Frequently found diseases	Rare diseases
Localized	Regional lymphadenitis	Lymphatic filariasis
	HIV infection	Lymphogranuloma inguinale, chancroid, granuloma inguinale
	Mycobacterial adenitis	Rubella

(Continued)

	Frequently found diseases	Rare diseases
Generalized	HIV infection CMV and EBV infection Measles Toxoplasmosis	Trypanosomiasis[a] Leprosy[b] Plague[c] Brucellosis Histoplasmosis Secondary syphilis Tuberculosis Rickettsiosis[d]

[a]Typically enlargement of posterior cervical lymph nodes (Winterbottom's sign).
[b]As part of reactional state in erythema nodosum leprosum.
[c]Bubonic plague—plague lately reported in DRC, outbreaks in Ituri subregion.
[d]See footnote b in table below.

Chronic adenopathy

Tuberculosis, filariasis, and brucellosis should be considered. Kala-azar patients present signs of parasitic invasion of the reticuloendothelial system, such as enlarged spleen and liver, but also enlarged lymph nodes (more frequent in Africa than in India).

Fever without focal symptoms

Acute fever with less than 4 weeks of symptoms

Frequently found diseases	Rare diseases	Very rare diseases
Malaria Typhoid fever Sepsis Unspecific viral infection Endocarditis	Amebic liver abscess[a] Rickettsiosis[b] CMV, EBV, acute HIV	Relapsing fever Trypanosomiasis Viral hemorrhagic fever[c]

[a]Rarely without pain in the upper abdomen.
[b]Rickettsioses (also called typhus) in Central Africa mainly from spotted fever group, predominantly *Rickettsia africae* [7]. Disease occurs in rural setting and in international travelers returning from safari, hunting, camping, etc. Symptoms include fever, but also eschars, maculopapular or vesicular rash, and lymphadenopathy. Few data concerning other rickettsial diseases. In Cameroon, human mono-cytotropic ehrlichiosis (HME) caused by *Ehrlichia chaffeensis* has been described [8].
[c]Can begin with monosymptomatic fever.

Chronic fever with more than 4 weeks of symptoms in immunocompetent and immunocompromised patients

The differential diagnosis of prolonged pyrexia is long: malaria, tuberculosis, enteric fever, visceral leishmaniasis, pneumonia, urinary tract infection, abscesses, infective endocarditis, secondary syphilis, trypanosomiasis. Noninfectious causes should be considered especially malignancies and autoimmune diseases.

Eosinophilia

	Frequently found diseases	Rare diseases
Asymptomatic	Intestinal worms Schistosomiasis Filariasis	
With fever	Katayama syndrome	Acute *Fasciola hepatica* infection[a] Trichinosis
With subcutaneous swellings	Loiasis	*M. perstans* infection Paragonimiasis

With abdominal pain	Intestinal worms (*A. lumbricoides*,
	  hookworms, *T. trichiuria*)
	Toxocariasis (*Toxocara canis,
	  Toxocara cati*)	

With elevated transaminases	Toxocariasis (*T. canis, T. cati*) Strongyloidiasis	Fascioliasis[a]
With pulmonary infiltrate	Löffler's syndrome Katayama syndrome	Paragonimiasis

[a]Practically no data from Central Africa, maybe to be expected in northern areas with livestock breeding.

Children

Diarrhea (19%), pneumonia (18%), malaria (16%), other infections (9%), and AIDS (4%) are estimated to be the most important killers in children in Central Africa [9]. All of these diseases may lead to delays in child development which may, in turn, result in increased susceptibility to childhood diseases. Malnutrition, commonly found in young children, can additionally aggravate these conditions.

The childhood vaccination program in the region is not achieving complete coverage, especially for measles, mumps, and rubella (MMR). Outbreaks of measles have been reported from the DRC as well as most other countries in the region. This means that rubella and mumps may be prevalent and a risk to nonimmunized travelers. The countries in the region are working toward a third diphtheria-tetanus-pertussis vaccination, DT3, coverage of 70%, which means that tetanus both neonatal and in adults may be encountered (http://www.who.int/immunization/GIN_August_2010.pdf).

Antibiotic resistance

In Central Africa, resistance of common pathogens to antibiotics is alarmingly widespread. Though data are limited and of mixed quality since blood cultures are rarely done, they, however, allow to sketch the current situation [10].

Methicillin-resistant *Staphylococcccus aureus* (MRSA) was found in up to 66% of hospitalized patients and 23% of outpatients in Kinshasa; in Cameroon, MRSA was found in 21% of the surveyed samples. Panton-Valentine leukocidin genes are highly prevalent in Cameroon [11]. Data on *S. pneumoniae* are very limited, while resistance to penicillin appears to be rare, resistance to chloramphenicol and sulfamethoxazole/trimethoprim exceeds 50%. In *Shigella* and *Salmonella*, high resistance rates to ampicillin, chloramphenicol, streptomycin, sulfonamides, trimethoprim, and tetracycline were noted. Other Enterobacteriaceae appear to be increasingly resistant to commonly used antibiotics like amoxicillin/clavulanic acid and first-generation cephalosporins. Reports on antibiotic resistance of *Vibrio cholerae* 01 El Tor from Chad and Cameroon show nearly no resistance while in the DRC and Angola, multidrug resistance to first-line drugs like ampicillin, tetracycline, doxycycline, sulfamethoxazole/trimethoprim, nalidixic acid, and chloramphenicol was highly prevalent during the reported outbreaks.

Drug resistance in *Mycobacterium tuberculosis* is common. A study from 2007 found that the primary resistance rate reached 43.5%; the multidrug resistance rate (MDR-TB) notified as resistant to both rifampicin and isoniazid was 5.3% [12]. XDR strains have been reported from Central Africa.

Demographic data

Basic economic and demographic data

Country	GNI per capita (USD)[a]	Life expectancy at birth (total, years)[b]	School enrollment primary (% net)[c]
Angola	3,340	53	ND
Cameroon	1,150	52	88
Central African Republic	410	48	66
Chad	540	46	59 (data from 2002)
Democratic Republic of Congo	150	52	32 (data from 1999)
Republic of Congo	1,790	55	ND
Equatorial Guinea	14,980	53	69 (data from 2002)
Gabon	7,320	59	ND
Sao Tomè and Principe	1,790	61	97

Source: United Nations Educational, Scientific, and Cultural Organization (UNESCO) Institute for Statistics. 2009. World Education Indicators. Paris: UNESCO.
GNI, gross national income; ND, no data.
[a]World Bank, 2008.
[b]WHO, 2009.
[c]Primary gross school enrollment in 2008.

Causes of death in children under 5 years—regional average

Causes	×1000 (%)
HIV/AIDS	1651/11248 (14.7%)
Respiratory infections	1437/11248 (12.8%)
Cardiovascular diseases	1175/11248 (11.4%)
Diarrheal diseases	1005/11248 (8.9%)
Perinatal conditions	977/11248 (8.7%)
Malaria	806/11248 (7.2%)
Injuries	769/11248 (6.8%)
Measles	182/11248 (1.6%)
Others	29.7%

Source: World Health Organization. The global burden of disease: 2004 update. Geneva, WHO, 2008. Available at www.who.int/evidence/bod.

Ten most common causes of death (%) in all ages in two countries selected for a regional low (Chad) and middle (Gabon) GNI per capita

Chad	Gabon
Respiratory infections 23.3/168.3 (13.8%)	HIV/AIDS 2.7/13.8 (19.6%)
Malaria 16.7/168.3 (9.9%)	Cardiovascular diseases 2.5/13.8 (18.1)
Cardiovascular diseases 16.0/168.3 (9.5%)	Perinatal conditions 0.9/13.8 (6.5%)
Diarrhea 15.9/168.3 (9.4%)	Respiratory infections 0.9/13.8 (6.5%)
Perinatal conditions 15.8/168.3 (9.4%)	Malaria 0.8/13.8 (5.8%)
Malignant neoplasms 6.8/168.3 (4.0)	Injuries 0.8/13.8 (5.8%)
Maternal conditions 5.0/168.3 (3.0)	Respiratory diseases[a] 0.6/13.8 (4.3%)
Respiratory diseases[a] 4.4/168.3 (2.6)	Diarrheal diseases 0.5/13.8 (3.6%)
Injuries 3.6/168.3 (2.1%)	Digestive diseases 0.4/13.8 (2.9%)
Digestive diseases 3.2/168.3 (1.9%)	Diabetes mellitus 0.3/13.8 (2.2%)

Source: World Health Organization. The global burden of disease: 2004 update. Geneva, WHO, 2008. Available at www.who.int/evidence/bod.
None of the countries is classified as "high income."
[a]COPD and Asthma.

References

1. Gonçalves DU, Proietti FA, Ribas JG, et al. Epidemiology, treatment, and prevention of human T-cell leukemia virus type 1-associated diseases. Clin Microbiol Rev 2010;23:577–89.

2. Zheng H, Wolfe ND, Sintasath DM, et al. Emergence of a novel and highly divergent HTLV-3 in a primate hunter in Cameroon. Virology 2010;401:137–45.

3. Nkinin SW, Daly KR, Walzer PD, et al. Evidence for high prevalence of *Pneumocystis jirovecii* exposure among Cameroonians. Acta Trop 2009;112:219–24.

4. Cunin P, Tedjouka E, Germani Y, et al. An epidemic of bloody diarrhea: *Escherichia coli* O157 emerging in Cameroon? Emerg Infect Dis 1999;5:285–90.

5. Gonzalez JP, Josse R, Johnson ED, et al. Antibody prevalence against haemorrhagic fever viruses in randomized representative Central African populations. Res Virol 1989;140:319–31.

6. Rimoin AW, Mulembakani PM, Johnston SC, et al. Major increase in human monkeypox incidence 30 years after smallpox vaccination campaigns cease in the Democratic Republic of Congo. Proc Natl Acad Sci USA 2010;107 (37):16262–7.

7. Ndip LM, Fokam EB, Bouyer DH, et al. Detection of Rickettsia africae in patients and ticks along the coastal region of Cameroon. Am J Trop Med Hyg 2004;71:363–6.

8. Ndip LM, Labruna M, Ndip RN, et al. Molecular and clinical evidence of *Ehrlichia chaffeensis* infection in Cameroonian patients with undifferentiated febrile illness. Ann Trop Med Parasitol 2009;103:719–25.

9. Black RE, Cousens S, Johnson HL, et al. and the Child Health Epidemiology Reference Group of WHO and UNICEF. Global, regional, and national causes of child mortality in 2008: a systematic analysis. Lancet 2010;375:1969–87.

10. Vlieghe E, Phoba MF, Tamfun JJ, et al. Antibiotic resistance among bacterial pathogens in Central Africa: a review of the published literature between 1955 and 2008. Int J Antimicrob Agents 2009;34:295–303.

11. Breurec S, Fall C, Pouillot R, Boisier P, et al. Epidemiology of methicillin-susceptible Staphylococcus aureus lineages in five major African towns: high prevalence of Panton-Valentine leukocidin genes. Clin Microbiol Infect 2010 Jul 29. [Epub ahead of print]

12. Kabedi MJ, Kashongwe M, Kayembe JM, et al. Résistance primaire de *Mycobacterium tuberculosis* aux anti-tuberculeux à Kinshasa, République Démocratique du Congo. Bull Soc Pathol Exot 2007;100:275–6.

Chapter 8
North Africa

Philippe Gautret,[1] Nadjet Mouffok[2] and Philippe Parola[1]
[1]Infectious Diseases and Tropical Medicine Unit, Hopital Nord, Marseille, France
[2]Infectious Diseases Department, University Hospital and Medical College, Oran, Algeria

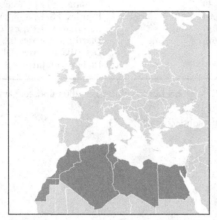

Algeria
Egypt
Libya
Morocco
Sudan
Tunisia
Western Sahara

Two regions should be individualized in North African area. In the region of the Maghreb (Morocco, Algeria, Tunisia, and Libya) and Egypt, due to climatic and socioeconomic conditions, the traveler is at risk of acquiring a number of infections common to other geographic areas. However, the traveler is also at risk of acquiring more exotic infections including Mediterranean spotted fever, typhus, rabies, intestinal parasitosis, visceral and cutaneous leishmaniasis, and hydatidosis. Schistosomiasis is present in Egypt. *Plasmodium vivax* is present in limited areas including El-Fayoum in Egypt, the area of Janet in the south of Algeria, the area of Khouribga in Morocco, and rare hearths in Libya in the valley of Senegal River. By contrast, in Sudan, the traveler is at risk of tropical diseases overrepresented in Africa as a whole, including *Plasmodium falciparum* malaria, dengue, Chikungunya, and yellow fever. Schistosomiasis is also a public health concern in Sudan. North Africa as a whole is a high risk area for traveler's diarrhea and other fecal–oral acquired infections such as hepatitis A and less commonly typhoid fever. HIV and tuberculosis dominate the spectrum of communicable diseases in the area.

Infectious Diseases: A Geographic Guide, First Edition.
Edited by Eskild Petersen, Lin H. Chen & Patricia Schlagenhauf.
© 2011 John Wiley & Sons, Ltd. Published 2011 by John Wiley & Sons, Ltd.

Central Nervous System (CNS) infections: meningitis and encephalitis

Acute infections with less than 4 weeks of symptoms

Besides cosmopolitan infections [1–3], local infections like Toscana virus infection [4], West Nile encephalitis [5], rabies, and typhus should be considered. Among enteroviruses [6], coxsackievirus is frequently responsible for meningitis [7]. *Brucella* is frequent in breeding areas and may be responsible for meningitis [8]. *Leptospira* is frequent in North Africa, but rarely responsible for meningitis.

Frequently found microorganisms	Rare microorganisms	Very rare microorganisms
Enteroviruses, coxsackievirus, herpes virus, varicella zoster virus, Toscana virus	Rabies virus, West Nile virus	Influenza
Neisseria meningitidis, Streptococcus pneumoniae, Haemophilus influenzae	Neurosyphilis, *Listeria*, *Mycobacterium tuberculosis*, *Brucella*, *Leptospira*, *Rickettsia prowazekii*, *Rickettsia conorii*	*Brucella*, *Klebsiella pneumoniae*, *Tropheryma whipplei*, *Rickettsia typhi* [9] *Naegleria* and other free-living ameba

Infection with symptoms for more than 4 weeks and in the immunocompromised host

Microorganisms with symptoms for more than 4 weeks	Microorganisms in the immunocompromised host
Human Immunodeficiency Virus (HIV) *M. tuberculosis* [10,11], neuroborreliosis	*M. tuberculosis* *Cryptococcus* spp., *Candida* spp., *Aspergillus* spp., *Rhodotorula*, *Nocardia*, *Toxoplasma*
Consider noninfectious causes like lymphoma.	

Ear, nose, and throat infections

Ear, nose, and throat infections with less than 4 weeks of symptoms

Frequently found microorganisms	Rare microorganisms and conditions	Very rare microorganisms
Rhinovirus, coronavirus, Respiratory Syncytial Virus (RSV), myxovirus, herpes virus, adenovirus, enterovirus (tonsillitis, rhinitis, otitis), Epstein–Barr virus (EBV) (tonsillitis)		
Streptococcus (tonsillitis, otitis), *Haemophilus*, *B. catarrhalis* (otitis)	*M. tuberculosis* (tonsillitis, otitis)	Diphtheria (tonsillitis)

Ear, nose, and throat infections with symptoms for more than 4 weeks and in the immunocompromised host

Microorganisms with symptoms for more than 4 weeks	Microorganisms in the immunocompromised host
Tuberculosis, syphilis (tonsillitis)	*Candida* spp.

Consider noninfectious causes like cancer.

Cardiopulmonary infections

Pneumonia with less than 4 weeks of symptoms

Frequently found microorganisms	Rare microorganisms and conditions	Very rare microorganisms
Influenza *S. pneumoniae, Mycoplasma pneumoniae, H. influenzae, Staphylococcus aureus, Chlamydia pneumoniae* [12], *Coxiella burnetii*	*Legionella pneumophila, Chlamydophila psittaci*	Diphtheria, *K. pneumoniae*

Endocarditis with less than 4 weeks of symptoms [13,14]

Frequently found microorganisms	Rare microorganisms and conditions	Very rare microorganisms
Staphylococcus and Streptococcus spp., *Bartonella* spp. [15]	*Neisseria gonorrhoeae, C. burnetii, Haemophilus* spp., *Actinobacillus actinomycetemcomitans, Capnocytophaga* spp., *Cardiobacterium hominis, Eikenella corrodens, Kingella kingae* (HACEK) group	*Brucella*

Pulmonary symptoms for more than 4 weeks and in the immunocompromised host

Microorganisms and diseases with symptoms for more than 4 weeks	Microorganisms in the immunocompromised host
Tuberculosis *Aspergillus*	Cytomegalovirus (CMV) *Coxiella* *Aspergillus, Candida, Pneumocystis*

Consider noninfectious causes like lung cancer, autoimmune lung fibrosis, Wegener's granulomatosis.

Endocarditis for more than 4 weeks and in the immunocompromised host

Microorganisms and diseases with symptoms for more than 4 weeks	Microorganisms in the immunocompromised host
Staphylococcus and *Streptococcus* spp., *Enterococcus*, *C. burnetii*, *Bartonella quintana*, *Brucella*	*Aspergillus, Candida*
Consider noninfectious causes like sarcoidosis.	

Gastrointestinal infections

Gastrointestinal infections with less than 4 weeks of symptoms

Frequently found microorganisms	Rare microorganisms and conditions	Very rare microorganisms
Adenovirus, norovirus and calicivirus, rotavirus, hepatitis A virus [16] *Escherichia coli, Salmonella typhi* and *nontyphi* [17], *Campylobacter, Shigella* *Giardia intestinalis, Trichomonas intestinalis, Entamoeba histolytica* [18]	*Cryptosporidia* spp.	Tuberculosis, Whipple *Cyclospora cayetanensis* [19]
Consider noninfectious causes like inflammatory bowel disease and intestinal malignancies like colon cancer.		

Diarrhea is often associated with infections with bacteria, virus, and parasites. Repeated negative bacterial cultures and microscopy for parasites should lead to the consideration that the symptoms may not be caused by an infection. Inflammatory bowel diseases like colitis and Crohn's disease are differential diagnosis and malabsorption and celiac disease must also be considered.

North Africa is one of the destinations from where traveler's diarrhea is very frequently reported.

Gastrointestinal infections with symptoms for more than 4 weeks and in the immunocompromised host

Microorganisms with symptoms for more than 4 weeks	Microorganisms in the immunocompromised host
Hepatitis A Whipple, tuberculosis	Herpes virus, CMV *Isospora*, Microsporidium *Candida*

(Continued)

Microorganisms with symptoms for more than 4 weeks	Microorganisms in the immunocompromised host
G. intestinalis, E. histolytica, cryptosporidia, *T. intestinalis*, helminths: *Ascaris lumbricoides, Trichuris trichiura, Hymenolepis nana, Strongyloides stercoralis, Echinococcus granulosus, Schistosoma mansoni* (Sudan and Egypt only) [18]	

Consider noninfectious causes like inflammatory bowel disease, intestinal malignancies like colon cancer, malabsorption, and celiac disease.

Infections of liver, spleen, and peritoneum

Acute infections of liver, spleen, and peritoneum with less than 4 weeks of symptoms

	Frequently found diseases	Rare diseases
Jaundice	Hepatitis A Hepatitis B EBV, CMV infection	Hepatitis C Hepatitis E Rickettsiosis Leptospirosis Syphilis II Crimean–Congo Hemorrhagic Fever
Space-occupying lesion in liver Splenomegaly	Bacterial liver abscess Typhoid fever Bacterial endocarditis Viral hepatitis EBV, CMV	Amebic liver abscess Visceral leishmaniasis Relapsing fever Brucellosis Tuberculosis

[a]Has not been described.

Chronic infections of liver, spleen, and peritoneum with more than 4 weeks of symptoms

	Frequently found diseases	Rare diseases
Jaundice	Chronic viral hepatitis Schistosomiasis[a]	Brucellosis Q fever hepatitis Toxocariasis Hepatic tuberculosis[b] Leprosy[b] Histoplasmosis
Space-occupying lesion in liver		Tuberculosis
Ascites	Tuberculous peritonitis	Schistosomiasis[a]
Splenomegaly	Hepatosplenic schistosomiasis	Tuberculosis Brucellosis

[a]Hepatic schistosomiasis is most often due to *S. mansoni* and only present in Sudan and Egypt.
[b]Hepatic TB may occur as miliary, nodular, and solitary abscess form.

Infections of liver, spleen, and peritoneum in the immunocompromised host

Infections in the immunocompromised host are no different from the immunocompetent host.

Genitourinary infections

Cystitis, pyelonephritis, and nephritis with less than 4 weeks of symptoms

Frequently found microorganisms	Rare microorganisms and conditions	Very rare microorganisms
E. coli, K. pneumoniae, Staphylococcus saprophyticus, Proteus mirabilis	*Pseudomonas aeruginosa, Enterococcus faecalis*	Tuberculosis

Consider noninfectious causes, especially malignancies like renal cell carcinoma.

Sexually transmitted infections with less than 4 weeks of symptoms

Frequently found microorganisms	Rare microorganisms and conditions	Very rare microorganisms
Chlamydia spp., *N. gonorrhoeae, Gardnerella vaginalis*, syphilis *Trichomonas vaginalis*	Lymphogranuloma venereum, *Ducrey Entamoeba dispar* and *E. histolytica*	

Cystitis, pyelonephritis, and nephritis with symptoms for more than 4 weeks and in the immunocompromised host

Microorganisms with symptoms for more than 4 weeks	Microorganisms in the immunocompromised host
Tuberculosis, *Schistosoma haematobium* [20]	*Candida*

Consider noninfectious causes, especially malignancies like renal cell carcinoma.

Sexually transmitted infections with symptoms for more than 4 weeks and in the immunocompromised host

Microorganisms with symptoms for more than 4 weeks	Microorganisms in the immunocompromised host
HIV, herpes virus, papilloma virus, hepatitis B virus Syphilis, *N. gonorrhoeae*	Syphilis *Candida*

Joint, muscle, and soft tissue infections

Joint, muscle, and soft tissue infections with less than 4 weeks of symptoms

Frequently found microorganisms	Rare microorganisms and conditions	Very rare microorganisms and conditions
S. aureus S. pneumoniae		Lice, scabies

Joint, muscle, and soft tissue infections with more than 4 weeks of symptoms and in the immunocompromised host

Microorganisms with symptoms for more than 4 weeks	Microorganisms in the immunocompromised host
Tuberculosis	*Candida*, dermatophytes

Skin infections

Skin infections with less than 4 weeks of symptoms

Frequently found microorganisms	Rare microorganisms and conditions	Very rare microorganisms and conditions
Erysipelas, *S. pneumoniae* *S. aureus* *Borrelia* spp. Dermatomycosis		

We have not listed a rash due to viral infections as this is not considered an infection limited to the skin.

Skin infections with more than 4 weeks of symptoms and in the immunocompromised host

Microorganisms with symptoms for more than 4 weeks	Microorganisms in the immunocompromised host
Syphilis, tuberculosis [21], leprosy Leishmania [22] Blastomycosis Scabies	*Candida* Dermatophytes [23]

Adenopathy

Adenopathy of less than 4 weeks' duration

Frequently found microorganisms	Rare microorganisms and conditions	Very rare microorganisms and conditions
EBV, CMV, parvovirus B19, HIV *Toxoplasma gondii*	Tularemia, *Bartonella*	*Ehrlichia, Yersinia pestis* [24]

Adenopathy of more than 4 weeks' duration and in the immunocompromised host

Microorganisms with symptoms for more than 4 weeks	Microorganisms in the immunocompromised host
Rubella, T. gondii Tuberculosis	Adenovirus, HIV, CMV

If the diagnosis is not made within a few days, biopsies should be performed to exclude malignancies like lymphoma and carcinomas.

Fever without focal symptoms

Fever for less than 4 weeks without focal symptoms

Frequently found microorganisms	Rare microorganisms and conditions	Very rare microorganisms and conditions
Dengue (Sudan only) [25], Chikungunya (Sudan only) [26], yellow fever (Sudan only) [26]	Rift Valley fever virus [27], West Nile virus, HIV	*Mycobacterium* (atypical)
Salmonella typhi, Meditteranean spotted fever (*R. conorii*) [28], *Rickettsia* spp. [29,30], *Brucella, Streptococcus* (endocarditis)	Tuberculosis, *C. burnetii*	Leishmania (visceral)
Malaria (Sudan only) [31], amebiasis	*Schistosoma*	

S. haematobium is present in the whole region, while *S. mansoni* is only present in Sudan and Egypt.

Fever for more than 4 weeks without focal symptoms and in the immunocompromised host

Microorganisms with symptoms for more than 4 weeks	Microorganisms in the immunocompromised host
C. burnetii [32], tuberculosis, *B. quintana* [33]	Leishmaniasis (visceral), tuberculosis, *Mycobacterium* (atypical)

Noninfectious causes should be considered from the beginning including malignancies like lymphoma and autoimmune diseases.

Noninfectious causes like lymphoma, other malignancies, and autoimmune diseases should be considered early.

Eosinophilia and elevated IgE

Eosinophilia and elevated IgE less than 4 weeks

Frequently found microorganisms	Rare microorganisms and conditions	Very rare microorganisms and conditions
A., T. trichiura, H. nana	Toxocara, Fasciola	Myiasis [34], filariasis, Trichinella

Eosinophilia and elevated IgE for more than 4 weeks and in the immunocompromised host

Microorganisms with symptoms for more than 4 weeks	Microorganisms in the immunocompromised host
S. stercoralis, E. granulosus, S. mansoni and S. haematobium, Dracunculus medinensis (Sudan only)	

S. haematobium is present in the whole region, while S. mansoni is only present in Sudan and Egypt.

Basic diagnostics in patients with eosinophilia and elevated IgE

Microorganisms	Diagnostics
Ascaris spp. Toxocara spp.	Fecal microscopy Serology

Antibiotic resistance

Multidrug-resistant *Salmonella enterica* have been isolated in Algeria [35]. *Shigella dysenteriae* and enteropathogenic *E. coli* show high resistance rates against ampicillin, chloramphenicol, tetracyclines, cotrimoxazol, nalidixic acid, sulfonamide, and neomycin in Sudan [36]. High degrees of penicillin resistance are observed in *S. pneumoniae* in North African countries, as well as dual resistance to penicillin and erythromycin [37,38]. Methicillin-resistant *Staphylococcus aureus* have been isolated in travelers returning from North Africa [39]. A high prevalence of multidrug-resistant tuberculosis was also described in Egypt [40]. In Sudan, *Plasmodium falciparum* exhibit a high level of resistance to antimalarials, leading the country to adopt artesunate+sulfadoxine/pyrimethamine combination as the first-line drug [41].

Vaccine-preventable diseases in children

According to WHO (http://www.who.int/immunization_monitoring/data/en/), the childhood vaccination program includes vaccination against tuberculosis, diphtheria, tetanus, poliomyelitis (oral polio vaccine), pertussis, measles, and hepatitis B in all North African countries. Vaccination against *H. influenzae* infection is provided in Algeria, Morocco, Sudan, and Libya. Vaccination against mumps is provided in Morocco, Egypt, and Libya, and vaccination against rubella in Morocco, Tunisia, Egypt, and Sudan. Finally, vaccination against meningitis A and C is provided in Egypt and against meningitis A, C, Y, and W135 in Libya. Of interest, cases of diphtheria and poliomyelitis are reported from Sudan only. Cases of tetanus, measles, rubella, and pertussis are reported from the entire North African area with local variations (WHO).

Basic economic and demographic data

Basic demographics*	GNI per capita (USD)	Life expectancy at birth (total, years)	School enrollment, primary (% net)
Algeria	4,260	72	95
Egypt	1,800	70	96
Libyan Arab Jamahiriya	11,590	74	NA
Morocco	2,580	71	89
Sudan	1,130	58	41
Tunisia	3,290	74	95
Western Sahara	NA	NA	NA

*World Bank.
GNI, gross national income; NA, not available.

Causes of death in children under 5 years—regional average

	%
Neonatal causes	26
Pneumonia	21
Diarrheal diseases	17
Malaria	17
HIV/AIDS	7
Measles	4
Injuries	2
Others	6

WHO, 2006 data.

Most common causes of death in all ages in three countries selected for a low (Sudan), middle (Morocco), and high (Libya) regional GNI per capita

	%		
	Sudan	Morocco	Libya
Ischemic and hypertensive heart disease	8	24	28
HIV/AIDS	6	NS	NS
Lower respiratory infections	NS	6	5
Cerebrovascular disease	5	7	8
Malaria	6	NS	NS
Perinatal conditions	5	7	4
Tuberculosis	5	NS	NS
Diarrhea	6	4	2
Measles	5	NS	NS
War	4	NS	NS
Road traffic accidents	3	4	4
Cirrhosis of the liver	NS	3	2
Chronic obstructive lung disease	NS	2	2
Nephritis and nephrosis	NS	3	3

NS, not stated.
WHO 2002.

References

1. Nakhla I, Frenck RW Jr, Teleb NA, et al. The changing epidemiology of meningococcal meningitis after introduction of bivalent A/C polysaccharide vaccine into school-based vaccination programs in Egypt. Vaccine 2005;23 (25):3288–93.

2. Selim HS, El-Barrawy MA, Rakha ME, Yingst SL, Baskharoun MF. Microbial study of meningitis and encephalitis cases. J Egypt Public Health Assoc 2007;82(1–2):1–19.

3. Afifi S, Karsany MS, Wasfy M, Pimentel G, Marfin A, Hajjeh R. Laboratory-based surveillance for patients with acute meningitis in Sudan, 2004–2005. Eur J Clin Microbiol Infect Dis 2009;28(5):429–35.

4. Bahri O, Fazaa O, Ben Alaya-Bouafif N, Bouloy M, Triki H, Bouattour A. [Role of Toscana virus in meningo-encephalitis in Tunisia.] Pathol Biol (Paris). 2010 Apr 6.

5. Schuffenecker I, Peyrefitte CN, el Harrak M, Murri S, Leblond A, Zeller HG. West Nile virus in Morocco, 2003. Emerg Infect Dis 2005;11 (2):306–9.

6. Bahri O, Rezig D, Nejma-Oueslati BB, et al. Enteroviruses in Tunisia: virological surveillance over 12 years (1992–2003). J Med Microbiol 2005;54(Part 1):63–9.

7. Rezig D, Ben Yahia A, Ben Abdallah H, Bahri O, Triki H. Molecular characterization of coxsackievirus B5 isolates. J Med Virol 2004;72 (2):268–74.

8. Guenifi W, Rais M, Gasmi A, et al. [Neurobrucellosis: description of 5 cases in Setif Hospital, Algeria]. Med Trop (Mars) 2010;70 (3):309–10 (French).

9. Letaïef AO, Kaabia N, Chakroun M, Khalifa M, Bouzouaia N, Jemni L. Clinical and laboratory features of murine typhus in central Tunisia: a report of seven cases. Int J Infect Dis 2005;9 (6):331–4.

10. Abdelmalek R, Kanoun F, Kilani B, et al. Tuberculous meningitis in adults: MRI contribution to the diagnosis in 29 patients. Int J Infect Dis 2006;10(5):372–7.

11. Youssef FG, Afifi SA, Azab AM, et al. Differentiation of tuberculous meningitis from acute

bacterial meningitis using simple clinical and laboratory parameters. Diagn Microbiol Infect Dis 2006;55(4):275–8.

12. Azzouzi N, Elhataoui M, Bakhatar A, Takourt B, Benslimane A. [Part of *Chlamydia pneumoniae* in atherosclerosis and exacerbation of chronic obstructive pulmonary disease and asthma]. Ann Biol Clin (Paris) 2005;63(2):179–84.

13. Hammami N, Mezghani S, Znazen A, et al. [Bacteriological profile of infectious endocarditis in the area of Sfax (Tunisia)]. Arch Mal Coeur Vaiss 2006;99(1):29–32 (French).

14. Letaief A, Boughzala E, Kaabia N, et al. Epidemiology of infective endocarditis in Tunisia: a 10-year multicenter retrospective study. Int J Infect Dis 2007;11(5):430–3.

15. Znazen A, Rolain JM, Hammami N, Kammoun S, Hammami A, Raoult D. High prevalence of *Bartonella quintana* endocarditis in Sfax, Tunisia. Am J Trop Med Hyg 2005;72(5):503–7.

16. Frank C, Walter J, Muehlen M, et al. Major outbreak of hepatitis A associated with orange juice among tourists, Egypt, 2004. Emerg Infect Dis 2007;13(1):156–8.

17. Ghenghesh KS, Franka E, Tawil K, et al. Enteric fever in Mediterranean north Africa. J Infect Dev Ctries 2009;3(10):753–61.

18. El Guamri Y, Belghyti D, Achicha A, et al. [Epidemiological retrospective survey intestinal parasitism in the Provincial Hospital Center (Kenitra, Morocco): review of 10 years (1996–2005)]. Ann Biol Clin (Paris) 2009;67(2):191–202.

19. Kansouzidou A, Charitidou C, Varnis T, Vavatsi N, Kamaria F. *Cyclospora cayetanensis* in a patient with travelers' diarrhea: case report and review. J Travel Med 2004;11(1):61–3.

20. Stothard JR, Chitsulo L, Kristensen TK, Utzinger J. Control of schistosomiasis in sub-Saharan Africa: progress made, new opportunities and remaining challenges. Parasitology 2009;136(13):1665–75.

21. Zouhair K, Akhdari N, Nejjam F, Ouazzani T, Lakhdar H. Cutaneous tuberculosis in Morocco. Int J Infect Dis 2007;11(3):209–12.

22. Pratlong F, Dereure J, Ravel C, et al. Geographical distribution and epidemiological features of Old World cutaneous leishmaniasis foci, based on the isoenzyme analysis of 1048 strains. Trop Med Int Health 2009;14(9):1071–85.

23. Mebazaa A, Oumari KE, Ben Said M, et al. Tinea capitis in adults in Tunisia. Int J Dermatol 2010;49(5):513–16.

24. Bitam I, Baziz B, Rolain JM, Belkaid M, Raoult D. Zoonotic focus of plague, Algeria. Emerg Infect Dis 2006;12(12):1975–7.

25. Adam I, Jumaa AM, Elbashir HM, Karsany MS. Maternal and perinatal outcomes of dengue in PortSudan, Eastern Sudan. Virol J 2010;7:153.

26. Gould LH, Osman MS, Farnon EC, et al. An outbreak of yellow fever with concurrent chikungunya virus transmission in South Kordofan, Sudan, 2005. Trans R Soc Trop Med Hyg 2008;102(12):1247–54.

27. Hassanain AM, Noureldien W, Karsany MS, Saeed el NS, Aradaib IE, Adam I. Rift Valley fever among febrile patients at New Halfa hospital, eastern Sudan. Virol J 2010;7:97.

28. Mouffok N, Parola P, Lepidi H, Raoult D. Mediterranean spotted fever in Algeria—new trends. Int J Infect Dis 2009;13(2):227–35.

29. Mouffok N, Benabdellah A, Richet H, et al. Reemergence of rickettsiosis in Oran, Algeria. Ann N Y Acad Sci 2006;1078:180–4.

30. Mouffok N, Parola P, Raoult D. Murine typhus, Algeria. Emerg Infect Dis 2008;14(4):676–8.

31. Mirghani SE, Nour BY, Bushra SM, Elhassan IM, Snow RW, Noor AM. The spatial-temporal clustering of *Plasmodium falciparum* infection over eleven years in Gezira State, The Sudan. Malar J 2010;9:172.

32. Kernif T, Aissi M, Doumandji SE, Chomel BB, Raoult D, Bitam I. Molecular evidence of *Bartonella* infection in domestic dogs from Algeria, North Africa, by polymerase chain reaction (PCR). Am J Trop Med Hyg 2010;83(2):298–300.

33. Bellazreg F, Kaabia N, Hachfi W, et al. Acute Q fever in hospitalised patients in Central Tunisia: report of 21 cases. Clin Microbiol Infect 2009;15(Suppl. 2):138–9.

34. Perez-Eid C, Mouffok N. [Human urinary myiasis caused by *Fannia canicularis* (Diptera, Muscidae) larvae in Algeria]. Presse Med 1999;28(11):580–1 (French).

35. Naas T, Bentchouala C, Lima S, et al. Plasmid-mediated 16S rRNA methylases among extended-spectrum-beta-lactamase-producing *Salmonella enterica* Senftenberg isolates from Algeria. J Antimicrob Chemother 2009;64(4):866–8.

36. Ahmed AA, Osman H, Mansour AM, et al. Antimicrobial agent resistance in bacterial isolates from patients with diarrhea and urinary tract infection in the Sudan. Am J Trop Med Hyg 2000;63(5–6):259–63.

37. Benouda A, Ben Redjeb S, Hammami A, Sibille S, Tazir M, Ramdani-Bouguessa N. Antimicrobial resistance of respiratory pathogens in North African countries. J Chemother 2009;21(6):627–32.

38. Shaban L, Siam R. Prevalence and antimicrobial resistance pattern of bacterial

meningitis in Egypt. Ann Clin Microbiol Antimicrob 2009;8:26.

39. Stenhem M, Ortqvist A, Ringberg H, et al. Imported methicillin-resistant *Staphylococcus aureus*, Sweden. Emerg Infect Dis 2010;16(2): 189–96.

40. Abbadi SH, Sameaa GA, Morlock G, Cooksey RC. Molecular identification of mutations associated with anti-tuberculosis drug resistance among strains of *Mycobacterium tuberculosis*. Int J Infect Dis 2009;13(6):673–8.

41. Menegon M, Talha AA, Severini C, et al. Frequency distribution of antimalarial drug resistance alleles among *Plasmodium falciparum* isolates from Gezira State, central Sudan, and Gedarif State, eastern Sudan. Am J Trop Med Hyg 2010;83(2):250–7.

Chapter 9
Southern Africa

Marc Mendelson,[1] Olga Perovic[2] and Lucille Blumberg[3]

[1]Division of Infectious Diseases and HIV Medicine, Department of Medicine, Groote Schuur Hospital, University of Cape Town, Cape Town, South Africa
[2]Microbiology External Quality Assessment Reference Unit, National Institute for Communicable Diseases, Johannesburg, South Africa
[3]Epidemiology Division (Travel and International Health), National Institute for Communicable Diseases, Johannesburg, South Africa

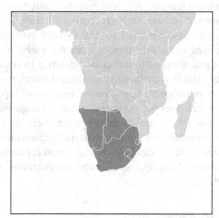

Namibia
Botswana
South Africa
Losotho
Sawisland

Southern Africa's burden of disease is dominated by the collision of two epidemics; HIV and tuberculosis. Malaria completes the triumvirate of major clinical infectious diseases, with endemic areas in all countries except Lesotho. The traveler to southern Africa is at risk of acquiring a number of infections either common to other geographic areas or those that are over-represented in Africa as a whole. These infections include vector-borne diseases such as African tick bite fever, the commonest cause of febrile syndrome in the returning traveler from South Africa, mosquito-borne West Nile virus and Sindbis and water-related infections such as schistosomiasis and leptospirosis. Southern Africa is an intermediate risk area for traveler's diarrhea, and other fecal–oral acquired infections, such as hepatitis A and less commonly typhoid fever, are important causes of morbidity in visiting travelers.

Infectious Diseases: A Geographic Guide, First Edition.
Edited by Eskild Petersen, Lin H. Chen & Patricia Schlagenhauf.
© 2011 John Wiley & Sons, Ltd. Published 2011 by John Wiley & Sons, Ltd.

Acute infections within 4 weeks of exposure

Three infections dominate the infectious diseases landscape of southern Africa; HIV, malaria, and tuberculosis. As the incubation period of tuberculosis even for primary infection is rarely <4 weeks, it will not be discussed further in this section.

Worldwide, southern Africa is the region most seriously affected by HIV. South Africa is home to the largest population of people living with HIV [1], its seroprevalence rate amongst 15- to 24-year-old antenatal clinic attendees being 29.3% [2]. This is eclipsed by Swaziland's antenatal seroprevalence rate of 42% in 2008, which has been steadily increasing since 1992 [1]. Overall, each country in southern Africa has adult seroprevalence rates exceeding 15% [2]. HIV seroconversion illness is clinically apparent in 40–90% of new HIV infections, with symptoms occurring within days–weeks of infection which generally last <14 days [3]. Although clinical features are often nonspecific, fever is the commonest symptom. A maculopapular rash is evident in 40–80% of patients and mucocutaneous ulceration and aseptic meningitis are frequently seen [4].

HIV seroconversion illness should be considered in any traveler returning from southern Africa with fever and nonspecific symptoms. Furthermore, pretravel advice should incorporate strong messaging around safe-sex practices, with particular reference to condom use.

Southern Africa has low rates of malaria transmission compared to other endemic regions in Africa and transmission is commonly seasonal. The summer months of September to May see the highest rates of transmission, which does not occur uniformly throughout each country, but is found in distinct geographic areas. Of the five countries in southern Africa, Lesotho, whose lowest point is 1,400 m, is the only country where malaria transmission does not occur. Chloroquine resistance is widespread and the drug is no longer used for malaria prophylaxis, or for treatment of *Plasmodium falciparum*. Mefloquine, atovaquone-proguanil, or doxycycline are recommended for chemoprophylaxis.

Malaria transmission in southern Africa

Country	Malaria-endemic areas	Malaria type	Seasonal transmission [5]
Botswana	North of 22°S in the northern provinces of Central, Chobe, Ghanzi, Ngamiland, and Okavango Delta area	*P. falciparum* 90%	September to May in northern provinces and Okavango Delta
		Plasmodium ovale 5% *Plasmodium vivax* 5%	
Lesotho	None	NA	NA
Namibia	Kunene, Ohangwena, Okavango, Omaheke, Omusati, Oshana, Oshikoto, Otjozondjupa provinces, and the Caprivi Strip	*P. falciparum* 90%	Year-round along the Kuene River, Caprivi and Kavango regions
		Plasmodium. malariae, P. ovale, and *P. vivax* 10%	September to May in other areas
Swaziland	Northern and eastern areas bordering Mozambique and South Africa including all of Lubombo district	*P. falciparum* 90%	Year-round in lowveld areas (Big Bend, Mhlume, Simunye, and Tshanen)

Country	Malaria-endemic areas	Malaria type	Seasonal transmission [5]
South Africa	Provinces of Mpumalanga, Limpopo, and northeastern KwaZulu-Natal as far south as the Tugela River	*P. ovale* 5% *P. vivax* 5% *P. falciparum* 90% *P. ovale* 5% *P. vivax* 5%	Seasonal risk September to May

Adapted from information from the CDC Malaria Map Application. Accessed August 12, 2010 at http://cdc-malaria.ncsa.uiuc.edu/index.php.

In addition to HIV and malaria, patients presenting with acute febrile illness from southern Africa within 4 weeks of exposure may have acquired an infection that is either particular to the African continent or tropical climes, or one that is common worldwide, for example, influenza and other upper respiratory tract viral infections. The latter will not be discussed further in this chapter.

Fever and rash

• *African tick bite fever* (ATBF) is the commonest cause of fever in travelers returning to their home country from South Africa [6] and travel to southern Africa is a recognized risk factor for acquiring *Rickettsia africae*, the causative organism [7]. Risk factors for exposure to the *Amblyomma* ticks which transmit *R. africae* in southern Africa include male sex, traveling for tourism, and travel during the summer months [7]. Interestingly, travel during winter was found to be a risk factor in multivariate analysis for those restricting their travel to South Africa [6]. ATBF should be suspected in any traveler returning with the classic triad of fever, eschar, and maculopapular rash, although in up to 45% of patients, the rash may be vesicular [8] and rash may be absent in a percentage of travelers with ATBF. Mediterranean Spotted Fever (MSF) rickettsiosis may also be acquired in southern Africa from *Rhipicephalus* spp. ticks (brown dog tick), which carry *R. conorii*. This infection presents with similar clinical features, although clinically apparent eschars and lymphadenopathy are less common. Diagnosis is primarily made on clinical features and risk exposure. Complications of bleeding and multisystem disease may occur in a small percentage of persons. Treatment is with doxycycline.

• *Acute schistosomiasis*, also known as Katayama fever, is endemic in southern Africa and follows swimming in inland waterways. Penetration of waterborne cercariae through the skin may lead to cercarial dermatitis hours after exposure; an itchy, localized rash, which resolves within hours. Katayama fever, an acute hypersensitivity reaction is thought to be a result of initial egg deposition by the adult female worm, and usually occurs 2–8 weeks after infection. It is characterized by fever, urticaria, and eosinophilia ± wheeze. *Schistosoma* ova may be absent from urine or stool at this stage and serological tests can take up to 3 months to become positive. Treatment is with prednisone to reduce the hypersensitivity reaction. If praziquantel is administered, the dose should be repeated at 3 months after last water contact in the endemic area, to ensure that adult worms are killed.

• *Typhoid fever* may become evident in a febrile patient with or without bowel disturbance who develops Rose spots, a discrete maculopapular rash, commonly localized to the abdomen and trunk. Rose spots are generally rare especially in dark-skinned patients. Leukopenia is characteristic and blood cultures should be sent with early instigation of antibiotic therapy.

• *Meningococcal meningitis or septicemia* occurs sporadically throughout southern Africa, but is more common in the winter months.

• *Viral exanthems* such as measles and rubella are common in southern Africa and may be acquired by nonimmune travelers.

• *West Nile fever* due to infection with the mosquito transmitted WNV is endemic in southern Africa. Although 80% of cases are asymptomatic, abrupt onset of high fever (often >39°C) headache, myalgia, and gastrointestinal symptoms occur in approximately 20%. A transient nonitchy maculopapular rash may occur, commonly affecting the trunk and extremities. West Nile neuroinvasive disease will occur in <1% of infected individuals and carries a mortality of up to 30% [9].

• *Sindbis and Chikungunya*, in keeping with other members of the alphavirus family, these viruses have a predilection for causing arthritis, but may also be characterized by rash in addition to fever. Sindbis is more commonly reported than Chikungunya in southern Africa, having a wider geographic distribution. Both are mosquito-borne and cause an abrupt onset of fever with polyarticular small joint arthralgia and chills. A maculopapular rash involving trunk, limbs, face, palms, and soles may occur early in the illness. Mild leukopenia with relative leukocytosis may be present. Treatment is supportive.

• *Strongyloidiasis* has a tropical and subtropical distribution and a prepatent period of 17–28 days. Patients may present with pruritus at the site of larval entry or pulmonary symptoms related to larval migration. If autoinfection ensues, signs of established infection such as larva currens may occur. Hyperinfection in immunocompromised patients may develop.

• *Viral hemorrhagic fevers* can present with a morbilliform rash, in particular Congo–Crimean Hemorrhagic Fever (CCHF), which is endemic in a number of areas throughout southern Africa, and the newly identified Lujo virus, a novel arenavirus that was the focus of an outbreak in Johannesburg, South Africa in 2008 [10].

Fever and jaundice

• *Hepatitis A*, manifesting 2–6 weeks after infection with the picornavirus, is commonly asymptomatic in children, but up to 70% of adults will experience jaundice. Fulminant hepatitis is rare and treatment is supportive. Vaccination for travelers to the region is recommended to prevent this infection.

• *Leptospirosis*, caused by the spirochete *Leptospira* spp., is a zoonosis transmitted by rats. Exposure to rat excreta in infected water increases the risk of acquisition in travelers undertaking water sports such as white-water rafting. Leptospirosis also occurs in urban areas where rats cohabit. It classically runs a biphasic course with initial bacteremia followed by an immune phase associated with antibody production and immune complex deposition. Abrupt onset of fever with nonspecific symptoms occurs. Conjunctival suffusion without purulent discharge and intense myalgia are common. Headache, retro-orbital pain, and aseptic meningitis may occur. Weil's disease describes the severe form of leptospirosis accompanied by hepatic (jaundice) and renal failure, carrying a mortality rate of up to 15%.

• *Hepatitis E* is far less common than its counterpart hepatitis A virus, yet can cause higher rates of severe disease.

Relapsing fever

• *Tick-Borne Relapsing Fever* (TBRF) is endemic to the southern Africa region, transmitted by members of the *Ornithodoros* soft tick species. *Borrelia duttonii* is the predominant cause of the abrupt febrile illness with nonspecific symptoms that last several days, followed by a crisis and cessation of fever. If untreated, the fever recurs on average 7 days later. Multiple relapses can occur, which tend to be milder as the number progresses [11].

Diarrhea ± fever

• *Travelers diarrhea* (TD): Southern Africa is classified as an intermediate risk region for acquiring TD; 8–20% of travelers experience TD associated with a stay of ≥2 weeks abroad [12]. A suggestion that South Africa is a low-risk country in contrast to its neighbors was not supported by a recent study [6]. The commonest cause of TD is enterotoxigenic *Escherichia coli*. Early treatment rather than prophylactic antibiotics is recommended for travelers to the region.

• *Amebiasis* caused by the protozoan *Entamoeba histolytica* has a clinical spectrum from asymptomatic to dysentery to fulminant colitis. Metronidazole or tinidazole is the treatment of choice.

• *Cholera* epidemics have been ongoing in southern Africa in recent years, including the spill over of the Zimbabwean cholera epidemic of 2009 to southern African countries. South Africa and Botswana were particularly affected. Sporadic cases and small clusters continue to occur, but the risk of acquiring cholera in the region is low.

CNS infections: meningitis, encephalitis, and other infections with neurological symptoms

Acute infections with less than 4 weeks of symptoms

Frequently found microorganisms	Rare microorganisms	Very rare microorganisms
P. falciparum	*Listeria monocytogenes*	Influenza
Streptococcus pneumoniae	*Haemophilus influenzae*	Measles
Neisseria meningitidis	*Treponema pallidum*	WNV
Enteroviruses	*Leptospirosis* spp.	*Brucella*
Herpes virus (type I)	Spotted fever group (SFG) rickettsioses	Rabies
HIV		*P. vivax* malaria

CNS infections: meningitis and encephalitis with symptoms for more than 4 weeks and in the immunocompromised host

Microorganisms with symptoms for more than 4 weeks	Microorganisms in the immunocompromised host
Tuberculosis	*Cryptococcus* spp.
Neurocysticercosis	Tuberculosis
Cryptococcus spp.	Toxoplasmosis
HIV	Cytomegalovirus (CMV)
	HIV
	Nocardia
	JC virus
	Aspergillus
	Varicella zoster virus (VZV)
	Epstein–Barr virus (EBV), EBV-driven primary CNS lymphoma

Consider noninfectious causes like lymphoma.

Ear, nose, and throat infections

Ear, nose, and throat infections with less than 4 weeks of symptoms

Frequently found microorganisms	Rare microorganisms and conditions	Very rare microorganisms
Streptococcal throat infection	Peritonsillar abscess[a]	*H. influenzae* type B (incidence reduced by vaccination program)
Viral infections; influenza A and B, parainfluenza, rhinovirus	Tuberculosis	*Neisseria gonorrhoeae*
EBV	Necrotizing fasciitis[a]	Diphtheria
Herpes virus (type I and II)	Lemierre's syndrome[a]	
	Vincent's angina	

[a]Requires acute ENT evaluation.

Ear, nose, and throat with symptoms for more than 4 weeks and in the immunocompromised host

Microorganisms with symptoms for more than 4 weeks	Microorganisms in the immunocompromised host
Tuberculosis	*Candida*
Pseudallescheria boydii	Herpes virus
	Human herpes virus 8 (Kaposi's sarcoma)
	Pseudomonas aeruginosa
	EBV, EBV-driven non-Hodgkin's lymphoma
	Cancrum oris

Consider noninfectious causes like vasculitis and lymphoma.

Cardiopulmonary infections

Pneumonia with less than 4 weeks of symptoms

Frequently found microorganisms	Rare microorganisms and conditions	Very rare microorganisms
S. pneumoniae	*Staphylococcus aureus*	*Chlamydia psittaci*
Legionella pneumophilia	Influenza	Histoplasmosis
Mycoplasma pneumoniae	Aerobic gram-negative bacilli (e.g., *Klebsiella pneumoniae*)	Diphtheria
Chlamydia pneumoniae	Loeffler's syndrome (e.g., *Ascaris lumbricoides* migration)	
Respiratory viruses		
H. influenzae		

Endocarditis with less than 4 weeks of symptoms

Frequently found microorganisms	Rare microorganisms and conditions	Very rare microorganisms

Nonhemolytic streptococci
S. aureus
Enterococci
Coagulase-negative staphylococci
  (*Staphylococcus epidermidis*)
	Bartonella spp.
	Coxiella burnetii
	HACEK group
	Nutritionally variant streptococci
	  (*Abiotrophia/Granulicatella* spp.)
	S. pneumonia
	N. gonorrhoeae
		P. aeruginosa
		Brucella

Pulmonary symptoms for more than 4 weeks and in the immunocompromised host

Microorganisms and diseases with symptoms for more than 4 weeks	Microorganisms in the immunocompromised host
Tuberculosis *Cryptococcus* spp. *Aspergillus* *Nocardia* Chronic obstructive pulmonary disease (COPD)	*Mycobacterium tuberculosis* *Pneumocystis jirovecii* *Cryptococcus* spp. CMV Nontuberculous mycobacteria
	Aspergillus, Candida, and other deep fungal infections *Rhodococcus equi* Lymphoid interstitial pneumonitis *P. aeruginosa*

In addition to opportunistic pathogens such as *Pneumocystis jirovecii*, the commonest organisms associated with pulmonary infection in HIV-infected patients are *S. pneumoniae* and *H. influenzae*. Consider noninfectious causes like lung cancer, autoimmune lung fibrosis, Wegener's granulomatosis.

Endocarditis for more than 4 weeks and in the immunocompromised host

As infective endocarditis is a recognized cause of pyrexia of unknown origin, all of the organisms listed above may cause a clinical illness that lasts for >4 weeks. In the immunocompromised host, *Aspergillus* must be considered, and very rarely, tuberculosis in high prevalent countries of southern Africa.

Basic diagnostics of pulmonary infections Fiber-optic bronchoscopy, bronchiolar lavage, and transbronchial biopsy are only available in specialist centers and CT is not routinely used for diagnosis of pneumonia in southern Africa.

Basic diagnostics of endocarditis High index of suspicion in any patient with fever, murmur ± extracardiac embolic phenomena such as Roth's spots, Osler's nodes, and so on. Echocardiography is limited to specialist centers in southern Africa; hence more reliance is made on clinical diagnosis and use of criteria such as the Duke criteria.

Gastrointestinal infections

Gastrointestinal infections with less than 4 weeks of symptoms

Frequently found microorganisms	Rare microorganisms and conditions	Very rare microorganisms
Salmonella (nontyphi) Shigella Campylobacter Enterotoxigenic E. coli S. aureus toxin Giardia intestinalis E. histolytica A. lumbricoides Enterobius vermicularis (threadworm)	Salmonella typhi Bacillus cereus toxin Anisakis spp.	Whipple's disease

Consider noninfectious causes like inflammatory bowel disease and intestinal malignancies like colon cancer.

Gastrointestinal infections with symptoms for more than 4 weeks and in the immunocompromised host

Microorganisms with symptoms for more than 4 weeks	Microorganisms in the immunocompromised host
A. lumbricoides Hookworm spp. Schistosoma mansoni Taeniasis (Taenia solium and Taenia saginata) Strongyloides stercoralis Trichuris trichura Fascioliasis (Fasciola hepatica) Visceral toxocariasis (visceral) Tuberculosis HIV	Candida Cryptosporidium Isospora belli Microsporidiosis Salmonella (nontyphi) CMV Tuberculosis Nontuberculous mycobacteria Histoplasmosis Herpes virus type 1 AIDS cholangiopathy Human herpes virus 8 (Kaposi's sarcoma) Lymphoma

Consider noninfectious causes like inflammatory bowel disease, intestinal malignancies like colon cancer, malabsorption, and celiac disease.

Infections of liver, spleen, and peritoneum

Acute infections of liver, spleen, and peritoneum with less than 4 weeks of symptoms

	Frequently found diseases	Rare diseases
Jaundice	Malaria Hepatitis A Hepatitis B EBV, CMV infection	Hepatitis C Hepatitis E Rickettsiosis Leptospirosis Syphilis II Relapsing fever Yellow fever
Space-occupying lesion in liver Splenomegaly	Bacterial liver abscess Malaria Typhoid fever Bacterial endocarditis Viral hepatitis EBV, CMV Tuberculosis	Amebic liver abscess Brucellosis Relapsing fever

Chronic infections of liver, spleen, and peritoneum with more than 4 weeks of symptoms

	Frequently found diseases	Rare diseases
Jaundice	Chronic viral hepatitis Schistosomiasis Hepatic tuberculosis	Brucellosis Q fever hepatitis Toxocariasis Histoplasmosis
Space-occupying lesion in liver Ascites Splenomegaly	Tuberculosis Tuberculous peritonitis Hepatosplenic schistosomiasis Hyperreactive malaria syndrome	*S. mansoni* Tuberculosis Brucellosis

Infections of liver, spleen, and peritoneum in immunocompromised host

Infections in the immunocompromised host are no different from the immunocompetent host.

Genitourinary infections

Cystitis, pyelonephritis, and nephritis with less than 4 weeks of symptoms

Frequently found microorganisms	Rare microorganisms and conditions	Very rare microorganisms
E. coli *K. pneumoniae*	*Enterococcus* spp. *P. aeruginosa*	

(Continued)

Frequently found microorganisms	Rare microorganisms and conditions	Very rare microorganisms
Proteus spp. Tuberculosis HIV-associated nephropathy	*S. aureus* Perirenal abscess Leptospirosis	

Consider noninfectious causes especially malignancies like renal cell carcinoma.

Sexually transmitted infections with less than 4 weeks of symptoms

Frequently found microorganisms	Rare microorganisms and conditions	Very rare microorganisms
Primary syphilis Herpes simplex type II *N. gonorrhoeae* Chancroid *Chlamydia* spp. *Trichomonas*	Lymphogranuloma venereum Granuloma inguinale	Tuberculosis

Cystitis, pyelonephritis, and nephritis with symptoms for more than 4 weeks and in the immunocompromised host

Microorganisms with symptoms for more than 4 weeks	Microorganisms in the immunocompromised host
Bacterial infections in patients with long-term catheters and renal stones *Schistosoma haematobium* Tuberculosis HIV-associated nephropathy	Tuberculosis *Candida* Human herpes virus 8 (Kaposi's sarcoma) *P. jirovecii* (extrapulmonary)

Consider noninfectious causes especially malignances like renal cell carcinoma.

Sexually transmitted infections with symptoms for more than 4 weeks and in the immunocompromised host

Syphilis and genital warts due to human papillomavirus may both persist for >4 weeks. Stigmatization in relation to any sexually transmitted infection that causes penile deformity may lead to delayed presentation in patients with penile edema secondary to lymphogranuloma venereum or tuberculosis.

Basic diagnostics of sexually transmitted infections

The majority of southern African countries employ a syndromic approach to management of sexually transmitted infection and therefore do not employ diagnostic tests, but rather treat individual syndromes.

Joint, muscle, and soft tissue infections

Joint, muscle, and soft tissue infections with less than 4 weeks of symptoms

Frequently found microorganisms	Rare microorganisms and conditions	Very rare microorganisms and conditions
S. aureus (including tropical pyomyositis)	Reiter's syndrome	*S. pneumoniae*
N. gonorrhoeae	Necrotizing fasciitis	Fournier's gangrene (perineum and urogenital)
	Group G streptococci	
	Viral arthritis (parvovirus, rubella, hepatitis B, enteroviruses)	Trichinosis
	Tuberculosis	
	Salmonella (nontyphi)	
	N. meningitidis	
	Sindbis and Chikungunya	

Joint, muscle, and soft tissue infections with more than 4 weeks of symptoms and in the immunocompromised host

Microorganisms associated with symptoms for >4 weeks include tuberculosis, HIV, and *Brucella*. In the immunocompromised host, candida and cryptococcal spp. are important causes.

Skin infections

Skin infections with less than 4 weeks of symptoms

Frequently found microorganisms	Rare microorganisms and conditions	Very rare microorganisms and conditions
S. aureus and Group A β-hemolytic streptococci (impetigo, boils, etc.)	Hidradenitis suppurativa	Gnathostomiasis[a]
Ringworm (*Tinea* spp.)	*S. pneumoniae*	
Herpes viruses (VZV and HSV)	*Bacillus anthracis*	
Spotted fever group rickettsioses (ATBF and MSF)		
Scabies		
Helminths (Acute schistosomiasis, hookworm-associated cutaneous larva migrans, strongyloidiasis)		
Tinea versicolor (*Malassezia furfur*)		

We have not listed a rash due to viral infections as this is not considered an infection limited to the skin.
[a]Reported cases after ingestion of raw bream in the Okavango Delta.

Skin infections with more than 4 weeks of symptoms and in the immunocompromised host

Microorganisms with symptoms for more than 4 weeks	Microorganisms in the immunocompromised host
Syphilis	Human herpes virus (Kaposi's sarcoma)
Tuberculosis	Deep fungal infection (histoplasmosis, blastomycosis, sporotrichosis, and cryptococcosis)
Sporotrichosis	Tuberculosis
Mycobacterium leprae	*Bartonella* (bacillary angiomatosis)
Mycetoma (actinomycosis, *Nocardia*)	*Candida*
Human herpes virus (endemic Kaposi's sarcoma)	

Adenopathy

Adenopathy of less than 4 weeks' duration

Frequently found microorganisms	Rare microorganisms and conditions	Very rare microorganisms and conditions
HIV	*Bartonella* (Cat scratch disease)—never seen here (very rare)	*Brucella*
Local suppurative disease (staphylococci, streptococci)	Parvovirus B19	
Infectious mononucleosis (EBV, CMV, and *Toxoplasma gondii*)		

Adenopathy of more than 4 weeks' duration and in the immunocompromised host

Microorganisms with symptoms for more than 4 weeks	Microorganisms in the immunocompromised host
HIV	HIV
Tuberculosis	Tuberculosis
Syphilis	Human herpes virus (Kaposi's sarcoma, Multicentric Castleman's disease)
	EBV (non-Hodgkin's lymphoma)
	Deep fungal infection (histoplasmosis, sporotrichosis, blastomycosis)
	Nontuberculous mycobacteria

Basic diagnostics of patients with adenopathy

Fine needle aspiration or Trucut biopsy should be performed on all suspicious lymph nodes, particularly those that are asymmetric, >1.5 cm or matted. Specimens should be sent for tuberculosis microscopy, culture (±histology), and cytology. If a diagnosis is not forthcoming, the node should be excised whenever possible and sent for the above-mentioned tests.

Fever without focal symptoms

Fever less than 4 weeks without focal symptoms

Frequently found microorganisms	Rare microorganisms and conditions	Very rare microorganisms and conditions
Malaria HIV Tuberculosis Endocarditis Pyogenic abscess Infectious mononucleosis (EBV, CMV, toxoplasmosis)	*Brucella*	

Fever for more than 4 weeks without focal symptoms and in the immunocompromised host

Microorganisms with symptoms for more than 4 weeks	Microorganisms in the immunocompromised host
Tuberculosis HIV	Tuberculosis EBV, EBV-associated lymphoma Cryptococcal spp. and other disseminated deep fungal infections

Noninfectious causes should be considered from the beginning including malignancies like lymphoma and autoimmune diseases.

Eosinophilia and elevated IgE

Eosinophilia and elevated IgE for less than 4 weeks

Frequently found microorganisms	Rare microorganisms and conditions	Very rare microorganisms and conditions
Ascaris spp. Hookworm spp. *Schistosoma* spp. Taeniasis (*T. solium* and *T. saginata*) *S. stercoralis* *T. trichura* Toxocariasis	Fascioliasis (*F. hepatica*)	

Eosinophilia and elevated IgE for more than 4 weeks and in the immunocompromised host

All of the above helminth infections can present with symptoms for >4 weeks. *S. stercoralis* hyperinfection syndrome must be considered in the immunocompromised host.

Antibiotic resistance

Antimicrobial resistance surveillance is lacking in the southern African region and the only national surveillance data available are from The Group for Enteric, Respiratory and Meningeal disease Surveillance program, South Africa (GERMS-SA). GERMS-SA is a national surveillance project with 25 enhanced surveillance sites using specific case definitions and standardized testing methods.

Methicillin-resistant **S. aureus**   Methicillin-resistant *S. aureus* (MRSA) is currently one of the most commonly identified resistant pathogens, documented in approximately 39% of public sector, hospitalized patients in blood isolates from sentinel sites. In the past decade, community-associated MRSA (CA-MRSA) without health-care associated risk factors has emerged in South Africa [13].

Multidrug-resistant **S. pneumoniae**   High-level resistance to β-lactams and multidrug resistance in *S. pneumoniae* are an ongoing concern [14]. Penicillin nonsusceptible isolates have increased in invasive pneumococci, with prevalence ranging between 32% and 52% in different provinces in South Africa, being common in children less than 5 years of age [15]. Likewise, ceftriaxone resistance in meningitis isolates was significant.

Multidrug-resistant gram-negative bacilli   Multidrug-resistant gram-negative bacilli are generally resistant to more than two classes of antimicrobial agents. However, some strains may also be resistant to the carbapenems, leaving colistin as the only agent available for treatment [16]. Fluoroquinolones (FQ) are used for treatment of invasive diarrheal disease in patients with *Salmonella*, which occurs more frequently in HIV-infected persons [17]. In South Africa FQ resistance is at low level in *Salmonella*. In contrast, extended spectrum beta-lactamases (ESBLs) were detected in 7% of isolates [17]. FQ use has been shown to be the only independent risk factor for FQ resistance in *E. coli* strains causing urinary tract infections [18,19]. FQ resistance rates of 23% have been reported from private health-care facilities, 5% of which were ESBLs.

Vaccine-preventable diseases in children

The childhood vaccination program will vary to some extent in southern African countries. While the basic expanded program for immunization (EPI) program is fairly uniform across the region, a number of new vaccines have been introduced in the past few years in South Africa as part of the EPI schedule.

Vaccine coverage is variable, both across the region and within countries and has a major impact on occurrence of disease and outbreaks, e.g. measles outbreaks have been reported quite widely in South Africa and Zimbabwe. A number of childhood vaccines are registered and available in some of the countries, but usage is, for the most part, restricted to the private sector because of resource limitations.

Additional vaccines to those listed in the EPI program, which are available and registered for use in children, include meningococcal vaccine (polysaccharide), seasonal influenza vaccine, human papillomavirus, and varicella zoster. Vaccines for special indications include rabies vaccine for postexposure prophylaxis.

EPI (SA) schedule as of April 1, 2009

Basic economic and demographic data

Age	Vaccine needed
At birth	OPV(0): Oral polio vaccine
	BCG: Bacillus Calmette–Guerin vaccine
6 weeks	OPV(1): Oral polio vaccine
	RV (1): Rotavirus vaccine
	DTaP-IPV//Hib (1): Diphtheria, tetanus, acellular pertussis/inactivated polio vaccine and *H. influenzae* type b
	Heb B(1): Hepatitis vaccine
	PCV(1): Pneumococcal conjugated vaccine
10 weeks	DTaP-IPV//Hib (2): Diphtheria, tetanus, acellular pertussis/inactivated polio vaccine and *H. influenzae* type b
	Heb B(2): Hepatitis vaccine
14 weeks	RV (2): Rotavirus vaccine
	DTaP-IPV//Hib (3): Diphtheria, tetanus, acellular pertussis/inactivated polio vaccine and *H. influenzae* type b
	Heb B(3): Hepatitis vaccine
	PCV(2): Pneumococcal conjugated vaccine
9 months	Measles vaccine (1)
	PCV(3): Pneumococcal conjugated vaccine
18 months	DTaP-IPV//Hib (4): Diphtheria, tetanus, acellular pertussis/inactivated polio vaccine and *H. influenzae* type b
	Measles vaccine (2)
6 years	Td vaccine: Tetanus and reduced amount of diphtheria vaccine
12 years	Td vaccine: Tetanus and reduced amount of diphtheria vaccine

Basic demographics	GNI[a] per capita, 2009 (USD)	Life expectancy at birth (total, years)	School enrollment, primary (% net)
Botswana	6,260	51	84
Lesotho	1,020	43	72
Namibia	4,310	53	87
South Africa	5,770	50	86
Swaziland	2,350	46	87

World Development Indicators database, World Bank, revised July 9, 2010 World Bank.
[a]Gross National Income (http://siteresources.worldbank.org/DATASTATISTICS/Resources/GNIPC.pdf).

Cause of death in children under 5 years expressed as percent of the total number of deaths

	Botswana	Lesotho	Namibia	South Africa	Swaziland	Regional average
Neonatal causes	40	33	39	35	27	26
Pneumonia	1	5	3	1	12	21
Diarrheal diseases	1	4	3	1	10	17

(Continued)

	Botswana	Lesotho	Namibia	South Africa	Swaziland	Regional average
Malaria	0	0	0	0	0	17
HIV/AIDS	54	56	53	57	47	7
Measles	0	0	0	0	0	4
Injuries	3	2	3	5	4	2
Others	0	0	0	1	1	6

WHO, regional average 2000–2003 (http://www.who.int/whosis/mort/profiles/en/#).

Top 10 causes of deaths in all ages in 2002

	Botswana	Lesotho	Namibia	South Africa	Swaziland
HIV/AIDS	80	63	51	52	64
IHD/hypertensive heart disease	2	3	4	4	2
Cerebrovascular disease	2	3	4	5	2
Lower respiratory tract infection	1	4	2	4	5
Tuberculosis	1	2	4	2	4
Measles	1	3	NS	2	NS
COPD	NS	2	NS	NS	1
Perinatal conditions	1	1	4	1	2
Violence	2	3	2	NS	NS
Road traffic accidents	NS	NS	2	3	1
Diabetes	1	1	NS	2	NS

NS, not stated; IHD, ischemic heart disease.

Expressed as percent of the total. World Health Organization, 2006 (http://www.who.int/whosis/mort/profiles/en/#).

References

1. UNAIDS, 2008. Report on the Global AIDS Epidemic. Geneva: UNAIDS.
2. Department of Health, 2009. 2008 National Antenatal Sentinel HIV and Syphilis Prevalence Survey, South Africa. Pretoria: Department of Health.
3. Kahn JO, Walker BD. Acute Human Immunodeficiency Virus type 1 infection. N Engl J Med 1998;339(1):33–9.
4. Schacker T, Collier AC, Hughes J, Shea T, Corey L. Clinical and epidemiological features of primary HIV infection. Ann Intern Med 1996;125:257–64.
5. World Health Organization. International Travel Health (2010). Accessed August 11, 2010 at http://www.who.int/ith/ITH2010countrylist.pdf.
6. Mendelson M, Davis XM, Jensenius M, et al. Health risks in travelers to South Africa: The GeoSentinel experience and implications for the 2010 FIFA World Cup. Am J Trop Med Hyg 2010;82(6):991–5.
7. Jensenius M, Davis X, von Sonnenburg F, et al. Muticenter GeoSentinel analysis of rickettsial diseases in international travelers, 1996–2008. Emerg Infect Dis 2009;15(11):1791–8.
8. Raoult D, Fournier PE, Fenollar F, et al. *Rickettsia africae*, a tick-borne pathogen in travelers to sub-Saharan Africa. N Engl J Med 2001; 344:1504–10.
9. Watson JT, Pertel PE, Jones RC, et al. Clinical characteristics and functional outcome of West Nile Fever. Ann Intern Med 2004;141 (5):360–5.

10. National Institute for Communicable Diseases, 2008. Arenavirus outbreak, South Africa. Communicable Diseases Communique 7:1–3. Accessed September 6, 2010 at http://www.nicd.ac.za.

11. Southern PM Jr, Sandford JP. Relapsing fever: a clinical and microbiological review. Medicine 1969;48:129–49.

12. Steffan R. Boppart I. Travellers' diarrhoea. In: Klaus E, Gyr GE (eds). Baillière's Clinical Gastroenterology, Vol. 1. London: Baillière Tindall, 1987:361–76.

13. Oosthuysen WF, Duse AG, Marais E. Molecular characterization of methicillin-resistant *Staphylococcus aureus* in South Africa. 17th ECCMID, Munich, March 31–April 3, 2007.

14. Rodríguez-Cerrato V, Gracia M, Del Gardo G, et al. Antimicrobial susceptibility of multidrug-resistant *Streptococcus pneumoniae* strains with penicillin MICs of 8 to 32 mg/L. Diag Microbiol Infect Dis 2010;66(3):336–8.

15. Group for Enteric, Respiratory and Meningeal disease Surveillance in South Africa. GERMS-SA Annual Report 2009. Accessed September 6, 2010 at http://www.nicd.ac.za/units/germs/germs.htm.

16. Aubron C, Poirel L, Ash RJ, Nordmann P. Carbapenemase-producing *Enterobacteriaceae*, U.S. Rivers. Emerg Infect Dis 2005. Available from http://www.cdc.gov/ncidod/EID/vol11no02/03-0684.htm.

17. Angulo FJ, Swerdlow DL. Bacterial enteric infections in persons infected with human immunodeficiency virus. Clin Infect Dis 1995; 2(Suppl. 1):S84–93.

18. Maslow JN, Lee B, Lautenbach E. Fluoroquinolone-resistant *Escherichia coli* carriage in long-term care facility. Emerg Infect Dis 2005;11(6):889–94.

19. Kassis-Chikhani N, Vimont S, Asselat K, et al. CTX-M b-lactamase-producing *Escherichia coli* in long-term care facilities, France. Emerg Infect Dis 2004;10(9):1697–8.

Chapter 10
West Africa

Joanna S. Herman[1] and Peter L. Chiodini[1,2]
[1]Hospital for Tropical Diseases, London, UK
[2]London School of Hygiene and Tropical Medicine, London, UK

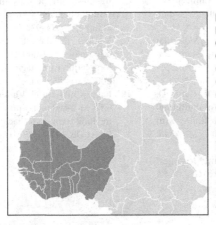

Benin
Burkina Faso
Cape Verde
Côte d'Ivoire
Gambia
Ghana
Guinea
Guinea-Bissau
Liberia
Mali
Mauritania
Niger
Nigeria
Senegal
Sierra Leone
Togo

West Africa occupies approximately one-fifth of Africa. The vast majority of this region is composed of plains lying less than 300 m above sea level, but the northern section is composed of a semiarid terrain known as the Sahel, a transitional zone between the Sahara and the savannahs and forests of western Sudan. Patterns of infectious diseases are determined by both landscape and socioeconomic factors. Like many parts of sub-Saharan Africa, adequate health-care infrastructures are lacking, and basic epidemiological data for many diseases are not available.

A broad spectrum of infections is seen in travelers from West Africa ranging from the short lived, easily detected, and treatable to the more exotic such as filarial infections. Whilst some of the common short-lived infections are regularly seen in the short-term

Infectious Diseases: A Geographic Guide, First Edition.
Edited by Eskild Petersen, Lin H. Chen & Patricia Schlagenhauf.
© 2011 John Wiley & Sons, Ltd. Published 2011 by John Wiley & Sons, Ltd.

traveler (e.g., gastrointestinal disorders or malaria), the more exotic tropical diseases are more likely in those who spend prolonged periods abroad, particularly in rural endemic areas. Those presenting to physicians in industrialized countries include Western tourists/businessmen, Africans resident in industrialized countries who return to their country of origin to visit friends and relatives (VFRs), and migrants of African origin who have become resident outside endemic areas but came harboring initially asymptomatic tropical infections. VFRs comprise a significant proportion of travelers to West Africa, and as a group have particular health risks, especially in respect of malaria and other tropical infections prevalent in rural areas [1]. Some infections may be acquired during short-term visits (e.g., malaria, typhoid, hepatitis A and B), but others with long incubation periods may have been acquired well before their migration and only become manifest with time, presenting some years after arrival in their newly adopted countries (e.g., filariasis, strongyloidiasis, chronic schistosomiasis) [1,2].

Three main conditions are seen in returning travelers from the tropics: fever, gastro-enterological disorders, and dermatological problems [2,3]. Data from the Hospital for Tropical Diseases in London on returnees from West Africa show the most common infections seen in VFRs are schistosomiasis, *Plasmodium falciparum* malaria, strongyloides infection, filariasis, and onchocerciasis. In comparison, the most common diagnoses seen in Western travelers visiting the region are schistosomiasis, infectious diarrhea, *P. falciparum* malaria, giardiasis, undiagnosed fever, and bacterial skin infections. Viral hemorrhagic fever (VHF) is very rarely seen in returning travelers, but is endemic in many areas of this region, having significant mortality and major public health implications if the diagnosis is missed.

It is helpful to categorize infections according to symptoms and average time of presentation from last exposure. Most infections acquired in the tropics present within 21 days of leaving an endemic region, and almost always within 6 months. However, some infections, such as those due to helminths (e.g., strongyloidiasis, schistosomiasis, filariasis), and HIV may not present for years. Initial assessment of returnees from this region must focus on those diseases which are life-threatening, treatable, and of public health importance, and include malaria, VHF, and enteric fever. Most tropical infections can be easily treated if identified early enough.

Fever

About 3–11% of travelers report occurrence of fever, with up to 50% presenting within the first week of return and 96% within 6 months [4,5]. The key elements in the diagnostic approach to the investigation of imported fever are precise travel history, including assessment of risk factors for acquisition, and the time lapse between exposure and onset of symptoms. The most frequent causes of fever in a traveler returned from West Africa are malaria (85% *P. falciparum*, 5–10% *Plasmodium ovale*, *Plasmodium vivax* rare), common bacterial infections such as pneumonia or urinary tract infection (not necessarily specific to the area), nonspecific viral infections, and infectious diarrhea. If travel has included the meningitis belt during the epidemic season (see later), meningitis due to *Neisseria meningitidis* group A must be considered. VHF is rare, but must be excluded in any traveler returning with fever from an endemic region within 21 days (Figure 10.1). It is important to remember that acute febrile infections in travelers may be due to cosmopolitan organisms, which are not exclusive to the region visited [6].

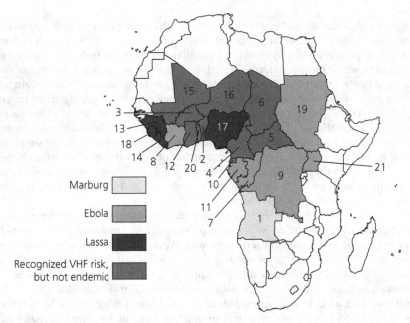

1. Angola, 2. Benin, 3. Burkino Faso, 4. Cameroon, 5. Central African Republic,
6. Chad, 7. Congo, 8. Cote d'Ivoire, 9. Democratic Republic of Congo (Zaire),
10. Equitorial Guinea, 11. Gabon, 12. Ghana, 13. Guinea, 14. Liberia, 15. Mali,
16. Niger, 17. Nigeria, 18. Sierra Leone, 19. Sudan, 20. Togo, 21. Uganda.

Fig. 10.1 Map depicting risk areas for VHF. (Created by Margaret Armstrong for the Hospital for Tropical Diseases (HTD) London, VHF guidelines. Copyright HTD.)

In many infections where fever is the predominant symptom, diagnostic features are often lacking. Symptoms at initial presentation may be nonspecific and physical findings unremarkable ("undifferentiated" fever), thus making it difficult to guide investigation and to distinguish between different causes. However before embarking on extensive investigations, it is important to establish the true presence of fever, as some patients complaining of "fever" are not actually febrile.

Causes of undifferentiated fever

Undifferentiated fever <4 weeks	Undifferentiated fever >4 weeks
Malaria	Malaria
Nonspecific viral infections	Katayama fever
VHF (must be <21 days)	HIV seroconversion[a]
Enteric fever	Brucella
Rickettsial infections	Amebic liver abscess[b]
Arbovirus infection	Trypanosomiasis

Undifferentiated fever <4 weeks	Undifferentiated fever >4 weeks
Leptospirosis	Histoplasmosis
	Noninfectious causes (e.g., malignancy, hematological conditions, autoimmune diseases)

[a]West Africa has been less affected by HIV and AIDS than other parts of sub-Saharan Africa, with prevalence rates varying between <2% (e.g., Benin, Sierra Leone) and 6% (e.g., Gabon), compared with approximate rates of 20% in parts of Southern Africa.
[b]Right upper quadrant pain common, but may be asymptomatic apart from fever.

Of the fevers presenting within 4 weeks of return, malaria and VHF have the greatest mortality and morbidity and therefore need rapid exclusion.

Malaria

Malaria is endemic throughout much of West Africa, and has high transmission rates particularly in the forested regions. However, rates are not uniform in the region, with some areas having endemic and perennial transmission, while others have epidemic and strongly seasonal transmission. Transmission peaks during the rainy season, which falls roughly between April and August with a second peak between October and November. Many VFRs do not take prophylaxis as they may incorrectly assume themselves to have some degree of residual immunity. Of the cases recorded by the UK Health Protection Agency (HPA) Malaria Reference Laboratory in 2009, where ethnicity was recorded, nearly 1,000 (999) were reported as Africans or of African descents compared with 123 white and 173 Asian or South Asian descents (HPA Malaria Reference Laboratory, personal communication). Over half (54%) of people with malaria were recorded as having traveled to or arrived from West Africa (813/1,495). Furthermore, epidemiological studies have shown that children of VFRs account for 15–20% of all imported cases [7], which is due to a lack of prophylaxis and preventative measures, implying that the message of malaria prevention is not reaching those in greatest need. *P. falciparum* malaria may have protean manifestations, often mimicking other infections (e.g., gastroenteritis, respiratory tract infections, or nonspecific viral infections), which may cause fatal delay in diagnosis and treatment. Chloroquine resistance is widespread and this drug should not be used for either treatment or prophylaxis of falciparum malaria in Africa. Quinine or artesunate should be used for treatment, and the use of mefloquine or doxycycline or atovaquone–proguanil is recommended for chemoprophylaxis. *P. ovale* causes significantly less morbidity, and remains sensitive to chloroquine.

Viral hemorrhagic fever

VHF needs rapid exclusion in any traveler returning with fever from an endemic region within 21 days. Ebola virus is endemic in Cote d'Ivoire, Lassa fever in Guinea, Sierra Leone, Liberia, and Nigeria. Benin, Mali, Togo, Burkina Faso, Ghana, Liberia, and Niger all have a risk of VHF, with occasional outbreaks (Figure 10.1). Symptoms include fever, headache, myalgia, pharyngitis, diarrhea, vomiting, retrosternal pain, purpuric rash, and bleeding diatheses. VHF is very rarely seen in travelers, but infection results in serious morbidity and mortality with a significant risk of human to human and nosocomial transmission. The probability of VHF can be assessed by a structured questionnaire, based on exposure risk and symptoms, which categorizes suspected patients into low, medium, and high risk, with the latter two groups needing rapid further investigation and high-level isolation [8].

Fever associated with specific signs and/or symptoms

Fever with rash

Many infections may have a rash as part of multiple presenting features, but this section will discuss those in which rash is the predominant feature in addition to fever.

Viral exanthems: Measles and rubella are common in West Africa and are not confined to children. They may be acquired in travelers who have not been vaccinated in childhood. Other common exanthemata such as Parvovirus B19 may be seen.

Meningococcal meningitis or septicaemia: Much of West Africa lies in the meningitis belt, which stretches from Senegal in the west to Ethiopia in the east. Large epidemic waves occur every 5–12 years due predominantly to serotype A. In 2009 there were over 4,000 deaths and 78,000 suspected infections (WHO statistics). Incidence is highest during the dry season between December and June. A polysaccharide vaccine is available for serotypes A, C, Y, and W 135, but a conjugate vaccine providing superior immunogenicity has recently become available.

Rickettsial infections: These are less common than in other parts of Africa but do occur.

Arbovirus infections: For example, Dengue, West Nile Virus, Chikungunya (occasionally seen, with outbreak reported from Senegal).

Epstein–Barr virus (EBV) or related viral infections: For example, cytomegalovirus (CMV) or the protozoan *Toxoplasma*.

Sexually transmitted infections: For example, secondary syphilis.

HIV seroconversion: This usually occurs 2–4 weeks after exposure with a similar picture to EBV infection (fever, lymphadenopathy and fine macularpapular erythematous rash). A high viremia and marked fall in CD4 count is seen, but HIV antibodies may be negative or indeterminate.

Katayama fever: Acute schistosomiasis may develop 4–8 weeks after initial infection with a large cercarial load. More common in travelers; it is rarely seen in residents of endemic areas, and represents an acute hypersensitivity reaction to initial egg deposition by the adult female worm. Symptoms include fever, urticaria, diarrhea, hepatosplenomegaly, cough, wheeze, and eosinophilia. Serology may be negative at first, and schistosoma ova may be absent from stool and urine. Treatment is with praziquantel under steroid cover. Individuals may remember that some weeks before they had had an initial itchy rash ("swimmer's itch" or cercarial dermatitis) which develops within 12h after exposure.

Fever with respiratory symptoms

Upper and lower respiratory tract infections are diagnosed in 7–24% of febrile returning travelers [1,4,6]. Few have specific tropical infections, more commonly having etiologies similar to those infections seen in the industrialized countries, for example, *Streptococcus pneumoniae*, *Haemophilus influenzae*, group A streptococcus, atypical organisms, and respiratory viruses including influenza. Of causes more common in the tropics, tuberculosis and pulmonary eosinophilia may be seen.

Tuberculosis (TB) is more commonly seen in VFRs and in health-care workers who have been resident in endemic regions. The estimated incidence rate is 3.5 infections per 1,000 person-months of travel, and of active disease 0.6 per 1,000 person-months of travel [9]. Thus the risk in long-term travelers to highly endemic regions is similar to that of the local population. Short-term Western travelers have little risk of infection. At present, West Africa is not known to have a significant amount of multidrug-resistant tuberculosis (MDRTB), with only two to four cases reported annually over the past 5 years, and no cases of extensively drug-resistant tuberculosis (XDRTB) (Laura Anderson, Enhanced Surveillance System, Health Protection Agency, London, personal communication).

Loeffler's syndrome/pulmonary eosinophilia may occur with certain helminth infections resulting in fever, cough, and wheeze. Pulmonary infiltrates are usually evident on chest radiograph, and a peripheral eosinophilia is invariably present. *Ascaris, Strongyloides*, hookworm, and acute schistosomiasis (Katayama fever) are potential causes, and appropriate serology and stool examination should be done. Loeffler's is more frequent in nonimmune travelers than VFRs.

It is important to remember that nonrespiratory infections may additionally present with pulmonary symptoms, for example, malaria (ARDS), amebic liver abscess (diaphragmatic irritation), and typhoid, so they must be included in the differential diagnosis for targeting investigations.

Fever with gastrointestinal symptoms

Both infectious and noninfectious gastroenterological conditions may present with fever and a variety of gastrointestinal symptoms, for example, diarrhea, vomiting, abdominal pain, and jaundice. Diarrheal illness and jaundice are discussed further in the following section. Several systemic infections may also have diarrhea as a part of their initial presentation, for example, malaria, atypical pneumonia, measles, and VHF. Noninfectious conditions unrelated to travel must also be considered as they may present in a similar fashion (e.g., appendicitis, pancreatitis, cholecystitis, and inflammatory bowel disease). Amebic liver abscess typically presents with fever and right upper quadrant pain, and a history of previous dysentery is not always evident.

Fever with jaundice

Hepatic causes include severe *P. falciparum* malaria, enteric fever, severe sepsis, acute hepatitis (A, B, E), leptospirosis, yellow fever, and VHF. Hemolytic causes include malaria, mycoplasma pneumonia, *Shigella*, or *E. coli* associated hemolytic-uremic syndrome, and hemoglobinopathies, for example sickle cell disease or β thalassemia which are common in this region.

Leptospirosis is a zoonosis transmitted predominantly by rats. There should be an exposure history of direct contact with urine of infected animals or contact with contaminated water. Infection may result in fever, rash, severe myalgia, aseptic meningitis, bleeding diatheses, mental confusion, myocarditis, and pulmonary symptoms. In the severe form (Weil's disease), hepatorenal failure occurs, carrying a mortality rate of up to 15%. The majority of cases in endemic regions are subclinical or mild, and are therefore often undiagnosed. The majority originate in rural areas, with peak incidence in the rainy season. Average incubation period is 10 days (range 4–19 days).

Fever with neurological symptoms

Causes include both infections specific to the tropics and those also seen in industrialized countries. Acute infections include *P. falciparum* malaria, rabies, bacterial meningitis (*N. meningitidis, S. pneumoniae*, or *H. influenzae* type b in children <5 years of age), viral meningitis (enteroviruses, herpesviruses), encephalitis (for example Herpes simplex virus type 1, Enterovirus, Varicella zoster virus), and secondary syphilis. Infections that may result in prolonged symptoms (>4 weeks) include TB meningitis/cerebral TB, neurocysticercosis. Additional organisms should be considered in immunocompromised individuals and include *Cryptococcus neoformans, Toxoplasma gondii*, CMV, JC virus, *Aspergillus*, as well as noninfectious causes such as non-Hodgkin's lymphoma.

Gastrointestinal disorders

In the tropics diarrhea causes over 6 million deaths per year, with 80% in children. Travelers' diarrhea is the main cause of morbidity in short-term travelers to the tropics, with incidence varying from 25% to 90% in the first 2 weeks of travel [1]. The risk is less in travelers originating from highly endemic countries as they have some degree of immunity. The main pathogens are enterotoxigenic *Escherichia coli* (ETEC) (up to 50% of cases), *Salmonella* spp., *Shigella* spp., and *Campylobacter*. Viral infections (rotavirus and noroviruses) and protozoa (*Giardia lamblia* and *Cryptosporidium* spp.) may also be a cause. However, in up to 50% of patients no pathogen will be identified [1,10]. Travelers' diarrhea usually starts on the third day after arrival abroad, and if untreated the mean duration is 4 days (average 3–5). Typically, there are less than 6 motions in 24 h. It is usually self-limiting, but the duration can be shortened by antibiotics. However, in 8–15% diarrhea persists for >1 week, and in 2% for >1 month [11]. Occasionally diarrhea may persist for many months with the development of a postinfective irritable bowel syndrome. Inflammatory bowel disease and celiac disease should also not be forgotten.

It is helpful to remember that the more common bacterial and viral causes of gastroenteritis tend to present early in the first few weeks of travel or return, whereas parasitic causes, for example giardiasis, tend to become evident later. Fever may occur, but is not invariable.

Skin conditions

The main dermatological problems travelers to West Africa encounter are insect/arthropod bites (often with secondary bacterial infection), pyogenic infections, dermatophyte infections, cutaneous larva migrans, allergic reactions, and myiasis (e.g., tumbu fly). Less commonly seen tropical diseases that manifest in the skin particular to West (and Central) Africa include loiasis, onchocerciasis, lymphatic filariasis, dracunculiasis (guinea worm) and mansonellosis (*Mansonella streptocerca* and *Mansonella perstans*). These infections tend to be seen only in VFRs or people who have spent prolonged periods in rural areas. Buruli ulcer (due to *Mycobacterium ulcerans*) is endemic in parts of West Africa, and causes extensive destructive and disfiguring ulceration predominantly on the distal extremities. However it is hardly ever seen in the West, and is confined to people who originate from those regions.

The climate of the region predisposes to lack of healing of superficial wounds and insect bites which frequently develop a secondary bacterial infection. The humidity is also ideal for development of dermatophyte infections.

Loiasis is a chronic filarial disease transmitted by a deer fly of the genus *Chrysops*, characterized by transient subcutaneous (or deeper) swellings caused by migration of the adult worm through the body. These "Calabar swellings," several centimeters in diameter, may occur on any part of the body and may be preceded by pain and associated with pruritus. Occasionally, the host mounts a marked allergic response with giant urticaria and fever. The worms may also migrate under the conjunctivae with resultant pain and edema. Diagnosis is made by the presence of microfilariae (larvae) in daytime peripheral blood, found after membrane filtration. Eosinophilia is frequent and history of travel to an endemic area essential. The incubation period is long, with symptoms usually appearing more than a year after infection, but may occur as early as 4 months. Microfilariae may appear in the peripheral blood 6 months after infection, and the adult worm may persist as long as 17 years. Treatment is with diethylcarbamazine (DEC), but if microfilariae are present steroids should be given in addition to DEC starting the day before to reduce the inflammatory response to dying larvae.

Onchocerciasis or "river blindness" is caused by the filarial worm *Onchocerca volvulus*. It is a major cause of both blindness and skin disease. It is transmitted by blackfly of the genus *Simulium* which breed in and bite people near to rapidly flowing freshwater. The symptoms are caused almost entirely by immunological reactions to dying microfilariae, which live for about 1 year. The adult worms cause few symptoms and may live up to 15 years (12 years on average).

Lymphatic filariasis due to *Wuchereria bancrofti* is often asymptomatic but a significant proportion of infections result in elephantiasis. The incubation period is usually 8–16 months, and symptoms include recurrent episodes of fever associated with lymphangitis that classically radiates distally from an enlarged tender lymph node. Secondary bacterial infection is a significant risk. The usual areas affected are groin and thigh, axilla and upper arm, breast in women and spermatic cord in men. It tends to be seen mainly in people originating from that region.

There are also many cutaneous manifestations of systemic febrile illnesses, often with nonspecific erythematous macular rashes, for example dengue, leptospirosis. However, the majority of dermatological conditions are easily diagnosed and treatable. Many will also be self-limiting and frequently resolve once the traveler has returned to his normal environment.

Antibiotic resistance

Data are very limited on antibiotic resistance patterns from West Africa. Several studies have been done by the Survey of Antibiotic Resistance (SOAR) Study Group investigating resistance patterns in three common organisms: *S. pneumoniae*, *Streptococcus pyogenes*, and *H. influenzae* [12]. Their findings show variable resistance rates across West Africa: for *S. pneumoniae* resistance rates to penicillin, amoxicillin, and erythromycin are very low and vary between none in Cote d'Ivoire to 3.3% in Nigeria [12]. Importantly, bacteremia due to *S. pneumoniae* remains sensitive to penicillin. Rates of macrolide/azalide resistance are similar (<4%). However, high-level resistance has been found to co-trimoxazole (e.g., 17% Cote d'Ivoire, 83% Nigeria), which poses a major problem for its use in many treatment protocols for empiric therapy of both upper and lower respiratory infections [12,13]. Beta-lactamase production by *H. influenzae* is variable (5% Cote d'Ivoire, 26% Senegal) [14]. Gonococcus resistance has been well documented, with a dramatic increase in both West and Central African penicillinase-producing strains, for example 73% of organisms in Abidjan, and 65% of strains resistant to tetracycline [15]. Enteric organisms still appear to remain sensitive to ciprofloxacin and this is still recommended as first-line treatment, in contrast to Asian strains [16].

Children

Infections causing the greatest mortality in children under 5 years of age include pneumonia (21%), diarrheal disease (17%), malaria (17%), HIV/AIDS (7%), and measles (4%). These are linked directly to socioeconomic status, but for pneumonia and measles appropriate vaccine coverage would significantly reduce mortality and morbidity. Education and distribution of insecticide treated bednets (ITBN) has been shown to significantly reduce deaths from malaria [17]. The Extended Program on Immunization (EPI) cover in the region is variable, for example 84–98% in Ghana, 39–50% in Nigeria. Rates vary within countries and with vaccine, for example greater uptake for BCG than MMR (WHO statistics).

Basic economic and demographic data

Basic demographics	GNI[a] per capita (USD)	Life expectancy at birth (total, years)	School enrollment, primary (% net)
Benin	690	62	80
Burkina Faso	480	52	58
Cape Verde	3,130	71	85
Côte d'Ivoire	980	58	55
Gambia	390	56	67
Ghana	670	57	73
Guinea	390	58	74
Guinea-Bissau	250	48	45
Liberia	170	58	31
Mali	580	54	63
Mauritania	840	64	80
Niger	330	57	45
Nigeria	1,160	47	64
Senegal	970	56	72
Sierra Leone	320	48	NA
Togo	400	63	77

World Bank.

NA, not available.

[a]Gross national income.

Causes of death in children under 5 years—regional average

	%
Neonatal causes	26
Pneumonia	21
Diarrheal diseases	17
Malaria	17
HIV/AIDS	7
Measles	4
Injuries	2
Others	6

WHO, 2002 data.

Most common causes of death in all ages in three countries selected for a low (Sierra Leone), middle (Senegal), and high (Cape Verde) regional GNI per capita

	%		
	Sierra Leone	Senegal	Cape Verde
HIV/AIDS	4	3	NS
Lower respiratory infections	13	16	3
Diarrhea	NS	7	11

	%		
	Sierra Leone	Senegal	Cape Verde
Cerebrovascular disease	10	4	11
Perinatal conditions	10	9	NS
Malaria	7	13	NS
Measles	4	NS	NS
Tuberculosis	3	5	11
Syphilis	2	NS	NS
Ischemic and hypertensive heart disease	2	4	4
Road traffic accidents	2	3	NS
Asthma	NS	NS	2
Whooping cough	NS	2	NS
Diabetes mellitus	NS	NS	2
Chronic obstructive lung disease	NS	NS	3

WHO, 2006.
NS, not stated.
Gross national income.

References

1. Ansart S, Perez L, Vergely O, Danis M, Bricaire F, Caumes E. Illnesses in travellers returning from the tropics: a prospective study of 622 patients. J Trav Med 2005;12:312–18.
2. Bottieau E, Clerinx J, Schrooten W, et al. Etiology and outcome of fever after a stay in the tropics. Arch Int Med 2006;166:1642–8.
3. Freedman DO, Weld LH, Kozarsky PE, et al., for the GeoSentinel Surveillance Network. Spectrum of disease and relation to place of exposure among ill travellers. N Eng J Med 2006;354:119–30.
4. O'Brian D, Tobin S, Brown GV, Torresi. Fever in returned travellers: review of hospital admissions for a 3-year period. Clin Infect Dis 2001;33:603.
5. Steffen R, Rickenbach M, Wilhelm U, Helminger A, Schar M. Health problems after travel to developing countries. J Infect Dis 1987;156:84–91.
6. Doherty JF, Grant AD, Bryceson ADM. Fever as the presenting complaint of travellers returning from the tropics. Q J Med 1995;88:277–81.
7. Ladhani S, Aibara RJ, Riordan FA, Shingadia D. Imported malaria in children: a review of clinical studies. Lancet Infect Dis 2007;7:349–57.
8. Woodrow CJ, Eziefula AC, Agranoff D, et al. Early risk assessment for viral haemorrhagic fever: experience at the Hospital for Tropical Diseases, London, UK. J Infect 2007;54:6–11.
9. Cobelens FG, van Deutekom H, Draayer-Jansen IW, et al. Risk of infection with *Mycobacterium tuberculosis* in travellers to areas of high tuberculosis endemicity. Lancet 2000; 356:461–5.
10. Jiang ZD, Lowe B, Verenkar MP, et al. Prevalence of enteric pathogens among international travellers with diarrhoea acquired in Kenya (Mombasa), India (Goa), or Jamaica (Montego Bay). J Infect Dis 2002;185:497–502.
11. Manson P. Tropical Diseases, 21st edn, London: Saunders, 2002.
12. Sievers, J, The SOAR Study Group. Antibacterial Resistance Among *Streptococcus pneumoniae* from Ten Countries in Africa and the Middle East: Results from the Survey of Antibiotic Resistance (SOAR) 2004–2006. Presented at the 46th Interscience Conference on Antimicrobial Agents and Chemotherapy, San Francisco, 2006. Abstract No: C2-425.
13. Hill PC, Onyeama CO, Ikumapayi UN, et al. Bacteraemia in patients admitted to an urban hospital in West Africa. BMC Infect Dis 2007;7:2.
14. O'Brien, D, The SOAR Study Group. Antibacterial Resistance Among *Streptococcus pneumoniae, Haemophilus influenzae* and *Streptococcus pyogenes* from 9 Countries in Africa and Middle East: Results from the Survey of Antibiotic Resistance (SOAR) 2007–2009. Presented at the 49th Interscience Conference on Antimicrobial

Agents and Chemotherapy, San Francisco, 2009. Abstract No: C2-140.

15. Van Dyck E, Crabbé F, Nzila N, Bogaerts J, Munyabikali JP, Ghys P et al. Sex Transm Dis. Increasing resistance of *Neisseria gonorrhoeae* in west and central Africa. Consequence on therapy of gonococcal infection. Sex Transm Dis 1997;24:32–7.

16. Patel TA, Armstrong M, Morris-Jones SD, Wright SG, Doherty T. Imported Enteric Fever: Case Series from the Hospital for Tropical Diseases, London, United Kingdom. Am J Trop Med Hyg 2010;82:1121–6.

17. Nevill CG, Some ES, Mung'ala VO, et al. Insecticide-treated bednets reduce mortality and severe morbidity from malaria among children on the Kenyan coast. Trop Med Int Health 1996;1:139–46.

Chapter 11
Eastern Asia

Susan MacDonald,[1] Yasuyuki Kato[2] and Annelies Wilder-Smith[3]

[1]Northern Health Authority, University Hospital of Northern British Columbia, Prince George, BC, Canada
[2]Disease Control and Prevention Center, National Center for Global Health and Medicine, Tokyo, Japan
[3]Institute of Public Health, University of Heidelberg, Germany

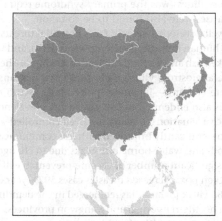

People's Republic of China
Mongolia
Republic of Korea (North)
Japan
Republic of Korea (South)
Taiwan

Eastern Asia consists of a large, highly diverse region with marked differences in climate, environment, population density, and cultures. Standards of hygiene as well as access to medical care and advanced diagnostics for infectious diseases may vary between and within countries, in particular, urban as compared to rural areas. Respiratory infections, hepatitis, and diarrheal diseases predominate in many regions; however, there is also a wide range of vector-borne diseases such as Japanese encephalitis, tick-borne encephalitis, dengue fever, and malaria. Added to this are the many diseases frequently associated with poverty including tuberculosis, sexually transmitted infections, and soil-, water-, and food-borne helminthiases. Emerging and reemerging infectious diseases remain a high risk in many areas; effective surveillance systems and infection control measures are inconsistent in some regions of Eastern Asia.

Infectious Diseases: A Geographic Guide, First Edition.
Edited by Eskild Petersen, Lin H. Chen & Patricia Schlagenhauf.
© 2011 John Wiley & Sons, Ltd. Published 2011 by John Wiley & Sons, Ltd.

Acute infections within 4 weeks of exposure

The geography of infectious diseases in Eastern Asia is diverse due to significant variations in climate (subtropical, temperate, and subarctic) as well as marked differences in environment, population density, and cultures. Socioeconomic changes have led to significant improvements in health care in Japan, South Korea, Taiwan, and China's major cities. Rural China and Mongolia continue to experience inequity in access to health care and public health measures, thus impacting the type and incidence of infectious diseases that occur in these areas.

In general, communicable diseases in Japan, South Korea, Taiwan, and urban China have decreased with a trend toward noncommunicable and chronic diseases [1]. A GeoSentinel study of travelers to China from 1998 to 2007 found that the most common infectious diseases were respiratory in nature and that respiratory illness was the primary syndrome requiring hospitalization during travel [2]. Diarrheal diseases were also found to be common.

Japan's health-care infrastructure is well developed yet still faces potential threats from emerging infections such as avian influenza, human immunodeficiency virus (HIV), and tuberculosis. Dietary preferences for raw or undercooked fish and seafood can lead to food-borne helminthiases such as anisakiasis, diphyllobothriasis, angiostrongyliasis, spiruroid larva migrans, and paragonimiasis. Three rickettsial diseases are endemic—Japanese spotted fever, scrub typhus, and Q fever [3]. Japanese encephalitis (JE) is also endemic but has a very low prevalence following preventive measures including pediatric vaccinations. Malaria has been controlled since 1961.

South Korea's medical system has also significantly improved with less communicable diseases reported. There is risk, however, for food- and water-borne outbreaks due to changes in dietary habits and increasing levels of travel. A significant number of vaccine-preventable illnesses occur (in 2007 more than 20,000 cases of chicken pox; increased measles cases 592% year on year; and 118% increase in mumps) [4]. Since 1986 vivax malaria has reemerged in the demilitarized zone and is currently limited to rural areas in northern Kyonggi and Kangwon provinces.

Taiwan has a well-developed health-care system with effective surveillance systems. It was the first country globally to initiate a hepatitis B vaccination program followed by a hepatitis A program with subsequent reduction in hepatitis cases and hepatocellular carcinoma [5]. Due to its subtropical climate and location, outbreaks of dengue fever as were reported in September 2010 by Taiwan CDC may occur. Respiratory infections including influenza, diarrheal diseases, food-borne helminthiases, and Japanese encephalitis also occur.

Data for infectious diseases in North Korea are limited; however, similar organisms endemic to South Korea and along the Chinese border are expected. Outbreaks of communicable diseases may be influenced by factors such as malnutrition and poverty. As with South Korea, vivax malaria reemerged in 1986 and is found in the southern part of the country and demilitarized zone.

Historically, Mongolia has a nomadic or seminomadic population with a close association with livestock. Recently, the rural population has been moving into the capital city, Ulaanbaatar. Respiratory and diarrheal diseases are common as is brucellosis [6]. Sexually transmitted infections (40.3%), viral hepatitis (23.7%), and tuberculosis (9.6%) are the most commonly reported infections [7]. Other important but less common diseases are echinococcosis, plague, tularemia, anthrax, and rabies [7].

China is the world's most populous country with over 1.3 billion persons. Recent socioeconomic changes have led to inequity in health care and a large migrant population of over 100 million persons. Migrants accounted for 37% of measles cases during the 2005 outbreak in all 31 provinces affecting 124,865 persons including 55 deaths [8].

Many different emerging disease threats exist for China such as human immunodeficiency virus/acquired immunodeficiency syndrome (HIV/AIDS), severe acute respiratory syndrome (SARS), and avian influenza. Since the SARS outbreak in 2003 (5,327 cases in China with 348 deaths), health-care infrastructure has improved in many regions; however, a wide range of infectious diseases such as viral hepatitis, typhoid fever, Japanese encephalitis, rabies, syphilis, neonatal tetanus, dengue fever, schistosomiasis, malaria, Crimean–Congo hemorrhagic fever, tick-borne encephalitis, clonorchiasis, and other food- and soil-borne helminthiases associated with poverty or lifestyle are found in different regions. China accounts for 90% of reported global hemorrhagic fever with renal syndrome cases [9] and 22% of the global burden of multidrug-resistant tuberculosis (MDR-TB) [10]. An outbreak of Chikungunya fever was reported in Dongguan city, Guangdong Province, in September 2010 with over 200 cases documented.

Vaccine-preventable infections such as hepatitis A and B, typhoid, rabies, measles, and influenza are common.

Japanese encephalitis is endemic and occurs in all areas except Qinghai province, Xinjiang, and Tibet. Major outbreaks occurred in 1966 (annual incidence >15/100,000) and in 1971 (174,932 cases and incidence of 20.92/100,000) [11]. A vaccination program has been in place since the 1980s; nonetheless, in 2008, there were 2,975 reported cases with 142 deaths in 25 provinces. High prevalence areas (JE incidence >1/100,000) include Shaanxi, Chongqing, Sichuan, Guizhou, Henan, and Yunnan. Although usually affecting mostly children under 15 years old, in the 2006 Yuncheng outbreak in Shanxi Province, 86% of patients were >30 years old with 28.8% fatality rate. Detection of Japanese encephalitis virus (JEV) genotype also changed from the more common genotype 3 to both genotypes 3 and 1 [11,12].

Malaria has decreased since the 1950s (30 million cases/year) to an annual incidence rate of 3.38/100,000 in 2008 (26,868 cases with 95% vivax) [13]. *Plasmodium falciparum* is only found in southern China in Yunnan and Hainan (considered an unstable malaria area along the Myanmar, Laos, and Vietnam borders with imported cases of drug-resistant falciparum malaria). *Plasmodium vivax* is the predominant species in China and is reemerging in central China where only vivax malaria is found.

The following tables outline many of the infectious diseases in Eastern Asia. It is important to keep in mind the changing nature of this region and the impact this may have on infectious disease patterns.

Central nervous system infections: encephalitis, meningitis, and other infections with neurological symptoms

Acute infections with less than 4 weeks of symptoms

Frequently found microorganisms	Less common microorganisms and diseases
Enteroviruses[a]	*Treponema pallidum*
Streptococcus pneumoniae	*Brucella* spp.[b]
Streptococcus agalactiae[c]	*Listeria monocytogenes*[d]
Haemophilus influenzae type b[e]	Rabies[f]
Neisseria meningitidis[g]	Influenza viruses
Japanese encephalitis virus[h]	Tick-borne encephalitis[i]
Herpes simplex I and II	*Angiostrongylus cantonensis*[j]
Mycobacterium tuberculosis	Cerebral malaria[k]

[a]Leading cause of aseptic meningitis. Outbreaks of acute encephalitis due to EV-71 in China and Taiwan.
[b]High incidence in Mongolia, sporadic cases in South Korea and Japan.
[c]Most common type of bacterial meningitis in neonates.
[d]Rare in Japan.
[e]Most common childhood meningitis in Mongolia [14].
[f]Japan and Taiwan considered rabies-free; 2,500 cases reported by China CDC in 2007.
[g]Rare in Japan, Taiwan.

[h]Highly endemic in China. Low annual incidence in Japan and South Korea but high reported prevalence of JEV-positive pigs. Not endemic in Mongolia.
[i]Northeast China, Japan (Hokkaido). First reported case in US traveler 2007 in Tianjin, China [15].
[j]Associated with ingestion of raw fish and snails in China, Taiwan, south Japan, and Korea. Outbreak in Beijing (2006).
[k]*P. falciparum* endemic in Yunnan and Hainan, China.

Central nervous system infections: meningitis and encephalitis with symptoms for more than 4 weeks and in the immunocompromised host

Microorganisms with symptoms for more than 4 weeks	Microorganisms in the immunocompromised host
HIV	*Nocardia*
M. tuberculosis	Polyomavirus
Cysticercus cellulosae	*Cryptococcus neoformans*
	JC virus
	Toxoplasma gondii

Ear, nose, and throat infections

Ear, nose, and throat infections with less than 4 weeks of symptoms

Frequently found microorganisms	Less common microorganisms and diseases
Enterovirus (rhinovirus, coxsackie virus, echovirus, EV-71)	Peritonsillar abscess
Adenovirus, coronavirus	Necrotizing fasciitis
Influenza A and B, parainfluenza	*M. tuberculosis*
Respiratory syncytial virus (RSV)	*Staphylococcus aureus*
Measles virus[a]	*Corynebacterium diphtheriae*
Rubella virus[b]	*Neisseria gonorrhoeae*
Epstein–Barr virus	*Chlamydia trachomatis*
Varicella zoster virus	*Legionella* spp.
H. influenzae type b[c]	Cytomegalovirus
Moraxella catarrhalis	HIV
Mycoplasma pneumoniae	
Chlamydophila	
Streptococcal spp.	
Herpes simplex I and II	

[a]Measles epidemics in Japan every 6–7 years since 1999 due to suboptimal vaccine coverage.
[b]Rubella not included in all regions of China's national vaccination program with epidemics every 6–8 years.
[c]More common in China, Mongolia, North Korea, and Japan due to lack of vaccination against *H. influenzae* type b.

Ear, nose, and throat infections with symptoms for more than 4 weeks and in the immunocompromised host

Microorganisms with symptoms for more than 4 weeks	Microorganisms in the immunocompromised host
M. tuberculosis Epstein–Barr virus Cytomegalovirus	*Candida* spp. *Aspergillus* spp. Herpes simplex I and II Cytomegalovirus Human herpes virus 8[a]

[a]Associated with Kaposi's sarcoma.

Cardiopulmonary infections

Pneumonia with symptoms for less than 4 weeks

Frequently found microorganisms	Less common microorganisms and diseases
S. pneumoniae *Klebsiella pneumoniae* *H. influenzae* *M. catarrhalis* *S. aureus* *M. pneumoniae* *Chlamydophila pneumoniae* Influenza virus, parainfluenza, RSV	*Legionella* spp. *Burkholderia pseudomallei*[a] *S. aureus* *Orientia tsutsugamushi*[b] (scrub typhus) *Leptospira interrogans*[c] *Paragonimus westermanii*[d] *Gnathostoma spinigerum*[e] *Bacillus anthracis* (anthrax) RSV *M. tuberculosis* *Yersinia pestis* (pneumonic plague)[f] Dengue hemorrhagic fever[g] Nontuberculous mycobacteria (*Mycobacterium kansasii*)[h] *M. tuberculosis* *Salmonella* spp.[i] *Acinetobacter baumannii*[a] SARS-corona virus *Coxiella* spp.[j]

[a]Southern China and Taiwan.
[b]Caused by bite of infected chigger mites in China, Korea, and Japan.
[c]Increased incidence in China; decreasing in Taiwan and Korea.
[d]Food-borne trematode, endemic in southern Japan, Korea, Taiwan, and central China.
[e]Japan, Korea, and China.
[f]Mongolia and China (Qinghai Province, Xinjiang, and Yunnan).
[g]Rare cases reported in south China [16].
[h]Korea.
[i]China.
[j]Less than 10 indigenous cases reported in Japan.

Endocarditis with less than 4 weeks of symptoms

Frequently found microorganisms	Less common microorganisms

S. aureus
Nonhemolytic streptococci
Coagulase-negative staphylococci
  (S. epidermidis)
S. pneumoniae
Enterococcus
	N. gonorrhoeae
	Bartonella quintana
	Coxiella burnetii
	
	Brucella
	Propionibacterium acnes
	Haemophilus species, Actinobacillus actinomycetemcomitans,
	  Cardiobacterium hominis, Eikenella corrodens,
	  and Kingella species (HACEK group)
	Pseudomonas aeruginosa
	Candida spp.

Pulmonary symptoms for more than 4 weeks and in the immunocompromised host

Microorganisms and diseases with symptoms for more than 4 weeks	Microorganisms and diseases in the immunocompromised host
S. pneumoniae M. catarrhalis (sinuses) H. influenzae S. aureus M. tuberculosis M. kansasii Mycobacterium avium complex P. aeruginosa Aspergillus spp. H. capsulatum[a] Cryptococcus spp.[b] Echinococcosis	Pneumocystis jirovecii Cytomegalovirus Deep mycoses (Candida, Cryptococcus, Mucormycosis, Aspergillus, Nocardia, Actinomycosis) Histoplasma capsulatum[a] M. tuberculosis Nontuberculous mycobacteria Rhodococcus equi P. aeruginosa Nocardia spp.

[a]Southeast China, Taiwan.
[b]71% of clinical strains in China (1985–2006) were from patients with no apparent risk factors [17].

Endocarditis for more than 4 weeks and in the immunocompromised host

The causative organisms can be any of those listed in the table for endocarditis with less than 4 weeks of symptoms. This may occur most commonly in cases of subacute endocarditis as progressive symptoms may develop over weeks to months.

Gastrointestinal infections

Gastrointestinal infections with less than 4 weeks of symptoms

Frequently found microorganisms and diseases	Less common microorganisms and diseases
Norovirus and calicivirus Rotavirus	Entamoeba histolytica Giardia lamblia[a]

Frequently found microorganisms and diseases	Less common microorganisms and diseases
Enterotoxigenic *Escherichia coli* (ETEC)[a] Shiga toxin-producing *E. coli* (STEC) *Shigella* spp.[c] *Salmonella*, nontyphi[d] *Vibrio parahaemolyticus* *Salmonella typhi* and *S. paratyphi*[f] *Campylobacter* *Bacillus cereus* toxin[i] *S. aureus* toxin *Ascaris lumbricoides* *Enterobius vermicularis*, other helminths Hookworm (*Ancylostoma duodenale, Necator americanus*) *Taenia solium*	Cryptosporidia spp. *Diphyllobothrium* spp.[b] *Anisakis* *M. tuberculosis* *Streptococcus suis*[e] *Vibrio cholerae*[g] *V. parahaemolyticus*[h] *Fasciolopsis* (giant intestinal fluke)[j] *Strongyloides stercoralis* *Taenia saginata*

[a]Rare in Japan.

[b]Cestode acquired by ingesting raw or undercooked fish, more common in Japan.

[c]*Shigella flexneri* is a common bacterial pathogen in Mongolia.

[d]Common in Mongolia during summer months.

[e]Outbreak in Sichuan, China (2005) with 215 reported cases.

[f]More common in China; infrequent in Mongolia, Japan.

[g]Endemic in China, Korea. Outbreak in Selenge Province, Mongolia, 1996.

[h]Sporadic cases, common source outbreaks in Japan.

[i]Commonly associated with improperly stored cooked rice.

[j]China and Taiwan.

Gastrointestinal infections with symptoms for more than 4 weeks and in the immunocompromised host

Microorganisms with symptoms for more than 4 weeks	Microorganisms in the immunocompromised host
A. lumbricoides *Trichuris trichiura* Hookworm spp. (*N. americanus* and *A. duodenale*)[a] *Helicobacter pylori*[b] *T. solium* and *T. saginata* *S. stercoralis* *M. tuberculosis* *Tropheryma whipplei* (Whipple's disease) *G. lamblia* *Fasciolopsis* (giant intestinal fluke)[c]	*Candida* spp. Herpes simplex I *Cryptosporidium parvum* and *Cryptosporidium hominis* Cytomegalovirus *M. tuberculosis* *Isospora belli* Microsporidia *E. histolytica* *S. stercoralis* *Cyclospora cayetanensis*[d]

[a]39 million reported cases in China in 2006; associated with poverty and tropical/subtropical climates.

[b]Decreased prevalence with improved socioeconomic conditions; associated with gastric carcinoma and peptic ulcer disease.

[c]China and Taiwan.

[d]Endemic in China; rare cases reported in Japan.

Infections of liver, spleen, and peritoneum

Acute infections of liver and biliary tract with less than 4 weeks of symptoms

Frequently found microorganisms	Less common microorganisms and diseases
Hepatitis A	Hepatitis D
Hepatitis B[a]	Hepatitis E
Hepatitis C	Amebic liver abscess
Epstein–Barr virus	Dengue virus[b]
Cytomegalovirus	*Leptospira*
Clonorchis sinensis[c]	Herpes simplex virus
Brucella[d]	Crimean–Congo hemorrhagic fever[e]

[a]High incidence in China and Mongolia; decreasing in Taiwan, Korea with vaccination programs.
[b]Southern China.
[c]Estimated 30 million persons infected worldwide, mostly in China; more than 2 million cases in Korea from 1974 to 1982; decreasing in Japan; associated with cholangiocarcinoma.
[d]1,000–1,500 cases reported per year in Mongolia.
[e]Xinjiang, China.

Chronic infections of the liver and biliary tract

Frequently found microorganisms	Less common microorganisms and diseases
Chronic hepatitis B or C	*Brucella*
Schistosoma japonicum[a]	*C. burnetii* (Q fever)
C. sinensis	*Echinococcus* spp.[b]
Toxocara canis and *Toxocara cati*	

[a]Common in Yangtze River basin; decreased by 90% in past 50 years; still endemic in 110 counties (up to 1% prevalence) [18].
[b]China Mongolia, and northern Japan.

Infections of liver and biliary tract in immunocompromised host

Similar microorganisms can be found in both immunocompetent and immunocompromised individuals.

Genitourinary infections

Cystitis, pyelonephritis, and nephritis with less than 4 weeks of symptoms

Frequently found microorganisms	Less common microorganisms and diseases
E. coli	Hantavirus (hemorrhagic fever with renal syndrome)[a]

Frequently found microorganisms	Less common microorganisms and diseases
K. pneumoniae	Enterococcus spp.
S. aureus	Ureaplasma
P. aeruginosa	Mycoplasma
	M. tuberculosis
	L. interrogans
	Adenovirus

[a]20,000–50,000 reported cases per year in China; 1,000 cases per year in South Korea; rare in Taiwan and Japan; not found in Mongolia.

Sexually transmitted infections with less than 4 weeks of symptoms

Frequently found microorganisms and diseases	Less common microorganisms
C. trachomatis	Haemophilus ducreyi
N. gonorrhoeae	Lymphogranuloma venereum
Primary syphilis[a]	E. histolytica
Mycoplasma spp.	Pediculosis pubis
Herpes simplex II	
Human papillomavirus	
Trichomonas vaginalis	
Molluscum contagiosum virus	

[a]Syphilis nearly eliminated in China (1950s); 10-fold increase in last decade with 278,215 reported cases and 9,480 reported cases congenital syphilis (2008). Most commonly reported communicable disease in Shanghai (2008) [19]; increasing in Mongolia (2008) [6].

Cystitis, pyelonephritis, and nephritis with symptoms for more than 4 weeks and in the immunocompromised host

Microorganisms with symptoms for more than 4 weeks	Microorganisms in the immunocompromised host
Proteus spp.	Candida spp.
Enterobacter spp.	M. tuberculosis
P. aeruginosa	Corynebacterium spp.
Mycoplasma spp.	
M. tuberculosis	

Sexually transmitted infections with symptoms for more than 4 weeks and in the immunocompromised host

Microorganisms with symptoms for more than 4 weeks	Microorganisms in the immunocompromised host
Human papillomavirus *T. pallidum* HIV[a]	Human papillomavirus Molluscum contagiosum virus HIV

[a]Low prevalence (820 HIV positive, 2009) in Mongolia but at increased risk due to changes in travel, lower age population, and increased sexually transmitted infections. Estimated 740,000 HIV positive in China (2009) with 70–80% in Yunnan, Guangxi, Henan, Sichuan, Xinjiang, and Guangdong; almost 9,000 HIV positive in Japan and 13,000 in South Korea 2008 (UNAIDS). Taiwan CDC reported 19,565 HIV cases from 1984 to September 2010. No report available for North Korea.

Joint, muscle, and soft tissue infections

Joint, muscle, and soft tissue infections with less than 4 weeks of symptoms

Frequently found microorganisms and diseases	Less common microorganisms and diseases
S. aureus *S. pneumoniae* *Streptococcus* spp. Hepatitis B Parvovirus B19 Rubella	Cysticercosis[a] *Trichinella spiralis* *N. gonorrhoeae* *H. influenzae* Human sarcocystis *Salmonella* spp. *Brucella* *Clostridium tetani*[b]

[a]China and Mongolia.
[b]More common in rural China, mostly neonatal tetanus.

Joint, muscle, and soft tissue infections with more than 4 weeks of symptoms and in the immunocompromised host

Microorganisms and diseases with symptoms for more than 4 weeks	Microorganisms in the immunocompromised host
Borreliosis (Lyme disease)[a] *M. tuberculosis* *Brucella*	*Candida* spp.

[a]Endemic in Japan, China, Taiwan, and Mongolia.

Skin infections

Skin infections with less than 4 weeks of symptoms

Frequently found microorganisms	Less common microorganisms and diseases

S. aureus
Group A streptococcus
Tinea spp.
 	
Scabies
Herpes viruses
Candida spp.
S. pneumoniae
	Cutaneous bacillus anthracis
	Borrelia spp.
	Spirillum minus and *Actinobacillus muris*
	   (rat-bite fever)[a]
	Cutaneous leishmaniasis[b]
	Mycobacterium ulcerans
	O. tsutsugamushi (scrub typhus)[c]
	Sparganum mansoni (sparganosis)[d]
	Cutaneous larva migrans[e]
	Rickettsia heilongjiangensis (Far Eastern
	   spotted fever)[f]
	Rickettsia japonica (Japanese spotted fever)[g]
	Rickettsia siberica (North Asian tick typhus)[h]
	Rickettsia typhi (murine typhus)

[a]Japan.
[b]Uygur Autonomous Region Xinjiang, China.
[c]Seasonal autumn outbreaks in north China, Korea; summer in south China; summer and autumn in Japan.
[d]Associated with ingestion of raw fish in Japan.
[e]Southern China.
[f]Northeast China and rarely Japan.
[g]135 reported cases in Japan (2008).
[h]North China and Mongolia.

Skin infections with more than 4 weeks of symptoms and in the immunocompromised host

Microorganisms and diseases with symptoms for more than 4 weeks	Microorganisms and diseases in the immunocompromised host
T. pallidum *M. tuberculosis* Human herpes virus 8 (Kaposi's sarcoma) *Mycobacterium leprae*[a] *Wuchereria bancrofti* (lymphatic filariasis)[b]	*Candida* spp. Human herpes virus 8 (Kaposi's sarcoma) Nontuberculous mycobacteria Deep fungal infections *M. tuberculosis*

[a]Approximately 10 cases reported per year in Japan.
[b]Lymphatic filariasis has recently been eliminated in China; South Korea close to elimination [1].

Adenopathy

Adenopathy for less than 4 weeks

Frequently found microorganisms and diseases	Less common microorganisms and diseases
Epstein–Barr virus Cytomegalovirus Parvovirus B19 HIV *T. gondii* Suppurative staphylococcal or streptococcal infections	*Francisella tularensis* (tularemia) *B. quintana* *Ehrlichia*[a] *Babesia*[b]

[a]China.
[b]Korea.

Adenopathy for more than 4 weeks and in the immunocompromised host

Microorganisms and diseases with symptoms for more than 4 weeks	Microorganisms and diseases in the immunocompromised host
T. gondii *M. tuberculosis* HIV	Adenovirus Cytomegalovirus Epstein–Barr virus HIV *M. tuberculosis* Nontuberculous mycobacteria Deep fungal infections

Fever without focal symptoms

Fever for less than 4 weeks without focal symptoms

Frequently found microorganisms and diseases	Less common microorganisms and diseases
Endocarditis Epstein–Barr virus Cytomegalovirus *T. gondii* HIV Parvovirus B19	*Brucella* *M. tuberculosis* Pyogenic abscess *C. burnetii* Dengue virus[a] *Plasmodium* spp.[b] *F. tularensis* *Babesia* *Ehrlichia* *O. tsutsugamushi* *R. japonica*[c] *S. typhi* and *S. paratyphi* A Bunya virus (Severe fever with thrombocytopenia syndome) [20]

[a]Southern China, Taiwan.
[b]Southern China, Korea.
[c]Western Japan, Korea.

Fever for more than 4 weeks without focal symptoms and in the immunocompromised host

Microorganisms with symptoms for more than 4 weeks	Microorganisms in the immunocompromised host
T. gondii	Cytomegalovirus
M. tuberculosis	Epstein–Barr virus
HIV	M. tuberculosis

Eosinophilia and elevated IgE

Eosinophilia and elevated IgE for less than 4 weeks

Frequently found microorganisms	Less common microorganisms
A. lumbricoides and A. suum	S. japonicum
Hookworm spp. (N. americanus and A. duodenale)	G. spinigerum[a]
T. solium and T. saginata	S. stercoralis
Toxocara spp.	A. cantonensis
T. trichiura	Anisakis
C. sinensis	Paragonimus spp.

[a]Korea, Japan, and China.

Eosinophilia and elevated IgE for more than 4 weeks and in the immunocompromised host

All of the organisms listed in the table "Eosinophilia and elevated IgE for less than 4 weeks" except for *A. cantonensis* may cause an eosinophilia with elevated IgE for more than 4 weeks. All organisms listed could cause this in an immunocompromised host.

Antibiotic resistance

Antimicrobial resistance is increasing with some variability between and within countries. As most regions worldwide, Methicillin-resistant *Staphylococcus aureus* (MRSA) is a significant public health problem with 60–80% resistant strains and up to 90% resistance reported for hospital-acquired infections (HAIs) in China [21]. A study of resistance patterns in 1999 and 2001 in China found 23–77% mean prevalence of resistance among HAI and 15–39% for community-acquired infections. Average growth rate of resistance was 22% in one study from 1994 to 2000 [21].

In a study of nosocomial infections in Chinese intensive care units (2003 and 2007), *E. coli* was the most common cause of urinary tract infections as well as a frequent cause of lower respiratory tract infections with 79.3% resistance to trimethoprim-sulfamethoxazole and 80% to ciprofloxacin [22]. All *S. aureus* were sensitive to vancomycin; *P. aeruginosa* isolates had 66.9% resistance to levofloxacin. China established the Guidelines for Surveillance and Prevention of Nosocomial Infections in 1994; however, uptake of these guidelines was inconsistent in many regions.

China's burden of disease due to tuberculosis is high. The first nationwide drug resistance survey confirmed 5.7% MDR-TB for new cases and 25.6% for previously treated cases with total estimates of 100,000 MDR-TB cases annually [10].

In Mongolia, antimicrobial resistance is also common. Some potential factors include frequent, routine usage of antibiotics for 3 days postsurgery; drug susceptibilities often not available; and antibiotics available without prescription and used inappropriately. Studies in *N. gonorrhoeae* isolates have found 48–50% resistance to penicillin; 15% resistance to tetracycline; and 25% resistance to ciprofloxacin [6].

In South Korea, the resistance rate to erythromycin was reported as 2% in 1994 but increased to 41.3% in 1998 and 51% in 2002 in throat group A streptococci isolates [23]. The KONSAR 2001 study found increasing prevalence of vancomycin-resistant *Enterococcus faecium*, expanded-spectrum cephalosporin-resistant *K. pneumoniae*, and imipenin-resistant *P. aeruginosa* [24].

Vaccine-preventable diseases in children

All countries in East Asia have pediatric vaccination programs; however, few programs include a vaccine against *H. influenzae* type b (unavailable in China, Japan, South Korea, or North Korea programs but available in Mongolia). Vaccines against *S. pneumoniae* are also generally unavailable. Japanese encephalitis vaccine is an important part of childhood immunizations in China, Japan, Taiwan, and South Korea and has greatly impacted on the incidence rate of this potentially fatal disease. Many Eastern Asian countries are hyperendemic for hepatitis B with the majority of transmission at birth. The hepatitis B vaccine series is included in the pediatric vaccination schedules in China, South Korea, North Korea, Taiwan, and Mongolia. Taiwan was the first country worldwide to offer routine hepatitis B vaccinations followed by the addition of hepatitis A vaccinations with a significant reduction in hepatitis B cases.

Varicella, human papillomavirus, influenza, and meningococcal vaccines also vary between country programs but are generally not included except for meningococcal A or meningococcal A and C in China and meningococcal ACWY in Mongolia. All countries give a dose of BCG following birth to reduce the risk of meningeal or miliary tuberculosis and all give at least one measles dose. Mumps vaccine is not offered in North Korea.

Despite the availability of these programs, there can be inconsistent uptake of vaccines in some populations (such as the "floating" or migrant population in China) leading to significant outbreaks of vaccine-preventable illnesses. Outbreaks of measles (2005 China; 2000, 2002, and 2007 Japan; 2007 South Korea) and mumps (2007 South Korea) have been recorded regularly. In addition, major outbreaks of influenza occur seasonally.

The World Health Organization has targeted 2012 for measles elimination in Eastern Asia. In order to accomplish this and also to decrease the burden of disease caused by vaccine-preventable illnesses, there is a significant need for strengthening of infectious diseases surveillance and better access to pediatric immunizations within many parts of this region.

Basic economic and demographic data

	GNI per capita (USD)	Life expectancy at birth (total, years)	School enrollment, primary (% net)
China	2,940	73	NA
Japan	38,210	83	99

	GNI per capita (USD)	Life expectancy at birth (total, years)	School enrollment, primary (% net)
Korea (North)	NA	67	NA
Korea (South)	21,530	79	98
Mongolia	1,680	67	89
Taiwan	NA	NA	NA

World Bank.

GNI, gross national income; NA, not available.

Causes of death in children under 5 years—regional average

	%
Neonatal causes	47
Pneumonia	14
Diarrheal diseases	12
Malaria	0
HIV/AIDS	0
Measles	1
Injuries	7
Others	18

WHO, 2000–2003 data.

Most common causes of death in all ages in Mongolia, China, and Japan

	%		
	Mongolia	China	Japan
Cerebrovascular diseases	13	18	14
Chronic obstructive lung diseases	NS	14	NS
Tuberculosis	5	3	NS
Lower respiratory infections	4	3	9
Diarrheal diseases	4	NS	NS
Perinatal conditions	5	3	NS
Ischemic and hypertensive heart diseases	9	8	10
Road traffic accidents	6	NS	NS
Self-inflicted injuries	NS	3	3
All cancers	12	13	21
Urogenital diseases	NS	NS	2

NS, not stated, i.e. not included in the 10 most common causes of death.

WHO, 2006.

References

1. World Health Organization. Western Pacific Region. Accessed September 1, 2010 at http://www.wpro.who.int/countries/countries.htm.
2. Davis X, MacDonald S, Borwein S, et al. Short report: Health risks in travelers to China: the GeoSentinel experience and implications for the 2008 Beijing Olympics. Am J Trop Med Hyg 2008;79(1):4–8.
3. Mahara F. Rickettsioses in Japan and the Far East. Ann N Y Acad Sci 2006;1078:60–73.
4. World Health Organization. Western Pacific Region. Accessed September 1, 2010 at http://www.wpro.who.int/countries/2009/kor/health_situation.htm.
5. Chien YC, Jan CF, Kuo HS, Chen CJ. Nationwide hepatitis B vaccination program in Taiwan: effectiveness in the 20 years after it was launched. Epidemiol Rev 2006;28(1):126–35.
6. Ebright JR, Altantsetseg T, Oyungerel R. Emerging infectious diseases in Mongolia. Emerg Infect Dis 2003;9(12):1509–15.
7. World Health Organization. Western Pacific Region. Accessed September 1, 2010 at http://www.wpro.who.int/countries/2009/mog/health_situation.htm.
8. Ji Y, Zhang Y, Songtao X, et al. Measles resurgence associated with continued circulation of genotype H1 viruses in China, 2005. Virol J 2009;6:135.
9. Arikawa J, Yoshimatsu K, Thang TU, Ninh TU. Hantavirus infection—typical rodent-borne viral zoonosis. Trop Med Health 2007;35:55–9.
10. WHO. Multidrug and Extensively-Drug Resistant TB (M/XDR-TB): 2010 Global Report on Surveillance and Response. Geneva: WHO, 2010.
11. Gao X, Nasci R, Liang G. The neglected arboviral infections in mainland China. PLoS Negl Trop Dis 2010;4(4):e624.
12. Wang LH, Fu SH, Wang HY, et al. Japanese encephalitis outbreak, Yuncheng, China, 2006. Emerg Infect Dis 2007;13(7):1123–5.
13. Guan Y. National Institute of Parasitic Diseases, China CDC. Available from http://www.actmalaria.net/downloads/pdf/info/2009/China.pdf.
14. Mendsaikhan J, Watt JP, Mansoor O, et al. Childhood bacterial meningitis in Ulaanbaatar, Mongolia, 2002–2004. Clin Infect Dis 2009:1 (48, Suppl. 2):141–6.
15. Tick-Borne Encephalitis among U.S. Travelers to Europe and Asia 2000–2009. MMWR. Case 4. Accessed August 5, 2010 at http://www.cdc.gov/mmwr/preview/mmwrhtml/mm5911a3.htm.
16. Tsang K, File T. Respiratory infections unique to Asia. Respirology 2008;13(7):937–49.
17. Chen J, Varma A, Diaz M, Litvintseva A, Wollenberg K, Kwon-Chung K. *Cryptococcus neoformans* strains and infection in apparently immunocompetent patients, China. Emerg Infect Dis 2008;14(5):755–62.
18. Zhou XN, Guo JG, Wu XH, et al. Epidemiology of schistosomiasis in the People's Republic of China, 2004. Emerg Infect Dis 2007;13(10):1470–6.
19. Tucker J, Chen XS, Peeling R. Syphilis and social upheaval in China. N Engl J Med 2010;362:1658–61.
20. Yu XJ, Liang MF, Zhang SY, et al. Fever with thrombocytopenia associated with a novel Bunyairus in China. N Engl J Med 2011 (in press).
21. Zhang R, Eggleston K, Rotimi V, Zeckhauser R. Antibiotic resistance as a global threat: evidence from China, Kuwait and the United States. Global Health 2006;2:6.
22. Ding JG, Sun QF, Li KC, et al. Retrospective analysis of nosocomial infections in the intensive care unit of a tertiary hospital in China during 2003 and 2007. BMC Infect Dis 2009;9:115.
23. Kim S, Lee NY. Epidemiology and antibiotic resistance of group A streptococci isolated from healthy schoolchildren in Korea. J Antimicrob Chemother 2004;54(2):447–50.
24. Lee K, Jang SJ, Lee HJ, et al. Increasing prevalence of vancomycin-resistant *Enterococcus faecium*, expanded-spectrum cephalosporin-resistant *Klebsiella pneumoniae*, and imipenem-resistant *Pseudomonas aeruginosa* in Korea: KONSAR Study in 2001. J Korean Med Sci 2004;19:8–14.

Chapter 12
South Central Asia

Prativa Pandey,[1] Holly Murphy[1,2] and Ashish Bhalla[3]
[1]CIWEC Clinic Travel Medicine Center, Kathmandu, Nepal
[2]Patan Academy of Health Sciences, Kathmandu, Nepal
[3]Post Graduate Institute of Medical Education and Research, Chandigarh, India

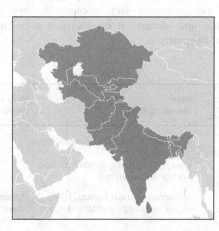

Afghanistan
Bangladesh
Bhutan
India
Kazakhstan
Kyrgyzstan
Nepal
Pakistan
Sri Lanka
Tajikistan
Turkmenistan
Uzbekistan

The South Central Asian region varies vastly in geography (from sea level to Mt. Everest), climate, language, and culture. All of these are developing countries with gross national income (GNI) varying from USD 400 (Nepal) to 6,140 (Kazakhstan) per capita. Life expectancy is as low as 44 years in Afghanistan to 72 in Sri Lanka. Infectious diseases account for significant mortality and morbidity in this region.

Infectious Diseases: A Geographic Guide, First Edition.
Edited by Eskild Petersen, Lin H. Chen & Patricia Schlagenhauf.
© 2011 John Wiley & Sons, Ltd. Published 2011 by John Wiley & Sons, Ltd.

Acute infections within 4 weeks of exposure

CNS infections: meningitis and encephalitis

Acute infections with symptoms for less than 2 weeks Among CNS infections, acute bacterial meningitis is most common, followed by Japanese encephalitis and other viral encephalitis [1]. In patients with bacterial meningitis *Streptococcus pneumoniae*, beta-hemolytic streptococci and *Staphylococcus aureus* are common among adults. *S. pneumoniae*, *Escherichia coli*, *Klebsiella pneumoniae*, *Pseudomonas* species, and *S. aureus* are common in the pediatric age group. *Haemophilus influenzae* remains a concern in Bangladesh and Nepal [1].

Japanese encephalitis is the most common viral encephalitis seen among adults in India though herpes simplex virus and adenovirus are also common. Encephalitis due to Chikungunya and influenza occur in epidemics.

Frequently found microorganisms	Rare microorganisms	Very rare microorganisms
Meningitis: *S. pneumoniae*, *H. influenzae*, *Neisseria meningitidis*, group B streptococcus, *Listeria monocytogenes*	*E. coli*, *Klebsiella*, and *Pseudomonas aeruginosa* coxsackie viruses, echovirus, and other enterovirus	
Encephalitis: Japanese encephalitis, herpes simplex virus, adenovirus, rabies virus, malaria	Influenza, parainfluenza, HIV, Chikungunya, measles, dengue	Poliomyelitis, *Naegleria fowleri*, anthrax, *Angiostrongyliasis*
Focal lesions: Streptococcal spp. (viridans), *S. aureus*, anaerobes (*Bacteroides*), oral anaerobes, tuberculosis (TB), neurocysticercosis (*Taenia solium*)	Leptospirosis Brucellosis Rickettsiosis: *Orientia tsutsugamushi*, *Rickettsia conorii*	Nocardiosis Blastomycosis

CNS infections: meningitis and encephalitis with symptoms for more than 2 weeks and in the immunocompromised host The leading cause of chronic CNS infections in the region is TB among immunocompetent and immunocompromised hosts. All other etiologies are significantly less common.

Microorganisms with symptoms for more than 2 weeks	Microorganisms in the immunocompromised host
TB Neurocysticercosis (*T. solium*) Nocardiosis	TB, nocardiosis, syphilis Toxoplasmosis Fungus (*Aspergillus*, *Cryptococcus neoformans*, zygomycetes, histoplasmosis) JC virus, CMV

Ear, nose, and throat infections

Ear, nose, and throat infections with symptoms for less than 4 weeks

Acute ear, nose, throat, and sinus infections in adults and children are mostly due to viruses. Predominant bacterial pathogens include streptococci, *H. influenzae*, and *Moraxella catarrhalis* [2]. Outbreaks of *Corynebacterium diphtheriae* have occurred in India associated with high mortality [3].

Frequently found microorganisms	Rare microorganisms and conditions	Very rare microorganisms
Streptococcus pyogenes or group A streptococci *Neisseria gonorrhoeae*	*Arcanobacterium haemolyticum*, group C and G streptococci	Diphtheria
H. influenzae, M. catarrhalis, Chlamydia pneumoniae	Actinomyces, fusariosis	Retropharyngeal abscess[a]
EBV, CMV, adenovirus, coxsackie	Peritonsillar abscess[a]—group A strep, *S. aureus*, mixed anaerobic or gram-negative bacteria [4]	Tularemia
	Parotitis (mumps), Ludwig's angina, HSV	Filariasis

[a]Require acute ear, nose, and throat evaluation.

Ear, nose, and throat infections with symptoms for more than 4 weeks and in the immunocompromised host

Chronic infections are common in the region due to lack of proper hygiene, education, and access to medical care. Organisms isolated in chronic suppurative otitis media (CSOM) are mostly *P. aeruginosa, S. aureus, Proteus* sp., and *Aspergillus* [5]. Chronic sinusitis in the immunocompromised patient is commonly due to mixed bacterial flora or fungal infections, especially *Aspergillus*. Tuberculosis often presents as cervical adenopathy and rarely as TB of the larynx, ear, oropharynx, or retropharyngeal abscess [6].

Microorganisms with symptoms for more than 4 weeks	Microorganisms in the immunocompromised host
CSOM—*P. aeruginosa, S. aureus, Proteus*, anaerobes	*Candida* sp., aspergillosis, rhinosporidiosis, and mucormycosis
TB of the nose, sinus, ear, or retropharyngeal abscess (rare)	TB
Sinusitis—mixed bacterial flora	Sinusitis—mixed bacterial or fungal: aspergillosis, *Rhizopus arrhizus* (rare)
Nose: TB, leprosy, blastomycosis (rare)	Syphilis

Cardiopulmonary infections

Pneumonia with symptoms for less than 4 weeks

Common causes of acute pneumonia include *S. pneumoniae, S. aureus*, influenza A, B, H1N1, and respiratory syncytial virus (RSV). Although rare, outbreaks of plague caused by *Yersinia pestis* are being reported from this region. *Pseudomonas* and *Acinetobacter* are emerging as important causes for hospital-acquired infections.

Frequently found microorganisms	Rare microorganisms and conditions	Very rare microorganisms
S. pneumoniae Hospital-acquired (*P. aeruginosa, Acinetobacter* sp., *Legionella*) *S. aureus* *K. pneumoniae, E. coli* *Mycoplasma pneumoniae, H. influenzae, Moraxella* sp. Influenza A, B, and H1N1, parainfluenza, RSV	Group A, C, and G streptococcus *Burkholderia pseudomallei*	Diphtheria *S. pyogenes* *Y. pestis*

Endocarditis/myocarditis with symptoms for less than 4 weeks

The most common predisposing condition for endocarditis in the Indian subcontinent is rheumatic heart disease, and *Streptococcus viridans* is the most common organism isolated [7]. Congenital heart disease is a common predisposing condition among children. The rate of culture-negative endocarditis in resource-poor areas of the region is significantly higher than among more developed countries—at 48% in Pakistan [8] and up to 72% in India [9].

Frequently found microorganisms	Rare microorganisms and conditions	Very rare microorganisms
S. pyogenes (myocarditis/rheumatic heart disease) *S. viridans* and other species	*Candida albicans*	*Salmonella typhi, Salmonella paratyphi*
Group C and G streptococci	Gram-negative bacilli—HACEK group	Brucellosis
Coagulase-negative staphylococci	*N. gonorrhoeae*	Fungal: aspergillosis, zygomycetes, *Candida* sp., *Pseudallescheria boydii*
S. aureus (including MRSA)	*Coxiella burnetii, Bartonella quintana*	*Bartonella henselae*
Gram-negative (*E. coli, Klebsiella, Enterobacter*), *Enterococcus faecalis*	*Propionibacterium*	*Chryseobacterium meningosepticum*
Viral	Leptospirosis (myocarditis)	

Pulmonary symptoms for more than 4 weeks and in the immunocompromised host

Mycobacterium tuberculosis and fungal infections are important causes of nonresolving pneumonias and pneumonia in immunocompromised individuals.

Microorganisms and diseases with symptoms for more than 4 weeks	Microorganisms in the immunocompromised host
TB Aspergillosis Histoplasmosis	*S. pneumoniae* *Pneumocystis jarovecii*, *Nocardia* CMV, VZV Aspergillosis, histoplasmosis, cryptococcosis, blastomycosis (rare), melioidosis

Consider noninfectious causes like lung cancer, autoimmune lung fibrosis, Wegener's granulomatosis.

Endocarditis for more than 4 weeks and in the immunocompromised host

Microorganisms and diseases with symptoms for more than 4 weeks	Microorganisms in the immunocompromised host
Coagulase-negative staphylococci Nonhemolytic streptococci	Aspergillosis, *Candida* spp.

Consider noninfectious causes like sarcoidosis.

Gastrointestinal infections

Acute diarrhea is most often associated with bacterial infections and to a smaller extent with viruses and parasites. Viral pathogens are increasingly being recognized in acute childhood diarrhea by improved molecular techniques [10]. Outbreaks of cholera tend to occur during rainy season and in natural disasters like flooding [11]. Repeated negative bacterial cultures and microscopy for parasites should lead to the consideration that the symptoms may not be caused by an infection.

Gastrointestinal infections with symptoms for less than 4 weeks

Frequently found microorganisms	Rare microorganisms and conditions	Very rare microorganisms
Acute diarrhea—Enterotoxigenic *E. coli*, *Campylobacter*, *Shigella*, *Salmonella* (nontyphi)	*Entamoeba histolytica*	*Yersinia enterocolitica*, *Aeromonas*
S. aureus toxin causing food poisoning	*Vibrio cholerae*—common pathogen during rainy season and flooding	
Acute parasitic diarrhea—*Giardia intestinalis*, *Cyclospora cayetanensis*	*Cryptosporidium* spp., *Dientamoeba fragilis*	
	Tuberculosis	*Strongyloides stercoralis*
Rotavirus, noroviruses *Helicobacter pylori*		Whipple's disease

Gastrointestinal infections with symptoms for more than 4 weeks and in the immunocompromised host

The burden of chronic gastrointestinal infection is very heavy in the South Central Asia region. Symptoms range from chronic diarrhea to severe malnutrition in children. Chronic diarrhea is mostly parasitic in nature, most common of which is *Giardia*. Chronic diarrhea in immunocompromised persons is often due to coccidian parasites [12] and rarely due to *S. stercoralis* [13]. Tuberculosis remains an important pathogen in normal and in immunocompromised hosts.

Microorganisms with symptoms for more than 4 weeks	Microorganisms in the immunocompromised host
Protozoa: *Giardia, Cyclospora, E. histolytica, D. fragilis, Leishmania* spp. (visceral) Nematodes: *Ancylostoma duodenale, Ascaris lumbricoides, Enterobius vermicularis, Trichuris trichiura, S. stercoralis* Cestodes: *Diphyllobothrium latum, Taenia saginata, T. solium, Hymenolepis nana, Echinococcus granulosus* (hydatid cyst in liver) TB	*Isospora belli, Microsporidia, Cryptosporidium, Cyclospora S. stercoralis* TB

Infections of liver, spleen, and peritoneum

Acute infections of liver, spleen, and peritoneum with symptoms for less than 4 weeks

Enterically transmitted hepatitis A and E are important infections in this region with hepatitis E having high mortality in pregnant women [14].

Frequently found microorganisms	Rare microorganisms and conditions	Very rare microorganisms
Acute hepatitis—hepatitis A, B, D, and E Infectious mononucleosis (EBV, CMV)	*Fasciola hepatica*	*Clonorchis sinensis, Opisthorchis* spp., Crimean Congo hemorrhagic fever
Abscess/focal lesion—*E. histolytica*, pyogenic abscess, echinococcosis, TB *S. typhi* and *S. paratyphi* Leptospirosis Rickettsiosis Leishmaniasis (visceral)	Melioidosis	Histoplasmosis
Peritonitis—*E. coli, Klebsiella, Proteus, Pseudomonas* *S. aureus* *E. faecalis*, TB	*Aeromonas hydrophila*	*Cryptococcus*
Anaerobes—*Bacteroides, Peptostreptococcus,* mixed flora common	Fungal peritonitis—*Candida* spp. (peritoneal dialysis patients)	

Chronic infections of liver, spleen, and peritoneum with symptoms for more than 4 weeks

Frequently found microorganisms	Rare microorganisms and conditions	Very rare microorganisms
Hepatitis B and C Tuberculosis Leishmaniasis (visceral) Brucellosis	Melioidosis Ascariasis	

Infections of liver, spleen, and peritoneum in the immunocompromised host

Infections in the immunocompromised host are similar to the ones in the immunocompetent host.

Genitourinary infections

Cystitis, pyelonephritis, and nephritis with symptoms for less than 4 weeks

Frequently found microorganisms	Rare microorganisms and conditions	Very rare microorganisms
E. coli, S. aureus, K. pneumoniae, Proteus S. saprophyticus	Pseudomonas aeruginosa	Candida Perirenal abscess

Sexually transmitted infections with symptoms for less than 4 weeks

Frequently found microorganisms	Rare microorganisms and conditions
HSV-2, *Chlamydia trachomatis,* *Trichomonas vaginalis, N. gonorrhoeae*	*Lymphogranuloma venereum,* syphilis

Cystitis, pyelonephritis, and nephritis with symptoms for more than 4 weeks and in the immunocompromised host

Microorganisms with symptoms for more than 4 weeks	Microorganisms in the immunocompromised host

Chronic UTI with same organism
  as acute infection
TB
Candida albicans
	E. coli, S. aureus, Enterococcus, Pseudomonas,
	  K. pneumoniae
	Candida albicans, mucormycosis
	TB

Consider noninfectious causes especially malignancies like renal cell carcinoma.

Sexually transmitted infections with symptoms for more than 4 weeks and in the immunocompromised host

Microorganisms with symptoms for more than 4 weeks	Microorganisms in the immunocompromised host
Syphilis	HSV-2, syphilis [15], HIV
HIV	*Trichomonas vaginalis*

Joint, muscle, and soft tissue infections

Joint, muscle, and soft tissue infections with symptoms for less than 4 weeks

The most comment etiology of skin and soft tissue infections (SSTI), muscle and joint infections are *S. aureus* (including MRSA) and *S. pyogenes*, respectively. *Acinetobacter baumannii* is emerging as a cause of necrotizing SSSI in war-torn areas. *A. baumannii* infections usually occur among hosts with underlying comorbidities (e.g., trauma, cirrhosis); are often bacteremic, multidrug resistance (MDR), and associated with substantial mortality [16].

Frequently found microorganisms	Rare microorganisms and conditions	Very rare microorganisms and conditions
S. aureus	Necrotizing fasciitis	Fournier's gangrene (perineum and urogenital; polymicrobial)
Group A beta-hemolytic streptococcus	*A. baumannii*	*Aspergillus fumigatus*
E. coli	Group B, C, and G beta-hemolytic streptococci	*Clostridium perfringens, Clostridium tetani*
N. gonorrhoeae	*Burkholderia pseudomallei*	*Sporotrichum schenckii*

Joint, muscle, and soft tissue infections with symptoms for more than 4 weeks and in the immunocompromised host

Tuberculosis remains a common cause of chronic joint infections in the region. A resurgence of Chikungunya fever occurred in India, affecting at least 1.3 million cases in India alone. Symptomatology includes sudden onset of fever with arthralgia followed by often debilitating and prolonged arthralgia.

Microorganisms with symptoms for more than 4 weeks	Microorganisms in the immunocompromised host
TB	*Candida* sp.
Chikungunya virus	*S. typhi*
Borreliosis (Lyme disease)	Ecthyma gangrenosum (*Pseudomonas aeruginosa*)
Brucella melitensis	Actinomycotic mycetoma (*Actinomadura* spp., *Streptomyces* spp., and *Nocardia* spp.); eumycetoma

Skin infection

Skin infection is an important cause of morbidity in the region, especially so in children.

Amongst skin infections lasting >4 weeks, tuberculosis, leprosy, and dermal leishmaniasis are common infections in the region. Since treatment for these conditions is prolonged and toxic, it is imperative to establish a definitive diagnosis before embarking on therapy.

Skin infections with symptoms for less than 4 weeks

Frequently found microorganisms	Rare microorganisms and conditions	Very rare microorganisms and conditions
S. aureus, S. pyogenes	Pityriasis alba, tinea (*Trichophyton violaceum*, *Trichophyton mentagrophytes*, *Microsporum canis*)	Rickettsial species
Infestations (scabies, lice)		*Leishmania donovani* [17]

Skin infections with symptoms for more than 4 weeks and in the immunocompromised host

Microorganisms with symptoms for more than 4 weeks	Microorganisms in the immunocompromised host
TB (lupus vulgaris, scrofuloderma, and tuberculosis verrucosa cutis) [18]	Candidiasis
Leprosy, cutaneous leishmaniasis [17]	*Herpes simplex*, dermatophytosis of the skin, *Molluscum contagiosum*, genital warts, scabies

Adenopathy

Adenopathy of less than 4 weeks' duration

Most acute onset adenopathy is generally benign and often caused by tonsillopharyngitis and suppurative infections of ear, nose, throat, and skin, infectious mononucleosis or infestations, including head lice. HIV can cause lymphadenopathy of <4 weeks of duration.

Common	Rare	Very rare
Tonsillopharyngitis and suppurative infections (oral streptococci, *S. pyogenes*)	*Bartonella*	*S. stercoralis*
Infectious mononucleosis (EBV, CMV) and HIV	Kawasaki disease	*Yersinia pestis*
Reactive lymphadenitis	Rubella	Tularemia
	Lymphatic filariasis	

Adenopathy of more than 4 weeks' duration and in the immunocompromised host

Mycobacterial infections are the most common cause for chronic adenopathy in normal and in immunocompromised hosts.

Common microorganisms with symptoms for more than 4 weeks	Rare microorganisms with symptoms for more than 4 weeks	Microorganisms in the immunocompromised host
Mycobacteria (TB and other)	*Nocardia, Actinomyces* Brucellosis Rosai–Dorfman disease[a]	TB, suppurative lymphadenitis Reactive lymphadenopathy HIV, EBV, CMV *Cryptococcus*, histoplasmosis

[a]Sinus histiocytosis with lymphadenopathy. A rare, benign disorder of unknown etiology characterized by the overproduction of histiocytes, which accumulate in lymph nodes.

Fever without focal symptoms

Fever for less than 4 weeks without focal symptoms

Febrile illness without localizing symptoms in the region is most commonly salmonellosis and malaria in endemic areas. Other, less common infectious etiology include dengue, rickettsiosis, and leptospirosis. Acute infections occur as outbreaks during monsoon season. After 4 weeks of symptoms and in the immunocompromised host, tuberculosis is the single most common etiology.

Frequently found conditions	Rare microorganisms and conditions	Very rare microorganism
Salmonellosis	*Coxiella burnetii*	
Dengue	Tularemia	Hantaviruses
Rickettsiosis (*R. typhi, Orientia tsutsugamushi*)	Ehrlichia	Crimean Congo hemorrhagic virus
M. pneumoniae	Plague	West Nile virus
Leptospirosis	Babesiosis	Kyasanur forest virus
Malaria (*M. falciparum, M. vivax, M. malariae*)	*Rickettsia conorii*	Bagaza virus
Bacterial endocarditis	Parvovirus B19	Chandipura virus
Abdominal abscess (pyogenic/amebic)		
Viral hepatitis (hepatitis A, B, E)		
Infectious mononucleosis (EBV, CMV)		
Japanese encephalitis		
HIV		

Fever for more than 4 weeks without focal symptoms and in the immunocompromised host

Microorganisms with symptoms for more than 4 weeks	Microorganisms in the immunocompromised host
Tuberculosis	Tuberculosis
Toxoplasmosis	CMV
Brucellosis	Adenovirus
	Histoplasmosis, cryptococcosis, aspergillosis

Eosinophilia and elevated IgE

Eosinophilia in the region is most commonly infectious, especially due to helminths and filaria. The most common cause of eosinophilia with lung infiltrates is tropical pulmonary eosinophilia associated with filarial species; *Strongyloides* and *Ascaris* also cause similar syndromes. Eosinophilia with gastrointestinal symptoms is commonly due to helminthic infections. Eosinophilia is a less common presentation of the common infections tuberculosis and HIV. Flukes, protozoa, and fungi constitute rare causes. These organisms are likely to cause chronic symptoms if untreated.

Eosinophilia and elevated IgE for less than 4 weeks

Frequently found microorganisms	Rare microorganisms and conditions	Very rare microorganisms and conditions
Intestinal nematodes (*Ascaris lumbricoides* and *Ascaris suum*), hookworm (*Necator* sp.)	Nematodes (*Toxocara* spp., *Trichinella spiralis*, *Angiostrongyliasis cantonensis*, and *costaricensis*)	*Gnathostoma spinigerum* (eosinophilic meningitis)
Tissue nematodes (*Wuchereria bancrofti, Brugia malayi* (lymphatic filariasis and tropical pulmonary eosinophilia))	HIV	Phaeohyphomycosis
Cestodes (*Echinococcus,* cysticercosis (*Taenia* spp.), *Paragonimus westermani*)	Aspergillosis (allergic bronchopulmonary aspergillosis)	*Diphyllobothrium latum*
	Trematodes (*S. haematobium* and *S. mansoni*)	Trematodes (*Fasciolopsis buski, C. sinensis, Opisthorchis* spp., *F. hepatica*)

Noninfectious etiologies include Kimura's disease, allergy, vasculitis, and malignancy.

Eosinophilia and elevated IgE for more than 4 weeks and in the immunocompromised host

Microorganisms with symptoms for more than 4 weeks	Microorganisms in the immunocompromised host
S. stercoralis, A. lumbricoides, A. suum, Toxocara spp. (visceral larva migrans)	Toxocara spp.
	Protozoa (D. fragilis, Isospora belli, Cryptosporidium parvum, Sarcocystis) S. stercoralis Cryptococcus neoformans, P. jaroveci (rarely)
Tuberculosis	Tuberculosis

Antibiotic resistance

A potentially major global problem is the emergence in the Indian subcontinent of gram-negative Enterobacteriaceae with resistance to carbapenems conferred by the New Delhi metallo-β-lactamase 1 (NDM-1). These carbapenemases are highly resistant to many antibiotic classes leaving negligible options for treatment. In India, Pakistan, and Bangladesh, NDM-1 isolates were primarily *K. pneumoniae* and *E. coli*, were clonal—suggesting the potential for outbreaks, and were community-acquired [19]. Spread of NDM-1-positive isolates in the United Kingdom and Europe is epidemiologically linked to the region. Selection pressure for the NDM-1 isolates is likely due to the widespread nonprescription access to antibiotic medicines in the region.

Methicillin-resistant *S. aureus* is a growing concern in the Indian subcontinent and in war-torn areas of Afghanistan and Pakistan where MRSA and MDR *A. baumannii* infections are emerging problems. In a Pakistan-based study of patients with ventilator-associated pneumonia, 76% of isolates were *Acinetobacter* species and 43% were *P. aeruginosa*. All *Acinetobacter* and 72% *P. aeruginosa* were MDR [20].

Multi-drug resistance (MDR) and nalidixic-acid resistance (NAR) in *S. typhi* and *S. paratyphi* A have been problematic in the region with high-level ciprofloxacin resistance by the mid-2000s. Nearly 100% NAR among *Salmonella* and extended spectrum beta-lactamase producing *S. paratyphi* A have been reported from Nepal. Resistance to alternate regimens, including azithromycin and ceftriaxone, is a concern.

Antimicrobial resistance in *S. pneumoniae* varies widely in the region. Sri Lanka reports 90% of invasive pediatric isolates nonsusceptible to penicillin (PCN) and 50% nonsusceptible to third-generation cephalosporins [21]. Rates of PCN-resistance in India, Nepal, and Bangladesh are lower at 14% [22], 8% [23], and 7% [24], respectively. Co-trimoxazole resistance is 72% for Nepal, 63% for Sri Lanka [23], and exceeding 70% in Bangladesh [24]. Serotype coverage by the seven-valent pneumococcal conjugate vaccine (PCV7) varies from 30% in India, 45% in Nepal to 61% in Sri Lanka. Efforts underway to introduce PCV7 where relevant may attenuate the spread of resistance.

Vaccine-preventable diseases in children

Vaccine preventable diseases in children account for a significant number of childhood illnesses and deaths in the region. India alone had 48,000 cases of measles reported in 2008. India, Nepal,

Bangladesh, Afghanistan, Pakistan are among the 47 priority countries with high measles burden [25]. India, Pakistan, and Afghanistan are 3 of the 4 polio-endemic countries in the world where indigenous wild poliovirus transmission has never been interrupted. Spread of the virus to Tajikistan has led to a polio outbreak in 2010. Supplementary immunization and enhanced surveillance activities are being carried out in these countries. Diphtheria epidemic occurred from 1993 to 1996 in Uzbekistan, Tajikistan, Kazakhstan, and Kyrgyzstan, but strong control measures stopped this epidemic in 1996 whereas diphtheria continues to be reported in outbreaks from India. Most of the countries in the region are endemic for typhoid and hepatitis A with outbreaks occurring from time to time.

Childhood vaccination program reported by UNICEF for 2008 cites >95% coverage for Sri Lanka, Kazakhstan, Turkmenistan, Kyrgyzstan, Uzbekistan, and Bhutan for BCG, DPT ×3, polio ×3, measles ×1, and hepatitis B×3. Immunization uptake in Bangladesh is >95% for all these vaccines except for measles. Rates are lowest for India and Pakistan. Nepal, Afghanistan, and Tajikistan have rates >80%. *H. influenzae* b (Hib), pneumococcal conjugate (PCV7), hepatitis A, typhoid, and varicella vaccines are not offered in the national childhood immunization program of these countries, whereas mumps is offered in Uzbekistan, Kazakhstan, and Kyrgyzstan, and rubella in Sri Lanka. Second-dose measles, Hib, and PCV7 are being considered by countries in the region to be added in their national immunization programs. Japanese encephalitis (JE) vaccine was given to children in the endemic areas of Nepal in 2009 but this effort is not ongoing.

The following tables provide basic demographic and economic indicators as well as health-related information which list causes of deaths in all ages and in children under 5 years. This information coupled with information in the chapter should be valuable for medical practitioners and policy makers in caring for patients and in designing public health policy for the region. Many of the infections listed in this region can be prevented by strong yet simple public health measures.

Basic economic and demographic data

	GNI[a] per capita (USD)	Life expectancy at birth (total, years)	School enrollment, primary (% net)
Afghanistan	NA	44	NA
Bangladesh	520	66	87
Bhutan	1,900	66	87
India	1,070	65	89
Iran	3,540	71	94
Kazakhstan	6,140	66	90
Kyrgyzstan	740	68	85
Nepal	400	64	80
Pakistan	980	65	66
Sri Lanka	1,780	72	97
Tajikistan	600	67	98
Turkmenistan	2,840	63	NA
Uzbekistan	910	67	91

World Bank.
NA, not available.
[a]Gross national income.

Causes of death in children under 5 years—regional average

	%
Neonatal causes	44
Pneumonia	18
Diarrheal diseases	20
Malaria	1
HIV/AIDS	1
Measles	3
Injuries	2
Others	10

WHO, 2000–2003 data.

Most common causes of deaths in all ages in Nepal, India, and Kazakhstan (%)

	Nepal	India	Kazakhstan
Ischemic and hypertensive heart disease	13	15	28
Cerebrovascular disease	5	7	15
Chronic obstructive lung disease	3	5	3
Tuberculosis	3	4	3
Lower respiratory infections	10	11	2
Diarrheal diseases	7	4	NS
Perinatal conditions	10	7	NS
Measles	3	NS	NS
HIV/AIDS	NS	3	NS
Poisoning	NS	NS	5
Road traffic accidents	2	2	NS
Self-inflicted injuries	NS	2	3
All cancers	NS	NS	2
Cirrhosis of the liver	NS	NS	2

WHO, 2006.
NS, not stated, i.e., not included in the most common causes of death.

References

1. Singh RR, Chaudhary SK, Bhatta NK, Khanal B, Shah D. Clinical and etiological profile of acute febrile encephalopathy in Eastern Nepal. Indian J Pediatr 2009;76(11):1109–11.
2. Shamansurova EA. [The role of *Haemophilus influenzae* in pyoinflammatory diseases of the ear and paranasal sinuses]. Vestn Otorinolaringol 2006;3:11–12.
3. Jacob JT. Resurgence of diphtheria in India in the 21st century. Indian J Med Res 2008; 128(5):669–70.
4. Megalamani SB, Suria G, Manickam U, Balasubramanian D, Jothimahalingam S. Changing trends in bacteriology of peritonsillar abscess. J Laryngol Otol 2008;122(9):928–30.

5. Sharma S, Rehan HS, Goyal A, Jha AK, Upadhyaya S, Mishra SC. Bacteriological profile in chronic suppurative otitis media in Eastern Nepal. Trop Doct 2004;34(2):102–4.

6. Nalini B, Vinayak S. Tuberculosis in ear, nose, and throat practice: its presentation and diagnosis. Am J Otolaryngol 2006;27(1):39–45.

7. Garg N, Kandpal B, Tewari S, Kapoor A, Goel P, Sinha N. Characteristics of infective endocarditis in a developing country—clinical profile and outcome in 192 Indian patients, 1992–2001. Int J Cardiol 2005;98(2):253–60.

8. Tariq M, Alam M, Munir G, Khan MA, Smego RA, Jr. Infective endocarditis: a five-year experience at a tertiary care hospital in Pakistan. Int J Infect Dis 2004;8(3):163–70.

9. Balakrishnan N, Menon T, Fournier PE, Raoult D. *Bartonella quintana* and *Coxiella burnetii* as causes of endocarditis, India. Emerg Infect Dis 2008;14(7):1168–9.

10. Ramani S, Kang G. Viruses causing childhood diarrhoea in the developing world. Curr Opin Infect Dis 2009;22(5):477–82.

11. Harris AM, Chowdhury F, Begum YA, et al. Shifting prevalence of major diarrheal pathogens in patients seeking hospital care during floods in 1998, 2004, and 2007 in Dhaka, Bangladesh. Am J Trop Med Hyg 2008;79(5):708–14.

12. Gupta S, Narang S, Nunavath V, Singh S. Chronic diarrhoea in HIV patients: prevalence of coccidian parasites. Indian J Med Microbiol 2008;26(2):172–5.

13. Agrawal V, Agarwal T, Ghoshal UC. Intestinal strongyloidiasis: a diagnosis frequently missed in the tropics. Trans R Soc Trop Med Hyg 2009;103(3):242–6.

14. Navaneethan U, Al Mohajer M, Shata MT. Hepatitis E and pregnancy: understanding the pathogenesis. Liver Int 2008;28(9):1190–9.

15. Schneider JA, Lakshmi V, Dandona R, Kumar GA, Sudha T, Dandona L. Population-based seroprevalence of HSV-2 and syphilis in Andhra Pradesh state of India. BMC Infect Dis 2010;10:59.

16. Guerrero DM, Perez F, Conger NG, et al. *Acinetobacter baumannii*-associated skin and soft tissue infections: recognizing a broadening spectrum of disease. Surg Infect (Larchmt) 2010;11(1):49–57.

17. Siriwardana HV, Thalagala N, Karunaweera ND. Clinical and epidemiological studies on the cutaneous leishmaniasis caused by *Leishmania (Leishmania) donovani* in Sri Lanka. Ann Trop Med Parasitol 2010;104(3):213–23.

18. Ramesh V, Misra RS, Jain RK. Secondary tuberculosis of the skin. Clinical features and problems in laboratory diagnosis. Int J Dermatol 1987;26(9):578–81.

19. Kumarasamy KK, Toleman MA, Walsh TR, et al. Emergence of a new antibiotic resistance mechanism in India, Pakistan, and the UK: a molecular, biological, and epidemiological study. Lancet Infect Dis 2010;10(9):597–602.

20. Khan MS, Siddiqui SZ, Haider S et al. Infection control education: impact on ventilator-associated pneumonia rates in a public sector intensive care unit in Pakistan. Trans R Soc Trop Med Hyg 2009;103(8):807–11.

21. Batuwanthudawe R, Karunarathne K, Dassanayake M, et al. Surveillance of invasive pneumococcal disease in Colombo, Sri Lanka. Clin Infect Dis 2009;48(Suppl 2):S136–40.

22. Chawla K, Gurung B, Mukhopadhyay C, Bairy I. Reporting emerging resistance of *Streptococcus pneumoniae* from India. J Glob Infect Dis 2010;2(1):10–14.

23. Thomas K, Steinhoff MC, Lalitha MK, et al. Invasive pneumococcal disease in South Asia SAPNA Network. 5th International Symposium on Pneumococci and Pneumococcal Diseases; 2006; Alice Springs, Australia 2006.

24. Saha SK, Baqui AH, Darmstadt GL, et al. Comparison of antibiotic resistance and serotype composition of carriage and invasive pneumococci among Bangladeshi children: implications for treatment policy and vaccine formulation. J Clin Microbiol 2003;41(12):5582–7.

25. Global measles mortality, 2000–2008. MMWR Morb Mortal Wkly Rep 2009;58(47):1321–6.

Chapter 13
South-eastern Asia

Daniel H. Paris and Nicholas J. White

Mahidol-Oxford Tropical Medicine Research Unit (MORU), Bangkok, Thailand and Centre for Clinical Vaccinology and Tropical Medicine, Mahidol University, Oxford, UK

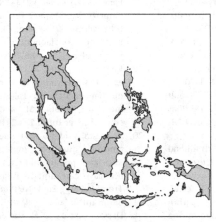

Brunei Darussalam
Cambodia
Indonesia
Lao PDR
Malaysia
Myanmar (Burma)
Philippines
Singapore
Thailand
Timor-Leste
Vietnam

Southeast Asia is the most populated area of the world and a global hot spot for the emergence of new infectious diseases and drug resistance. The emergence and spread of artemisinin-resistant malaria and multidrug resistant (MDR) TB and the widespread use of poor quality anti-infective drugs emanating from this region all pose serious global risks. Socioeconomic factors, tropical climate with vegetation ranging from paddy fields over scrublands to tropical jungle, as well as abundant domestic animal reservoirs (pigs, poultry) allow for a wide range of infectious diseases. Unfortunately epidemiological data on many of these infectious diseases remain limited, and their prevalence and incidence are often uncertain.

Infectious Diseases: A Geographic Guide, First Edition.
Edited by Eskild Petersen, Lin H. Chen & Patricia Schlagenhauf.
© 2011 John Wiley & Sons, Ltd. Published 2011 by John Wiley & Sons, Ltd.

Important regional infections within 4 weeks of exposure

Malaria

Ruling out malaria remains essential in the work up of a febrile traveler. Malaria transmission in Southeast Asia (SEA) is usually low, unstable, and seasonal, except for lowland areas of Papua New Guinea where higher and more stable transmission occurs. Malaria is therefore not a common infectious disease acquired in SEA. The prevalence of *Plasmodium falciparum* and *Plasmodium vivax* are similar, and malaria is largely found in forest and forest-fringe areas and some coastal areas.

Key symptoms: Fever, shivering, abdominal/bone/joint pain; Acute onset.

Typhus-like illness

Many infections present with flu-like symptoms, fever, variable skin rash, and nonspecific symptoms (myalgia, arthralgia, etc.) often accompanied by disorientation, confusion, and other CNS symptoms. Patients usually present with approximately 3–6 days of fever. The following diseases need to be considered.

Dengue fever   This is the most likely infection to be acquired by a traveler to SEA. Transmitted by the day-biting mosquitoes *Aedes aegypti*, which are prevalent in urban areas; it causes an acute flu-like illness affecting all age groups, but seldom causes death. The incubation phase of 3–8 days is followed by a sudden onset of fever, headache, muscle/joint pains, and variable CNS symptoms. A rash may develop within a few days of onset. Serious complications (shock syndrome, hepatitis, myocarditis, encephalitis) are uncommon.

Key symptoms: Acute systemic muscle and/or bone pain with high fever, petechial hemorrhages, usually lack of respiratory symptoms.

Chikungunya   This virus is an arbovirus transmitted by *A. aegypti* and *Aedes albopictus*, with monkeys as reservoirs. Outbreaks reported from SEA are sometimes associated with severe illness and symptoms. A prolonged arthralgia-dominated disease follows the initial acute febrile phase of 2–5 days, and disabling arthralgia can persist for weeks or months. Currently Chikungunya is of concern in Sri Lanka, Cambodia, Laos, and Eastern Thailand.

Key symptoms: Arthralgic pain with fever; Lack of other symptoms; Acute onset.

Scrub typhus and murine typhus   These are the two major rickettsial diseases in SEA. Scrub typhus is a predominantly rural disease with a seasonal pattern, caused by *Orientia tsutsugamushi* and transmitted by the larval stages of *Leptotrombidium* mites. It is often associated with an eschar at the mite-bite-site. Murine typhus is a more urban disease following no seasonality, caused by *Rickettsia typhi*, and transmitted by fleas depositing feces on the human skin, followed by self-inoculation through scratching (no eschar). Both diseases begin with a flu-like illness after a 3–10 day incubation period, and can develop serious complications if untreated. Currently rickettsial diseases are of general increasing concern throughout SEA.

Key symptoms: Fever, myalgia, sometimes skin rash; Scrub typhus often with lymphadenopathy, approximately half of cases with an eschar, history of rural activity; Murine typhus with urban activity, lymphadenopathy rare but potentially severe disease.

Leptospirosis   This is a biphasic infection with a 4 to 14-day incubation period. It begins with flu-like symptoms occasionally with sub-conjunctival hemorrhages, meningitis, jaundice, and renal failure. Leptospirosis is often misdiagnosed due to the wide range of symptoms.

Key symptoms: Acute onset with myalgia and jaundice; Exposure to contaminated environmental water.

Typhoid fever   This (*Salmonella typhi* serovar Typhi) is a slowly progressive febrile illness with sweating, gastrointestinal symptoms (abdominal discomfort, diarrhea, or constipation), sometimes accompanied by faint roseola and depressed sensorium. Complications around the third week include intestinal hemorrhage (bleeding into Peyer's Patches), perforation of the distal ileum with septicemia/peritonitis and metastatic abscesses (rarely CNS, endocarditis, osteitis, etc.). Currently typhoid is of general concern in India, Nepal, Bangladesh, Cambodia, Laos, and Indonesia.

Key symptoms: Slowly worsening fever with abdominal symptoms.

Melioidosis   This (*Burkholderia pseudomallei*) is an important serious systemic abscess-forming infection, which is prevalent in many parts of SEA and particularly in patients with diabetes and/or renal failure and/or thalassemia. It is transmitted via contact to contaminated soil and environmental water and can present either as an acute form (incubation approximately 1–3 weeks) or manifest after a latent period for up to 62 years.

Key symptoms: Acute fever with foci, usually in lungs, liver, spleen joints, or skin.

CNS infections

The most common causes of CNS infections in SEA include viral meningoencephalitis (enterovirus and flavivirus groups) and pyogenic meningitis caused by *Streptococcus pneumoniae*, *Haemophilus influenzae* B, *Neisseria meningitidis*, *Mycobacterium tuberculosis*, and *Streptococcus suis* (mainly Vietnam). Rare causes include:

Angiostrongylus cantonensis—Ingestion of undercooked snails or slugs and can cause meningoencephalitis with CSF eosinophilia in humans.

Gnathosthoma spp.—Humans become infected through ingestion of raw or undercooked paratenic hosts (fish, frogs, eels, pigs, and birds).

Zoonotic paramyxoviruses (Nipah, Hendra)—Rare causes of epidemic (often severe) encephalitis and aseptic meningitis associated with exposure to contaminated fruit from bats (flying fox or fruit bats). Reports are limited to Malaysia, Bangladesh, Singapore, and North Australia.

Rabies (lyssavirus, Rhabdoviridae)—Rabies with its uniformly fatal encephalitis in humans remains an important disease in SEA. Pre- and postexposure prophylaxis and vaccination are recommended.

Hepatitis

Hepatitis A is widespread throughout SEA. Chronic hepatitis B prevalence (HBsAg positivity) is high in SEA, about 70–90% of the population becomes HBV-infected before the age of 40, and up to 20% of people are HBV carriers (HBsAg positivity). Hepatitis E is acquired from contaminated drinking water and fecal–oral transmission throughout the region and is probably predominantly acquired from pigs. Special caution applies to pregnant women, as during the third trimester of pregnancy, hepatitis E can be severe with a case-fatality rate reaching 20%.

Parasitic disease

Trematodes: Schistosomiasis (*Schistosoma mekongi* and *Schistosoma japonicum*) occurs in Laos, Cambodia, Thailand, and the Philippines, but is rare and focal. Liver flukes (*Fasciola hepatica*) are common throughout SEA, but *Opisthorchis* and *Clonorchis* spp. are more limited to Laos, Cambodia, Thailand, and Vietnam. Lung flukes (*Paragonimus westermanii*—associated with freshwater crabs) may cause hemoptysis and are an important differential diagnosis to TB.

Cestodes: Due to widespread presence of domestic pigs and poor sanitary standards in slaughter houses, taeniasis is common in Laos and adjoining countries (*Taenia solium* and

Taenia saginata). Neurocysticercosis should be considered in cases of CNS symptoms in returning travelers.

Nematodes: The intestinal helminths *Necator americanus*, *Ancylostoma duodenalis* (hookworms), *Ascaris lumbricoides* (roundworm), *Trichuris trichiura* (whipworm), and *Strongyloides stercoralis* are all common. *Enterobius vermicularis* (threadworm) is common in young children.

While hookworm is prevalent in SEA, disease burden is low, but roundworm infestation is common. Disseminated strongyloidiasis may occur many years after exposure in immunocompromised patients.

Gnathostomiasis: *Gnathostoma* spp. are hosted in dogs and cats, and transmitted to humans by ingestion of larvae-containing meat. Although, they can comprise any organ system (eye, lung, GI tract, etc.), the most important are CNS complications due to larval migration leading to radiculomyelitis, encephalitis, and subarachnoid hemorrhages.

Influenza (H1N1)/avian influenza (H5N1)

SEA is a hotspot for pandemic influenza. It was the epicenter for H5N1 and was significantly affected by H1N1 influenza. Vaccination remains a key control strategy.

CNS infections: meningitis and encephalitis

Acute infections with less than 4 weeks of symptoms

Frequently found microorganisms	Rare microorganisms	Very rare microorganisms
Virus (enterovirus, JEV, dengue, Nipah, HSV, VZV, CMV, EBV, HIV, mumps, measles, rubeola)	*Staphylococcus aureus*[a]	Free-living amoebae (*Acanthamoeba*, *Balamuthia*, and *Naegleria* spp.)[b]
N. meningitidis	Influenza	*Listeria monocytogenes*
H. influenzae B	Eosinophilic meningoencephalitis[c]	Rabies
S. pneumoniae	Paramyxovirus (Hendra, Nipah)	*Echinococcus granulosus*
M. tuberculosis	*Toxoplasma gondii*	Poliomyelitis (abortive, paralytic, or nonparalytic)
S. suis	Postimmunization/vaccine[d]	
HIV/AIDS and opportunistic infections[e]	*B. pseudomallei*[f]	
P. falciparum, *P. vivax*	*Salmonella enterica* (nontyphoidal)	
Rickettsia spp.		
Cryptococcus neoformans var. *neoformans* and var. *gattii*		

[a]Dissemination often follows skin infections. Community-acquired MRSA is common in some areas.
[b]Granulomatous amebic encephalitis (GAE) and primary amebic meningoencephalitis (PAM).
[c]Most common: *A. cantonensis*, *Gnathostoma spinigerum* [1]. Fungal: Coccidiomycosis, *C. neoformans*.
Parasites: *T. solium*, *E. alveolaris*, *P. westermanii*, *S. japonicum*, *F. hepatica*, *T. canis*, *T. trichiura*, and *T. spiralis*.
[d]Yellow fever, measles, JEV, and rabies vaccines.
[e]HIV is neurotropic and may cause PML (progressive multifocal leukoencephalopathy); also IRIS (immune reconstitution inflammatory syndrome) may occur after starting antiretroviral therapy.
[f]In diabetics, patients with renal failure and immunocompromised.

CNS infections with symptoms for more than 4 weeks and in the immunocompromised host

Microorganisms with symptoms for more than 4 weeks	Microorganisms in the immunocompromised host
HIV/AIDS and opportunistic infections *M. tuberculosis* *Treponema pallidum* (neurosyphilis) *T. solium* (neurocysticercosis) *T. gondii*	*C. neoformans* *M. tuberculosis* (extrapulmonary TB) *T. gondii* *Nocardia, Actinomyces* spp. *Toxocara* spp. Free-living amoebae[a] (*Acanthamoeba, Balamuthia,* and *Naegleria* spp.) CMV Neurosyphilis (*T. pallidum*)

Consider noninfectious causes like vasculitis and lymphoma.
[a]GAE and PAM.

Ear, nose, and throat infections

Ear, nose, and throat infections with less than 4 weeks of symptoms

Frequently found microorganisms	Rare microorganisms and conditions	Very rare microorganisms
Group A streptococcal throat infection Otitis media and externa[b]	Melioidosis (parotid abscess)[a] *M. tuberculosis*	Diphtheria Nipah virus (outbreak)
Viral (HSV I and II, EBV, HIV, dengue, influenza)	Peritonsillar abscess[c]	Necrotizing stomatitis
Neisseria gonorrhoeae, HSV, syphilis, HPV	Necrotizing fasciitis[d]	
Candidia spp. (HIV, antibiotics, diabetes)		

[a]Melioid parotid abscess common in children.
[b]See resistance notes. *P. aeruginosa* and mycosis (*Aspergillus,* candidiasis) common in otitis externa.
[c]Requires acute ENT evaluation.
[d]Requires acute ENT or surgical evaluation.

Ear, nose, and throat infections with symptoms for more than 4 weeks and in the immunocompromised host

The main infection to consider in both immunocompetent and immunocompromised subjects is extrapulmonary TB. TB can affect nose, nasopharynx, oropharynx, middle ear, mastoid bone, larynx, deep neck spaces, and salivary glands. Leprosy targets nose, nasopharynx, and laryngopharynx, but is now rare. Further, candidiasis, HSV, and HIV-associated EBV are differential diagnoses in immunocompromised hosts. Consider noninfectious causes like vasculitis and lymphoma.

Cardiopulmonary infections

Cardiopulmonary infections with less than 4 weeks of symptoms

Frequently found microorganisms	Rare microorganisms and conditions	Very rare microorganisms
Pulmonary symptoms		
S. pneumoniae	Influenza	Diphtheria
H. influenza	*Legionella pneumophila*	Yersinia pestis
Mycoplasma pneumoniae	*C. neoformans*	*Coxiella burnetti*
S. aureus		
B. pseudomallei		
Klebsiella pneumoniae		
P. westermanii		
Leptospira spp.		
Endocarditis		
S. aureus	*N. gonorrhoeae*	*Bartonella* spp.
Viridans streptococci	*C. burnetti*	*Propionibacterium*
Enterococcus spp.	Coagulase-negative staphylococci (*S. epidermidis*)[a]	
Candidia spp.	HACEK group	
S. pneumoniae		

[a]Associated with prosthetic valves.

Pulmonary symptoms and/or endocarditis for more than 4 weeks and in the immunocompromised host

Microorganisms with symptoms for more than 4 weeks	Microorganisms in the immunocompromised host
Pulmonary symptoms[a]	
COPD	*Penicillium marneffei*
M. tuberculosis	*Pneumocystis jirovecii*
Aspergillus spp.	Aspergillus, candidiasis (neutropenic patients)
C. neoformans	*M. avium* complex (MAC)
B. pseudomallei	CMV
P. westermanii	*Bartonella henselae*, *Bartonella quintana*
	B. pseudomallei[b]
	Histoplasma capsulatum
Endocarditis, pericarditis[c]	
Coagulase-negative staphylococci (*S. epidermidis*)	*Aspergillus* spp.
Viridans streptococci	*T. trichiura*
Bartonella and *Rickettsia* spp.	*T. gondii*
Candidia spp. (IVDU)	Varicella Zoster Virus
Typhoid (*S. enterica* S. Typhi)	
Enterovirus	

[a]Consider noninfectious causes like lung cancer, autoimmune lung fibrosis, Wegener's granulomatosis.
[b]Diabetics, renal failure, and thalassemia.
[c]Rheumatic heart disease (RHD) remains a major predisposition for cardiac infections in SEA. The prevalence of RHD is estimated 21.5/1,000 [2]. Consider fever, cough, haemoptysis as a consequence of pulmonary hypertension and/or congestive heart failure with edema without infection.

Gastrointestinal infections

Gastrointestinal infections with less than 4 weeks of symptoms

Frequently found microorganisms	Rare microorganisms and conditions	Very rare microorganisms
E. coli (predominantly enterotoxigenic E. coli (ETEC), but also enteropathogenic E. coli (EPEC), enteroinvasive E. coli (EIEC), enterohemorrhagic E. coli(EHEC), enteroaggregative E. coli (EAEC))	Coccidiosis (*Isospora, Cryptosporidium, Cyclospora*)	*M. tuberculosis*
Salmonella spp. (nontyphoid)	*S. aureus* toxin	*Tropheryma whipplei*
Shigella spp.	*Bacillus cereus* toxin	*Yersinia enterocolitica*
Campylobacter spp.	*Vibrio cholerae*[a]	
Salmonella enterica S. Typhi[b]	*Capillaria philippinensis*	
Giardia intestinalis	*A. lumbricoides*	
E. vermicularis (threadworm)		
Norovirus, rotavirus		
Entamoeba histolytica (liver abscess)		
Clonorchis/Opisthorchis		

Repeated negative bacterial cultures and microscopy for parasites suggest noninfectious etiology. Consider inflammatory bowel diseases, malabsorption, celiac disease, or neoplasias. Also postinfectious malabsorption (tropical sprue).

[a]Reduced stomach acid production is associated with higher incidence of cholera (children, elderly, proton pump inhibitor, and histamine blocker use).

[b]Symptoms of headache, high fever with abdominal symptoms (diarrhea, constipation) [3].

Symptoms for more than 4 weeks and in the immunocompromised host

Microorganisms with symptoms for more than 4 weeks	Microorganisms in the immunocompromised host
Persistent diarrhea (*Giardia* spp., EAEC, *Cryptosporidium, Cyclospora, T. trichiura, C. philippinensis*)	Candidiasis
M. tuberculosis (extrapulmonary TB)	HSV
Dientamoeba fragilis[a]	Coccidiosis (*Isospora, Cryptosporidium*)
T. whipplei	*S. stercoralis* (hyperinfection syndrome)
Invasive schistosomiasis	*M. tuberculosis* (extrapulmonary TB)

Consider noninfectious causes like postinfectious malabsorption (tropical sprue), inflammatory bowel disease, intestinal malignancies like colon cancer, and celiac disease.

[a]Of uncertain pathogenicity in humans.

Infections of liver, spleen, and peritoneum

Acute infections of liver, spleen, and peritoneum with less than 4 weeks of symptoms

Hepatitis and jaundice[a]	Liver abscess or lesion	Granulomatous disease
Viral (hepatitis A–E viruses, CMV, EBV, HSV, measles, rubella, dengue)	*B. pseudomallei*[b,c]	*M. tuberculosis*
Leptospira spp.	*T. pallidum* (Gumma)	*S. japonicum* and *S. mekongi*
T. pallidum (acute)	*M. tuberculosis* (tuberculoma)	*P. marneffei*
F. hepatica[d]	*E. histolytica* (amebic abscess)	*Toxocara canis*
Clonorchis/Opisthorchis spp.[d]	Pyogenic abscess[e]	*S. stercoralis*
Salmonella typhi S. Typhi[c]	*Echinococcus* spp.	*P. westermanii*
P. falciparum[c]		
Rickettsia spp., *O. tsutsugamushi*		

[a]Noninfectious causes can include cholelithiasis/cholecystitis, drugs (INH, rifampicin, sulfonamides), alcohol, toxins (aflatoxins, mushrooms), or vaccine side effects (BCG).
[b]Melioidosis is commonly associated with hepatic abscesses.
[c]Commonly causes hepatosplenomegaly.
[d]Usually associated with eosinophilia, can cause cholangiocarcinoma.
[e]*Staphylococcus, Streptococcus, Salmonella enterica* Serovar Typhi.

Symptoms for more than 4 weeks and in the immunocompromised host

Microorganisms with symptoms for more than 4 weeks	Microorganisms in the immunocompromised host[a]
F. hepatica[b]	*P. marneffei*
Clonorchis/Opisthorchis spp.[b]	*P. jirovecii*
Disseminated *M. tuberculosis*	*Cryptosporidium* spp.
P. westermanii	CMV cholangitis
P. marneffei	*M. tuberculosis* or MAC
	Leishmania spp. (VL>CL)[c]
	Bartonella spp.[d]

Noninfectious etiologies include cholecystitis, neoplasias (HCC, cholangio- or pancreatic carcinoma).
[a]High frequency of granulomatous and/or cholangiosclerosing disease.
[b]Longstanding subclinical cholangitis can cause cholangiocarcinoma.
[c]Visceral forms more frequent than cutaneous forms.
[d]Bacillary hepatic peliosis.

Genitourinary infections

Symptoms with less than 4 weeks duration

Frequently found microorganisms	Rare microorganisms and conditions	Very rare microorganisms
Cystitis, pyelonephritis, and nephritis[a]		
E. coli (UPEC)[b,c] S. saprophyticus, S. epidermidis	Perirenal abscess	Hantavirus
K. pneumoniae[c]	M. tuberculosis	
Enterobacter spp.	B. pseudomallei (including prostatitis)	
Enterococcus spp.	S. mekongi	
Proteus mirabilis		
Chlamydia trachomatis (including urethritis, prostatitis)		
Pseudomonas aeruginosa (hospital-acquired)		
Sexually transmitted infections		
Chlamydia spp.	Lymphogranuloma venereum	
N. gonorrhoeae[d]	Entamoeba spp.	
Trichomonas vaginalis		
Syphilis (T. pallidum)		
Viral (HPV, HSV, HBV, HIV)		
Chancroid (H. ducreyi)		
Papillomata (HPV)		
Parasites (scabies and lice)		
Pyogenic bacteria (Staphylococcus spp., Streptococcus spp.)		

[a]Consider noninfectious causes especially malignancies like renal cell carcinoma.
[b]Throughout Asia E. coli can demonstrate multidrug resistant (MDR) to multiple antibiotics.
[c]E. coli and Klebsiella spp. associated with extended-spectrum β-lactamase (ESBL), increasingly common in Asia.
[d]See section on antibiotic resistance.

Symptoms for more than 4 weeks and in the immunocompromised host

Microorganisms with symptoms for more than 4 weeks	Microorganisms in the immunocompromised host
Cystitis, pyelonephritis, and nephritis[a]	
Bacterial infections (catheters and renal stones)	Candidiasis
M. tuberculosis (extrapulmonary TB)	Melioidosis (B. pseudomallei)
Melioidosis (B. pseudomallei)	M. tuberculosis (extrapulmonary TB)
Sexually transmitted infections	
Viral: HPV, HSV, HBV, HIV	Same panel as immunocompetent patients
Syphilis (all stages)	
Chancroid (H. ducreyi)	
T. vaginalis	
N. gonorrhoeae	
C. trachomatis	

[a]Consider noninfectious causes especially malignancies like renal cell carcinoma.

Joint, muscle, and soft tissue infections

Symptoms with less than 4 weeks duration

Frequently found microorganisms	Rare microorganisms and conditions	Very rare microorganisms and conditions
S. aureus (pyomyositis)	Necrotizing fasciitis (GAS, TSST, *Vibrio vulnificus, Clostridium perfringens, Bacterioides* spp.)	Fourniers gangrene (perineum and urogenital)
Chikungunya	*Echinococcus* spp.	*Sarcocystis*
Trichinella spiralis	S. pneumoniae[a]	*Sporothrix schenckii*
Melioidosis (*B. pseudomallei*)		
M. tuberculosis (extrapulmonary TB)		

GAS, group A streptococci; TSST, staphylococcal toxic shock syndrome, consider MRSA.
[a] Can cause cellulitis, soft tissue infection, scrotal/perineal abscess, and arthritis.

Symptoms with more than 4 weeks symptoms and in the immunocompromised host

Microorganisms with symptoms for more than 4 weeks	Microorganisms in the immunocompromised host
M. tuberculosis (extrapulmonary TB)	*Candidia* spp.
Viral (Influenza A and B, Chikungunya, dengue, HIV, enterovirus, hepatitis A and B)	*B. pseudomallei* (abscess-formation)
Melioidosis (*B. pseudomallei*)	*M. tuberculosis* (extrapulmonary TB)
Postviral myopathies/chronic fatigue syndrome	MAC

Skin infections

Skin infections with less than 4 weeks of symptoms

Frequently found microorganisms	Rare microorganisms and conditions	Very rare microorganisms and conditions
Erysipelas (*S. aureus*, group A streptococci, S. pneumoniae[a])	*Leishmania* spp.	Rat-bite fever (*Spirillum minus, Streptobacillus moniliformis*)
Furunculosis (*S. aureus*)	*C. neoformans*	*Erisipelothrix rusiopathiae*
Cutaneous and subcutaneous dermatophytoses	Leptospirosis	Yaws (*T. pallidum pertenue*)
N. gonorrhoeae	*S. stercoralis* (hyperinfection form)	*Leishmania* spp.

(Continued)

Frequently found microorganisms	Rare microorganisms and conditions	Very rare microorganisms and conditions
Syphilis (*T. pallidum*)	Melioidosis (*B. pseudomallei*)	
Candida spp.	*T. spiralis*	
Rickettsia spp. and *O. tsutsugamushi*[b]	*P. marneffei*[c]	
HIV/AIDS and opportunistic infections	Gnathostomiasis	
Sporothrix schenckii, Sporothrix globosa	Nontuberculous mycobacteria	
M. tuberculosis (extrapulmonary TB)	*S. suis*	
Lymphatic filariasis[d]		
Scabies (*S. scabiei*)		
Milaria (*S. aureus*, sweating)		

A rash due to viral infections was not considered an infection limited to the skin.

[a]Can cause cellulitis, soft tissue infection, scrotal/perineal abscess, and arthritis.

[b]An eschar is not always present. Consider differential diagnosis (DD): insect or spider bite (recluse spider), cutaneous anthrax, cat scratch disease, TB, tularemia, leishmaniasis, fungal lesion (sporotrichosis, aspergillosis, and mucormycosis).

[c]*P. marneffei* is endemic in Burma (Myanmar), Cambodia, Southern China, Indonesia, Laos, Malaysia, Thailand, and Vietnam.

[d]Common in Bangladesh, Burma (Myanmar), Indonesia, and Timor-Leste.

Skin infections with more than 4 weeks of symptoms and in the immunocompromised host

Microorganisms with symptoms for more than 4 weeks	Microorganisms in the immunocompromised host
Syphilis (*T. pallidum*)	*Candida* spp.
Extrapulmonary TB	*P. marneffei*[a]
Melioidosis (*B. pseudomallei*)	Extrapulmonary TB
Mycobacterium leprae	Scabies (*Sarcoptes scabiei* var. *hominis*)
Pityriasis versicolor	Melioidosis (*B. pseudomallei*)
Milaria (*S. aureus*, sweating)	MAC
Intertrigo (*Candida* spp., *Corynebacterium* spp., dermatophytes)	*S. schenckii, S. globosa*
Folliculitis (*S. aureus*)	Animal bites[b]

A rash due to viral infections was not considered an infection limited to the skin.

[a]*P. marneffei* is endemic in Burma (Myanmar), Cambodia, Southern China, Indonesia, Laos, Malaysia, Thailand, and Vietnam.

[b]Stray dogs are common throughout SEA and especially splenectomized travelers must beware of dog bites (*Pasteurella multocida* and *Capnocytophaga canimorsus*).

Lymphadenopathy

Lymphadenopathy of less than 4 weeks' duration

Frequently found microorganisms	Rare microorganisms and conditions	Very rare microorganisms and conditions
Regional LN		
Syphilis and other STDs	*Leishmania* spp.	Plague (*Y. pestis*)
Rickettsial diseases	Bartonella spp. (cat scratch disease)	*Babesia microti*
Skin lesions (fungal, secondary or superinfections)	Lymphatic filariasis (*W. bancrofti, B. malayi*)	Rat-bite fever[a]
Nontuberculous mycobacteria		
Systemic LN		
Viral infection (HIV, EBV, CMV, parvovirus B19, enterovirus, etc.)	MAC	
HIV (including primoinfection)	Leishmaniasis	
Rickettsial infections	Lymphatic filariasis	
Extrapulmonary TB	Melioidosis	
Toxoplasmosis (*T. gondii*)	Leptospirosis	

[a]Caused by *S. minus* or *S. moniliformis*.

Lymphadenopathy of more than 4 weeks duration and in the immunocompromised host

Microorganisms with symptoms for more than 4 weeks	Microorganisms in the immunocompromised host
T. gondii	*P. marneffei*
Extrapulmonary TB (*M. tuberculosis*)	CMV
Melioidosis (*B. pseudomallei*)	MAC
P. marneffei	*T. gondii*
	Extrapulmonary TB (*M. tuberculosis*)
	Melioidosis (*B. pseudomallei*)

If the diagnosis is not made within a few days, biopsies should be performed to exclude malignancies like lymphoma and carcinomas.

Fever without focal symptoms

Fever less than 4 weeks without focal symptoms

Frequently found microorganisms	Rare microorganisms and conditions	Very rare microorganisms
Viral infection (HIV, EBV, CMV, parvovirus B19, enterovirus, etc.)	Nontuberculous mycobacteria	*Neorickettsia sennetsu*
P. falciparum, P. vivax	*C. burnetti*	*B. microti*

(Continued)

Frequently found microorganisms	Rare microorganisms and conditions	Very rare microorganisms
Flaviviridae (dengue, Chikungunya, and JEV)	*P. marneffei*	Tularemia
Leptospira spp.	*Bartonella* spp.	Ehrlichiosis
Rickettsia spp., *O. tsutsugamushi*	*Brucella* spp.	
HIV/AIDS		
T. gondii		
Extrapulmonary TB		
B. pseudomallei		
S. enterica (typhoidal, nontyphoidal)		

Fever for more than 4 weeks without focal symptoms and in the immunocompromised host

Microorganisms with symptoms for more than 4 weeks	Microorganisms in the immunocompromised host
T. gondii	MAC
TB (*M. tuberculosis*)	*T. gondii*
M. leprae	Extrapulmonary TB
Typhoid, paratyphoid (*Salmonella* spp.)	*P. marneffei*
	Leishmaniasis (visceral > cutaneous forms)
	Microsporidia spp.
	B. microti (RF: CD4<200 and splenectomy)
	CMV

Noninfectious causes should be considered from the beginning, including malignancies like lymphoma and autoimmune diseases.

Eosinophilia and elevated IgE

Eosinophilia and elevated IgE less than 4 weeks

Frequently found microorganisms	Rare microorganisms and conditions	Very rare microorganisms and conditions
S. stercoralis[a]	*T. solium* (cysticercosis)	Hydatid disease (*E. granulosus*)
Hookworm (*Ancylostoma, Necator*)[a]	Streptococcal—scarlet fever	*Anisakis* spp.
E. vermicularis	*P. westermanii*	Influenza, SARS, and bird flu (outbreak settings)
Lymphatic filariasis (*W. bancrofti*, *B. malayi*, and *B. timori*)	*A. cantonensis*[a]	
Flukes (*Opisthorchis viverrini*, *Clonorchis sinensis, F. hepatica*)	*T. spiralis*	
S. mekongi, S. japonicum	*Gnathostoma* spp. Drug hypersensitivity syndrome (DHS)[b]	

Frequently found microorganisms	Rare microorganisms and conditions	Very rare microorganisms and conditions
T. trichiura *Dientamoeba fragilis*	Advanced HIV infection	

Consider "allergic"/hematological/dysplastic/immunological disorders and potential drug association before starting extensive parasitological examinations.
[a]Larval migration through lungs cause pulmonary symptoms and eosinophilia.
[b]DHS can be serious. It is characterized by fever, rash, and internal organ involvement. Ensure prompt identification of suspect responsible medicines and avoidance of reexposure. Caveat: cross-reactivity to structurally related medicines is common and first-degree relatives may be predisposed.

Eosinophilia and elevated IgE for more than 4 weeks and in the immunocompromised host

All helminthic infections mentioned above may cause eosinophilia after 4 weeks in subjects with adequate immune responses and in immunocompromised hosts. Advanced HIV infection itself (CD4<200/μL) can cause eosinophilia.

Antibiotic resistance in SEA

Malaria

SEA is the epicenter of drug resistance in *P. falciparum*, especially MDR and artemisinin resistance in Cambodia and adjacent countries, but risks to travelers are low. Highly chloroquine (CQ)-resistant strains of *P. vivax* are found in parts of Indonesia.

MDR *M. tuberculosis*

One-third (28%) of the world's MDR-TB cases are in the SEA region. The leading countries in SEA reporting first-line anti-TB drug resistance per 2010 are India with 2.3% MDR among new TB cases (95% CI) and 17.2% in previously treated TB cases, Myanmar with 4.2% and 10.0% and Thailand with 1.7% and 34.5%, respectively.

MDR *Salmonella* spp.

Typhoid: Plasmid-encoded resistance to chloramphenicol, ampicillin, trimethoprim–sulfamethoxazole in *S. enterica* serovar Typhi (MDRST) has been prevalent in SEA for many years. Chromosomal fluoroquinolone resistance (mutations of DNA gyrase *gyrA*) has spread widely in the past decade.

Nontyphoidal salmonellosis (NTS): An MDR strain of *Salmonella typhimurium* termed definitive phage type 104 (DT104) is emerging worldwide. It is resistant to ampicillin, chloramphenicol, streptomycin, sulfonamides, and tetracyclines, but not more virulent than the susceptible strains. Quinolone resistance in NTS strains is common in SEA, mainly due to DNA gyrase and topoisomerase alterations [4]. At present, reports of third-generation cephalosporin resistance are increasing for both typhoidal and nontyphoidal salmonelloses. Clinical management requires careful microbiological assessment.

Drug-resistant *S. pneumoniae*

Resistance of *S. pneumoniae* to β-lactams, macrolides, tetracyclines, chloramphenicol, and sulfonamides has been increasing rapidly in SEA. Vancomycin (with Rifampicin) has been required to treat patients with pneumococcal meningitis caused by strains resistant to extended-spectrum cephalosporins (e.g., cefotaxime and ceftriaxone). Korea has the highest frequency of nonsusceptible strains to penicillin with 80%, followed by Japan, Vietnam, and Thailand. SEA is the world leader in *S. pneumoniae* macrolide resistance (especially Vietnam, Korea, and Japan) [5,6].

Rickettsial disease

Reports of prolonged fever clearance times and resistance to doxycycline have been reported from Chiang Rai, North Thailand, South India, and Korea. Azithromycin is the alternative regimen, including pregnant women and children [7].

MDR Enterobacteriacae

The rates of MDR in Enterobacteriacae have risen drastically in SEA, mainly due to spread of ESBLs among isolates of Enterobacteriacae both from community and health-care settings. These enzymes confer resistance to third- and fourth-generation cephalosporins and mono-bactams, and are frequently associated with co-resistance to other antimicrobials, such as fluoroquinolones (emerging plasmid-mediated quinolone resistance, PMQR), co-trimoxazole, tetracyclines, and aminoglycosides. The most common organisms affected are *E. coli* and *K. pneumoniae*.

So far no evidence for importation of MDR Enterobacteriacae carrying the *bla*NDM-1 the gene (New Delhi metallobeta-lactamase) from India to SEA has been described (*E. coli, K. pneumoniae,* and *Enterobacter cloacae*). Awareness of MDR bacteria carrying NDM-1 is crucial, as they are resistant to most antibiotics, but still appear to respond to colistin and tigecycline.

Gonorrhea

MDR in *N. gonorrhoeae* (resistance to ciprofloxacin, tetracycline, spectinomycin, and penicillin) has increased rapidly in SEA in recent years, mainly due to high rates of gonorrhea and uncontrolled use of antibiotics. Many developed countries now recommend the use of third-generation cephalosporins instead of quinolones for the treatment of gonorrhea. Gonococcal resistance to third-generation cephalosporins given orally has already emerged in SEA.

HIV/AIDS and immunocompromised people

Antiretroviral therapy (ART) has been available in some SEA countries for almost two decades, but the HIV-incidence and ART-coverage rates in countries like Cambodia, Laos, and Bangladesh remain limited. In the more developed setting like Thailand, HIV drug resistance (HIVDR) threshold surveys based on blood bank and counseling centers show a low prevalence (<5%) of transmitted HIVDR [8]. Travel-associated prophylaxis and antimicrobial treatment may interfere with established HIV drug levels of patients under ART.

Vaccine-preventable diseases in children

Immunization is among the most successful and cost-effective public health interventions. Nonetheless, during 2002, approximately 1.9 million (76%) of the worldwide 2.5 million vaccine-preventable disease (VPD) deaths among children aged less than 5 years worldwide occurred in Africa or SEA. Through optimal use of currently existing vaccines alone, further significant reduction of mortality rates among children under 5 years can be achieved [9].

The major VPD in SEA are: diphtheria, tetanus, pertussis, poliomyelitis, hepatitis A and B, *H. influenzae* B, measles, meningococcal and pneumococcal disease, rabies, typhoid, and Japanese encephalitis. Strong emphasis on completing basic vaccination schedules is a required priority. In SEA the percent coverage of DPT (3 doses) in less than 1-year-old children was 72% (2010) and Hepatitis B coverage stands at 40% (2008) [10]. Although vaccination coverage is improving in some countries, measles transmission persists in SEA. Influenza infections can occur throughout the year in tropical areas. Polio resurfaced in Indonesia in 2005 and imported cases in neighboring countries have occasionally occurred. Unvaccinated people traveling or working in SEA should receive adequate counseling.

Background data on countries in SEA

Basic economic and demographic data

Country	GNI per capita (USD)[a]	Life expectancy at birth (total, years)[b]	School enrollment, primary (% net and year)[c]
Brunei Darussalam	12,196 or more	76	93 (2008)
Cambodia	650	60	89 (2008)
Indonesia	2,230	71	95 (2007)
Lao PDR	880	57	82 (2008)
Malaysia	7,230	73	98 (2006)
Myanmar (Burma)	995 or less	63	90 (2005)
Philippines	1,790	71	90 (2007)
Singapore	37,220	82	NA
Thailand	3,760	73	95 (2008)
Timor-Leste	2,460	67	76 (2008)
Vietnam	1,010	72	88 (2005)

NA, not available.

[a]Gross national income, World Development Indicators database, World Bank, per July 2010.
[b]The World Factbook, CIA, 2010 (https://www.cia.gov/library/publications/the-world-factbook/rankorder/2102rank.html).
[c]World Bank, School enrollment, primary (% net) (http://data.worldbank.org/indicator/SE.PRM.NENR).

Causes of death in children under 5 years in SEA—regional average

Causes of death (<5 years)	%
HIV/AIDS	0
Diarrhea	13
Measles	4
Malaria	1
Pneumonia	19
Prematurity	14

(Continued)

Causes of death (<5 years)	%
Birth asphyxia	11
Neonatal sepsis	7
Congenital abnormalities	3
Other diseases	23
Injuries	4

WHO Global Health Indicators 2010 report. Regional averages, data from 2008.

Globally, around 950,000 children less than 18 years old die due to injury and violence each year. Injury is a major cause of death in children more than 1 year in SEA. In 2004, SEA had the second highest rate of unintentional child injuries globally (49/100,000 children per year), following Africa. Road traffic injuries, drowning, burns, and self-inflicted injuries (intentional self-harm) are the leading causes of death among children in SEA.

The most common causes of deaths in all ages in three countries of SEA

Common causes of deaths[a]	%		
	Cambodia	Thailand	Singapore
HIV/AIDS	10	14	NS
TB	8	NS	NS
Diarrheal diseases	7	NS	NS
Perinatal conditions	7	NS	NS
Ischemic and hypertensive heart disease	7	7	25
Lower respiratory infections	5	3	10
Cerebrovascular disease	4	6	10
Chronic obstructive lung disease	NS	4	3
Road traffic accidents	NS	5	NS
Meningitis	4	NS	NS
Malaria	2	NS	NS
Diabetes mellitus	NS	5	4
All cancers	NS	5	17
Urogenital diseases	NS	2	NS
Measles	NS	NS	NS

Data summarized for a low (Cambodia), middle (Thailand), and high (Singapore) gross national income (GNI) per capita.
NS, not stated, i.e., not included in the most common causes of death.
WHO statistics, 2006. Mortality profile per country.
[a]WHO Fact Sheet. Child injury prevention.

References

1. Ramirez-Avila L, Slome S, Schuster FL, et al. Eosinophilic meningitis due to *Angiostrongylus* and *Gnathostoma* species. Clin Infect Dis 2009; 48(3):322–7.

2. Marijon E, Ou P, Celermajer DS, et al. Prevalence of rheumatic heart disease detected by echocardiographic screening. N Engl J Med 2007;357(5):470–6.

3. Parry CM, Hien TT, Dougan G, White NJ, Farrar JJ. Typhoid fever. N Engl J Med 2002;347 (22):1770–82.

4. Gunell M, Webber MA, Kotilainen P, et al. Mechanisms of resistance in nontyphoidal *Salmonella enterica* strains exhibiting a nonclassical quinolone resistance phenotype. Antimicrob Agents Chemother 2009;53(9):3832–6.

5. Song JH, Lee NY, Ichiyama S, et al. Spread of drug-resistant *Streptococcus pneumoniae* in Asian countries: Asian network for surveillance of resistant pathogens (ANSORP) study. Clin Infect Dis 1999;28(6):1206–11.

6. Song JH, Jung SI, Ko KS, et al. High prevalence of antimicrobial resistance among clinical *Streptococcus pneumoniae* isolates in Asia (an ANSORP study). Antimicrob Agents Chemother 2004;48(6):2101–7.

7. Kim YS, Yun HJ, Shim SK, Koo SH, Kim SY, Kim S. A comparative trial of a single dose of azithromycin versus doxycycline for the treatment of mild scrub typhus. Clin Infect Dis 2004;39(9):1329–35.

8. Sirivichayakul S, Phanuphak P, Pankam T, O-Charoen R, Sutherland D, Ruxrungtham K. HIV drug resistance transmission threshold survey in Bangkok, Thailand. Antivir Ther 2008;13(Suppl. 2):109–13.

9. WHO. Vaccine-preventable diseases: monitoring system. In: Global report, 2009.

10. WHO. Global health indicators. In: Global Health Indicators report, 2010.

Chapter 14
Western Asia and the Middle East: Part 1

Eyal Leshem and Eli Schwartz
The Center for Geographic Medicine and Tropical Diseases, The Chaim Sheba Medical Center,
Tel Hashomer and Sackler Faculty of Medicine, Tel Aviv University, Israel

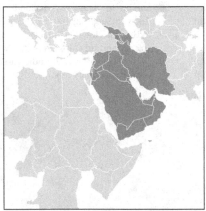

Armenia	Lebanon
Azerbaijan	Occupied Palestinian
Bahrain	Territory
Cyprus	Oman
Georgia	Qatar
Jordan	Saudi Arabia
Iran	Syrian Arab Republic
Iraq	United Arab Emirates
Israel	Yemen
Kuwait	

The West Asia and the Middle East region are both ethnically and geographically diverse area. The region stretches from arid deserts in its south to mountainous and temperate areas in the northern part. Nations in this area are characterized by a wide range of cultural backgrounds and religious history. Socioeconomic disparity is wide including industrialized affluent economies and developing economies.

As in most of the destinations, the most common infections in travelers are gastrointestinal infections. In a key GeoSentinel study published by Wilson et al. in 2007, the common causes of fever from this region were respiratory and diarrheal illnesses (16% each), while 31% of travelers with fever after traveling to the region remained undiagnosed [1].

Several specific infections that are endemic in this region including leishmaniasis, brucellosis, rickettsiosis, relapsing fever, and endemic viral diseases such as West Nile Fever will be discussed further. Chronic and latent infections which should be considered in immigrants from this region include echinococcosis and neurocysticercosis [2].

Infectious Diseases: A Geographic Guide, First Edition.
Edited by Eskild Petersen, Lin H. Chen & Patricia Schlagenhauf.
© 2011 John Wiley & Sons, Ltd. Published 2011 by John Wiley & Sons, Ltd.

Food- and water-borne infections

Diarrheal diseases caused by bacteria and parasites are common in this region. In an analysis of the GeoSentinel database the region had relative risk ratios of 45.4 and 30.1 for bacterial and parasitic diarrhea, respectively, compared with West and Northern Europe [3]. In this study the Middle East region was defined as moderate risk strata as compared with very high risk (relative risk ratio of 890) in the South Asia region. Another recently published analysis of the Geo-Sentinel database described the rates of different pathogens diagnosed in returning travelers from different regions. In this study, the following rates per 1,000 returning travelers from the Middle East region were found [4]:

1 Parasitic infections: *Giardia* 35/1,000, *Entamoeba histolytica* 17/1,000, *Dientamoeba fragilis* 8/1,000, tapeworms 1/1,000

2 Bacterial infections: *Campylobacter* 17/1,000, non-Typhi *Salmonella* 10/1,000

3 Hepatitis A 10/1,000

4 *Cryptosporidium* 4/1,000

Nondiarrheal enteric infections include several important pathogens as given below.

Hepatitis A is a common disease in this region. In Israel since the introduction of hepatitis A vaccine as a national vaccine (1999), a dramatic decline in its incidence occurred and the country became of a low-level country [5].

Hepatitis E is not known to be common although several reports describe seropositivity in Turkey, Israel, Iran, Saudi Arabia, Afghanistan, and other countries in the region and an outbreak has been reported in Jordan [6–8]. The reported seropositivity rates of hepatitis E range from 2% to 3% in different populations in Israel to 18% in adults >50 years old in Saudi Arabia [8,9].

Typhoid fever occurs mainly sporadically although outbreaks are sometimes reported [10,11]. A study from Sweden found a risk of acquiring *Salmonella typhi* and *Salmonella paratyphi* in the Middle East region was 5.91 and 3.64 per 100,000 travelers, respectively (second only to India and neighboring countries) [12]. Another study of typhoid fever among Swiss travelers found a decrease in the rates of typhoid fever in the West Asia region from 4/100,000 travelers between 1974 and 1981 to 0.07/100,000 travelers between 1999 and 2004 [13].

Polio outbreak has been reported in Yemen in 2005 following importation of the virus from Nigeria [14].

Vector-borne diseases

Malaria risk in this area is very low. Most of countries in the region are malaria free. *Plasmodium vivax* transmission occurs in some focal areas in Iraq, Syria, Turkey, and Saudi Arabia. Therefore, in our view, malaria prevention in this region should be based on personal protection by mosquito repellents only. In Yemen *Plasmodium falciparum* exists in all areas at altitude below 2,000 m as well as in some areas of Saudi Arabia. Thus, malaria prevention should be based on chemoprophylaxis (chloroquine resistance exists). Therefore, malaria is a rare cause of fever in travelers returning from West Asia [15]; however, since it is still endemic in several regions, it must be included in the differential diagnosis [16,17].

Malaria in the region (according to WHO)

Countries without malaria	*P. vivax* only	*P. falciparum* exists
Bahrain	Armenia	Iran (only eastern parts)
Cyprus	Azerbaijan	Oman
Israel	Georgia	Saudi Arabia (focal areas in Jazan
Jordan	Iraq	and Asir)
Kuwait	Syrian Arab Republic	Yemen (in all areas at altitude
Lebanon	Turkey	below 2,000 m)
Occupied Palestinian territory		
Qatar		
United Arab Emirates		

Leishmania: Both cutaneous and visceral leishmaniasis are endemic in vast areas of Western Asia [18–22]. Cutaneous leishmaniasis is widespread in the region. The majority of cases is due to *Leishmania major*, however *Leishmania tropica* is the major pathogen in Afghanistan and was recently reported to emerge in Israel and Jordan [23,24].

Visceral leishmaniasis occurs throughout the region and especially in small foci in Iraq, Saudi Arabia, Syria, and Turkey.

Filarial infection: (*Wuchereria bancrofti*) still endemic in some areas of Yemen.

Tick-borne infections such as *Rickettsia conorii* and relapsing fever (mainly due to *Borrelia persica*) are reported in most areas in the region [25,26].

Viral infection: Viral arthropod-borne diseases are also among the important pathogens endemic in all these countries. These include West Nile virus [27], Sindbis [28], Sandfly [29], and Crimean–Congo hemorrhagic fever (mainly in Turkey, Georgia, Iran, Iraq, and the Arabian Peninsula) [30]. Dengue fever is occasionally reported from East and North East countries in the region. Outbreaks were reported from Saudi Arabia [31], Afghanistan, and Yemen. It is important to note that *Aedes albopictus*, a mosquito vector capable of transmitting Dengue, Chikungunya and other pathogens, was introduced into many countries in the region during last few years. However, despite the existence of the vector, local transmission of Dengue and Chikungunya was not yet reported.

Soil- and water-associated diseases

While *Schistosoma mansoni* is only present in Yemen, Saudi Arabia, and Oman, *Schistosoma haematobium* has a wider distribution in Western Asia. Schistosomiasis may present as acute schistosomiasis in exposed travelers. Leptospirosis is pandemic and should be suspected in febrile travelers with a recent history of freshwater or soil exposure [32,33]. Geohelminthic infections (hookworm, strongyloidiasis, or ascariasis) may occur in exposed travelers.

Fever without focal symptoms

Frequently found pandemic microorganisms	Endemic microorganisms	Comments
Infectious mononucleosis-like syndromes (Epstein Barr virus (EBV), Cytomegalovirus (CMV), acute Human Immunodeficiency Virus (HIV))	Mumps	
Coxiella burnetii	West Nile virus	Highly endemic throughout the region, with proven cases from Israel, Iran, Iraq, Georgia, Jordan, Oman, Turkey, and United Arab Emirates. Outbreaks during late summer and early fall.
Bartonellosis—*Bartonella quintana*	Sindbis virus	Reported from Saudi Arabia, potentially endemic in Afghanistan, Iran, Israel, Kuwait, Syria, and Qatar.
Listeriosis	Sandfly virus	Reported from Afghanistan, Iran, Iraq, Israel, Jordan, and Turkey.
Leptospirosis	Spotted fever group rickettsia	*R. conorii* causes spotted fever throughout the region.
Endocarditis	Murine typhus	
Toxoplasmosis	Hantavirus—old world	Armenia, Georgia, Israel (seropositivity among dialysis patients), Kuwait, and Turkey.
	Crimean–Congo hemorrhagic fever	Reported from Afghanistan, Armenia, Georgia, Iran, Iraq, Kuwait, Oman, Saudi Arabia, and Turkey.
	North Asian tick typhus	Isolated from ticks in Armenia.
	Melioidosis	Reported from Iran and Oman.
	Enteric fever *S. typhi* or *S. paratyphi*	
	Brucellosis	
	Tuberculosis	
	Tick-borne relapsing fever—borreliosis	
	Malaria	See malaria in the region section above
	Visceral leishmaniasis	Cases reported from most countries in the region. Human disease may be caused by *Leishmania donovani* or *Leishmania infantum*.
	Amebic liver abscess	

Gastrointestinal infections

Gastrointestinal microorganisms causing diarrhea	Enterically transmitted microorganisms causing systemic illness	Enterically transmitted hepatic microorganisms
Norovirus and calicivirus	*S. typhi* and *S. paratyphi*	Hepatitis A
Rotavirus (pediatric)	Amebic lever abscess	Hepatitis E
Shigellosis	Neurocysticercosis	Amebic lever abscess
Salmonella (nontyphi)		*Echinococcus*
Campylobacteriosis		
ETEC		
Listeriosis		
Giardia intestinalis		
Bacillus cereus food poisoning		
Staphylococcal food poisoning		
Yersiniosis		
Hookworms		
Ascaris		
E. histolytica dysentery		
Ascaris lumbricoides		
Enterobius vermicularis (threadworm)		

Chronic posttravel diarrhea is best treated empirically with tinidazole even when *Giardia* was not found in stool samples. It is not uncommon for returning travelers to complain about "worms" found in their feces. This is essentially caused by three helminths: *Ascaris*, taeniasis, and *Trichuris*.

Hepatic infections

The main causes of hepatitis in West Asia include vaccine-preventable hepatitis A [5,6] and hepatitis B. Hepatitis E is often missed in both travelers and locally infected patients and should be considered [9,34]. Schistosomiasis may cause hepatic symptoms; however, chronic schistosomiasis is rare in travelers and almost never causes hepatic cirrhosis [35]. *Echinococcus* is a common cause of hepatic and intra-abdominal cysts throughout the region. Occasionally bone or pulmonary cysts are found. Amebic liver abscess may manifest months after infection has occurred.

Eosinophilia and elevated IgE

Eosinophilia is defined by ≥450 blood eosinophils/μL. Eosinophilia may occur in up to 10% of travelers. Eosinophilia and elevated IgE in travelers are usually caused by helminthic infections [36]. Other causes include allergies and asthma, drug hypersensitivity, infection, and neoplasm. The common causes in West Asia include strongyloidiasis, hookworm infection (during the acute phase), and *W. bancrofti*. Other possible causes include toxocariasis (visceral and ocular larva migrans), trichinosis, and *Ascaris* (during the acute phase). While *S. mansoni* is only present in Yamen, Saudi Arabia, and Oman, *S. haematobium* has a wider distribution in Western Asia. If acute schistosomiasis is suspected, it is important to inquire regarding freshwater exposure in these areas. Finally, echinococcosis may cause eosinphilia during spillage or cyst perforation.

Joint, muscle, and soft tissue infections

The most important endemic cause of osteomyelitis in the region is brucellosis. There are infrequent reports of bone cysts caused by echinococcosis.

Skin infections

Frequently found pandemic microorganisms	Endemic microorganisms and conditions
Group A streptococcus	Leishmaniasis (major and tropica)
Staphylococcus aureus	Anthrax
Gonococcus	
Syphilis	
Tuberculosis	
Actinomycosis	
Mycobacterium marinum	
Nocardia	
Sporothrix	
Leprosy	
Myiasis	

We have not listed a rash due to viral infections as this is not considered an infection limited to the skin. Cutaneous leishmaniasis is endemic in vast areas of Western Asia [21]. Both *L. major* and *L. tropica* are widely described in local populations, travelers, and soldiers [37].

Central nervous system (CNS) infections: meningitis, encephalitis, and other infections

Frequently found microorganisms	Rare microorganisms and conditions	Very rare microorganisms and conditions
Enterovirus infection	Mumps	Hantavirus
West Nile virus	Sindbis virus	Crimean–Congo hemorrhagic
Herpes simplex 1,2	Sandfly virus	fever
Meningococcal meningitis	Rabies[a]	Acute HIV[a]
Mycoplasma pneumoniae	Murine typhus	Poliomyelitis
Pneumococcal meningitis	Listeriosis	
Brucellosis	Enteric fever *S. typhi* or	
Spotted fever group rickettsia	*S. paratyphi*	
	Tuberculosis[a]	
	Leptospirosis	
	Malaria	
	Neurocysticercosis[a]	
	Acute schistosomiasis	

[a]Incubation may be longer than 4 weeks and patients may experience subacute symptom onset.

Ear, nose, and throat infections

Besides cosmopolitan causes, pertussis is a major causative agent reported with various incidence in the region [38–40]. The important factors determining risk of pertussis are population immunity levels determined by healthcare infrastructure of the different countries. Seasonal, pandemic, and avian flu all affect the region according to local and global parameters.

Cardiopulmonary infections

Frequently found cardiac microorganisms	Comments	Frequently found pulmonary microorganisms	Comments
Bacterial endocarditis	Usual pathogens such as *Staphylococcus aureus*, *Streptococcus viridans*	Pneumonia	Usual pathogens such as pneumococcus, *Mycoplasma pneumoniae*, *Legionella*
C. burnetii		Pulmonary echinococcosis	
Brucellosis		Acute schistosomiasis	
Tuberculous pericarditis		Loeffler's syndrome	
		Tuberculosis	

Adenopathy

Common causes of adenopathy in the region include cosmopolitan causes such as infectious mononucleosis-like syndromes (EBV, CMV, toxoplasmosis, and acute HIV), mumps, yersiniosis, cat scratch disease, and rickettsialpox. Tuberculosis although common only in some of the region, countries may cause scrofula. Contrary to New World leishmaniasis, cutaneous leishmaniasis in our region is a very rare cause of adenopathy.

Genitourinary infections

Important causes of genitourinary (GU) infections typical to the West Asia region include brucella epididymo-orchitis and *S. haematobium*. Interestingly, a recent report described sexual transmission of brucellosis in two couples in Israel [41]. Common cosmopolitan causes of GU disease in the region include tuberculosis, mumps, and sexually transmitted pathogens (herpes simplex 1,2, gonorrhea, chlamydia, mycoplasma, and syphilis).

References

1. Wilson ME, Weld LH, Boggild A, et al. Fever in returned travelers: results from the GeoSentinel Surveillance Network. Clin Infect Dis 2007;44 (12):1560–8.

2. Leshem E, Kliers I, Bakon M, Zuker T, Potasman I, Schwartz E. Neurocysticercosis in Israel. Harefuah 2010 Sep;149(9):576–9, 620.

3. Greenwood Z, Black J, Weld L, et al. Gastrointestinal infection among international travelers globally. J Travel Med 2008;15(4):221–8.
4. Swaminathan A, Torresi J, Schlagenhauf P, et al. A global study of pathogens and host risk factors associated with infectious gastrointestinal disease in returned international travellers. J Infect 2009;59(1):19–27.
5. Dagan R, Leventhal A, Anis E, Slater P, Ashur Y, Shouval D. Incidence of hepatitis A in Israel following universal immunization of toddlers. JAMA 2005;294(2):202–10.
6. Carmoi T, Safiullah S, Nicand E. Risk of enterically transmitted hepatitis A, hepatitis E, and *Plasmodium falciparum* malaria in Afghanistan. Clin Infect Dis 2009;48(12):1800.
7. Piper-Jenks N, Horowitz HW, Schwartz E. Risk of hepatitis E infection to travelers. J Travel Med 2000;7(4):194–9.
8. Arif M. Enterically transmitted hepatitis in Saudi Arabia: an epidemiological study. Ann Trop Med Parasitol 1996;90(2):197–201.
9. Karetnyi YV, Favorov MO, Khudyakova NS, et al. Serological evidence for hepatitis E virus infection in Israel. J Med Virol 1995;45(3):316–20.
10. al-Zubaidy AA, el Bushra HE, Mawlawi MY. An outbreak of typhoid fever among children who attended a potluck dinner at Al-Mudhnab, Saudi Arabia. East Afr Med J 1995;72(6):373–5.
11. Bahrmand AR, Velayati AA. Antimicrobial resistance pattern and plasmid profile of *Salmonella typhi* isolated from an outbreak in Tehran province. Scand J Infect Dis 1997;29(3):265–9.
12. Ekdahl K, de Jong B, Andersson Y. Risk of travel-associated typhoid and paratyphoid fevers in various regions. J Travel Med 2005;12(4):197–204.
13. Keller A, Frey M, Schmid H, Steffen R, Walker T, Schlagenhauf P. Imported typhoid fever in Switzerland, 1993 to 2004. J Travel Med 2008;15(4):248–51.
14. Dennis C. Polio fight falters as Yemen and Java report fresh cases. Nature 2005;435(7039):133.
15. Leder K, Black J, O'Brien D, et al. Malaria in travelers: a review of the GeoSentinel surveillance network. Clin Infect Dis 2004;39(8):1104–12.
16. Guerra CA, Howes RE, Patil AP, et al. The international limits and population at risk of *Plasmodium vivax* transmission in 2009. PLoS Negl Trop Dis 2010;4(8):e774.
17. Hay SI, Guerra CA, Gething PW, et al. A world malaria map: *Plasmodium falciparum* endemicity in 2007. PLoS Med 2009;6(3):e1000048.

18. Pratlong F, Dereure J, Ravel C, et al. Geographical distribution and epidemiological features of Old World cutaneous leishmaniasis foci, based on the isoenzyme analysis of 1048 strains. Trop Med Int Health 2009;14(9):1071–85.
19. Abdeen ZA, Sawalha SS, Eisenberger CL, et al. Epidemiology of visceral leishmaniasis in the Jenin District, West Bank: 1989–1998. Am J Trop Med Hyg 2002;66(4):329–33.
20. Mohebali M, Hamzavi Y, Edrissian GH, Forouzani A. Seroepidemiological study of visceral leishmaniasis among humans and animal reservoirs in Bushehr province, Islamic Republic of Iran. East Mediterr Health J 2001;7(6):912–17.
21. Postigo JA. Leishmaniasis in the World Health Organization Eastern Mediterranean Region. Int J Antimicrob Agents 2010;36(Suppl. 1):S62–5.
22. Peters W, Elbihari S, Liu C, et al. Leishmania infecting man and wild animals in Saudi Arabia. 1. General survey. Trans R Soc Trop Med Hyg 1985;79(6):831–9.
23. Shani-Adir A, Kamil S, Rozenman D, et al. *Leishmania tropica* in northern Israel: a clinical overview of an emerging focus. J Am Acad Dermatol 2005;53(5):810–15.
24. Klaus S, Axelrod O, Jonas F, Frankenburg S. Changing patterns of cutaneous leishmaniasis in Israel and neighbouring territories. Trans R Soc Trop Med Hyg 1994;88(6):649–50.
25. Assous MV, Wilamowski A. Relapsing fever borreliosis in Eurasia—forgotten, but certainly not gone! Clin Microbiol Infect 2009;15(5):407–14.
26. Jensenius M, Davis X, von Sonnenburg F, et al. Multicenter GeoSentinel analysis of rickettsial diseases in international travelers, 1996–2008. Emerg Infect Dis 2009;15(11):1791–8.
27. Aboutaleb N, Beersma M, Wunderink H, Vossen A, Visser L. Case report: West-Nile virus infection in two Dutch travellers returning from Israel. Euro Surveill 2010;15(34):pii19649.
28. Wills WM, Jakob WL, Francy DB, et al. Sindbis virus isolations from Saudi Arabian mosquitoes. Trans R Soc Trop Med Hyg 1985;79(1):63–6.
29. Ellis SB, Appenzeller G, Lee H, et al. Outbreak of sandfly fever in central Iraq, September 2007. Mil Med 2008;173(10):949–53.
30. Chinikar S, Ghiasi SM, Hewson R, Moradi M, Haeri A. Crimean–Congo hemorrhagic fever in

Iran and neighboring countries. J Clin Virol 2010;47(2):110–14.

31. Khan NA, Azhar EI, El-Fiky S, et al. Clinical profile and outcome of hospitalized patients during first outbreak of dengue in Makkah, Saudi Arabia. Acta Trop 2008;105(1):39–44.

32. Kariv R, Klempfner R, Barnea A, Sidi Y, Schwartz E. The changing epidemiology of leptospirosis in Israel. Emerg Infect Dis 2001;7(6):990–2.

33. Sebek Z, Bashiribod H, Chaffari M, Sepasi F, Sixl W. The occurrence of leptospirosis in Iran. J Hyg Epidemiol Microbiol Immunol 1987;31 (4 Suppl.):498–503.

34. Gunaid AA, Nasher TM, el-Guneid AM, et al. Acute sporadic hepatitis in the Republic of Yemen. J Med Virol 1997;51(1):64–6.

35. Meltzer E, Artom G, Marva E, Assous MV, Rahav G, Schwartz E. Schistosomiasis among travelers: new aspects of an old disease. Emerg Infect Dis 2006;12(11):1696–700.

36. Meltzer E, Percik R, Shatzkes J, Sidi Y, Schwartz E. Eosinophilia among returning travelers: a practical approach. Am J Trop Med Hyg 2008;78 (5):702–9.

37. Aronson NE, Wortmann GW, Byrne WR, et al. A randomized controlled trial of local heat therapy versus intravenous sodium stibogluconate for the treatment of cutaneous *Leishmania major* infection. PLoS Negl Trop Dis 2010;4(3):e628.

38. Rendi-Wagner P, Tobias J, Moerman L, et al. The seroepidemiology of *Bordetella pertussis* in Israel—estimate of incidence of infection. Vaccine 2010;28(19):3285–90.

39. Dilli D, Bostanci I, Dallar Y, Buzgan T, Irmak H, Torunoglu MA. Recent findings on pertussis epidemiology in Turkey. Eur J Clin Microbiol Infect Dis 2008;27(5):335–41.

40. Kakar RM, Mojadidi MK, Mofleh J. Pertussis in Afghanistan, 2007–2008. Emerg Infect Dis 2009;15(3):501.

41. Meltzer E, Sidi Y, Smolen G, Banai M, Bardenstein S, Schwartz E. Sexually transmitted brucellosis in humans. Clin Infect Dis 2010;51(2):e12–15.

Chapter 15
Western Asia and the Middle East: Part 2

Jaffar A. Al-Tawfiq[1] and Ziad A. Memish[2]
[1]Speciality Internal Medicine Unit, Dhahran Health Center, Dhahran, Kingdom of Saudi Arabia
[2]Ministry of Health, Riyadh, Kingdom of Saudi Arabia

Zoonotic infection

Several important zoonoses must be considered in returning travelers from the region. Febrile illness including endocarditis, osteomyelitis, and epididymo-orchitis are all common manifestations of brucellosis [1]. While Q fever is a pandemic cause of fever, it is increasingly recognized in travelers and local population in the region. Rabies is endemic throughout the region and several countries occasionally report outbreaks [2,3]. Anthrax must be considered in the setting of its classical presentation and is frequently reported from the region, especially from Turkey [4]. Echinococcosis is common in immigrants from the region but rarely reported in travelers. Echinococcosis is caused by the tapeworm *Echinococcus granulosus* and it is endemic in the Middle East and areas around the Mediterranean [5]. The most common sites of involvement are the lung the liver. The disease is slow and progressive in nature and is frequently discovered incidentally in patients presenting other unrelated complaints.

Another important zoonotic disease is brucellosis. The disease is caused by *Brucella* spp. and is transmitted from animals to humans by direct contact with infected animals or consumption of raw animal products such as unpasteurized milk or cheese [6]. Four species of the genus *Brucella* are pathogenic for humans and include *Brucella melitensis* (from sheep and goats), *Brucella abortus* (from cattle and other Bovidae), *Brucella suis* (from pigs), and *Brucella canis* (from dogs) [7]. It is estimated that the annual incidence of brucellosis in Saudi Arabia is between 9 and 21.4/100,000 population [6,8].

Antibiotic resistance

The rate of antimicrobial resistance in major human pathogens is increasing in many parts of the world and specifically in this region. Antimicrobial resistance is a major problem especially among gram-negative bacilli. For example, ciprofloxacin resistance of *Enterobacter cloacae* in Saudi Arabia has increased from 8.3% in 2000 to 17.4% in 2006 [9]. Similarly, other reports from the region documented the emergence of qnr-based quinolone resistance in *Enterobacter* and *Klebsiella* species. Fluoroquinolone resistance is a major concern with emerging problem in

Infectious Diseases: A Geographic Guide, First Edition.
Edited by Eskild Petersen, Lin H. Chen & Patricia Schlagenhauf.
© 2011 John Wiley & Sons, Ltd. Published 2011 by John Wiley & Sons, Ltd.

many countries in the Middle East. In one study, *Klebsiella pneumoniae* resistance to ciprofloxacin increased from 2.6% to 23% over time [10]. A high rate (31%) of resistance was also reported among community isolates of urinary isolates of *Escherichia coli* in Oman [11]. However, a much higher rate of ciprofloxacin resistance reaching 97.4% was reported from United Arab Emirates in *Pseudomonas aeruginosa* [12].

Resistance among *Streptococcus pneumoniae* is another concern. In a study of invasive pneumococcal disease, the rate of penicillin resistance reached up to 78% [13]. In addition, erythromycin resistance in this region is more prevalent in younger children, ranging from 8% in isolates of older children (under age 14) to 26% in isolates of children under 5 years of age. Cephalosporin resistance in invasive pneumococci reached 12% in children under age 12 in Qatar [13].

Acinetobacter baumannii is of particular importance due to the increasing number of bloodstream infections in patients at military medical facilities in which service members injured during Operation Iraqi Freedom [14]. Multidrug resistance among *A. baumannii* was documented in 14–35.8% of isolates [15,16]. Community-acquired methicillin-resistant *Staphylococcus aureus* (MRSA) has recently emerged in studies evaluating MRSA carriage among Palestinian population of the West Bank and Gaza [17].

Hajj—medical aspects

One of the unique aspects of the region is the Hajj pilgrimage. Every year millions of pilgrims from around the world gather under extremely crowded conditions in Makkah, Saudi Arabia, to perform the Hajj. Transmission of infectious diseases during the Hajj is a major concern during the extended stays at Hajj sites due to the physical exhaustion, extreme heat, and crowded accommodation. Two major outbreaks of meningococcal disease occurred in recent years associate with the annual Hajj pilgrimage to Makkah, Saudi Arabia. The first outbreak occurred in 1987 and was caused by *Neisseria meningitidis* serogroup A. The outbreak resulted in an attack rate of 640 per 100,000 American pilgrims. Subsequently, Saudi Arabia required vaccination against *N. meningitidis* serogroup A as a condition for receiving the Hajj visa. Serogroup W-135 was identified in 6.4% of 483 confirmed cases of meningococcal disease admitted to Mecca hospitals from 1987 through 1997. However, in the 2000 Hajj, more than 400 cases of W-135 infection in pilgrims and their close contacts were reported from 16 countries with an attack rate in returning pilgrims of 25–30 per 100,000 persons. Subsequently, quadrivalent vaccine has been required for entry into Saudi Arabia for the Hajj [18].

The number of pilgrims traveling to the Hajj, Saudi Arabia, 2006–2009 (1427H–1430H)

Year	Total number of international pilgrims
2006 (1427H)	1,653,912
2007 (1428H)	1,708,314
2008 (1429H)	1,729,669
2009 (1430H)	1,619,212

Data from Ref. [19].

Communicable diseases hazards at the Hajj

Communicable diseases
Meningococcal meningitis
Respiratory tract infections (upper and lower) including tuberculosis, viral infections, and community-acquired pneumonia
Poliovirus
Blood-borne diseases
Food poisoning
Zoonotic diseases

Data from Ref. [19].

The arbovirus that causes Alkhurma hemorrhagic fever emerged in the Kingdom of Saudi Arabia in the mid 1990s. Human and animal movements, especially those associated with the annual mass gathering event of Hajj (pilgrimage), may facilitate introduction into other continental masses, where it must be differentiated from dengue and other similar arboviral hemorrhagic fevers. In addition to dengue and Kadam viruses, which are known to be endemic in Saudi Arabia, it is thought that other flaviviruses exist in the region, though undetected [20].

A high incidence of respiratory infection, including influenza, has been reported at the Hajj in Makkah, Saudi Arabia. In a study of 260 pilgrims, 150 were from the United Kingdom and 110 were from Saudi; of those 38 (25%) UK pilgrims and 14 (13%) Saudi pilgrims had respiratory infections detectable by real time reverse transcriptase-polymerase chain reaction rtRT-PCR. Rhinovirus infection was present in 13% of the UK group and 3% of the Saudi group. The other isolated viruses included influenza virus, parainfluenza virus, and respiratory syncytial virus [21]. During the Hajj season, there is intense congestion, living in close proximity and the increasing number of elderly pilgrims. These factors may increase the risk of transmission of tuberculosis [19]. Moreover, many Muslims travel from countries of high tuberculosis endemicity. However, the risk of tuberculosis transmission during the Hajj season is not known. In a study from Singapore, 10% of 357 pilgrims showed a substantial rise in immune response to QuantiFERON TB assay antigens post-Hajj when compared to a pre-Hajj test [22].

Another respiratory illness that may be important during Hajj is pertussis. However, there is limited data on the prevalence of pertussis among Hajj pilgrims. One study showed that 1.4% of pilgrims acquired pertussis [23]. Thus, some authors recommended the administration of acellular pertussis vaccine to pilgrims before the Hajj season [23].

International spread of poliomyelitis through pilgrimage is a major concern for Saudi Arabia. Since poliomyelitis had not been eradicated in Afghanistan, India, Nigeria, and Pakistan, all pilgrims from these four countries, regardless of age and vaccination status, are required to show a proof of at least one dose of oral polio vaccine (OPV) 6 weeks or more prior departure in order to apply for an entry visa for Saudi Arabia. These travelers will also receive a dose of OPV at border points when arriving in Saudi Arabia [19].

Rift Valley fever (RVF) virus is a zoonotic virus causing severe disease, abortion, and death in domestic animals (especially young sheep, cattle, and goats) in Africa and the Arabian Peninsula. The first confirmed cases in the Arabian Peninsula occurred in September 2000 in the southwestern coastal Saudi Arabia and neighboring areas of Yemen. There were more than 120 human deaths and major losses in livestock populations from disease and slaughter [24,25]. Although there is a concern that increased rainfall in the Hajj area may lead to outbreak of RVF, there is no reported outbreaks of this disease among pilgrims.

Basic economic and demographic data

Basic demographics	GNI per capita (USD)	Life expectancy at birth (total, years)	School enrollment, primary (% net)
Armenia	3,350	74	85
Azerbaijan	3,830	67	95
Bahrain	17,390	76	98
Georgia	2,470	71	94
Iran	3,540	71	94
Iraq	NA	68	89
Jordan	3,310	73	89
Kuwait	38,420	78	88
Lebanon	6,350	72	83
Oman	12,270	76	73
Qatar	NA	76	93
Saudi Arabia	15,500	73	85
Syria	2,090	74	95
Turkey	9,340	74	92
United Arab Emirates	26,270	79	91
Yemen	950	63	75

World Bank (www.worldbank.org).
GNI, gross national income; NA, not available.

Causes of death in children under 5 years in Yemen, Armenia, and Saudi Arabia

	%		
	Yemen	Armenia	Saudi Arabia
Neonatal causes	33	48	100
Pneumonia	20	12	7
Diarrheal diseases	16	10	6
Malaria	7	0	0
HIV/AIDS	0	0	0
Measles	2	0	0
Injuries	4	6	14
Others	17	23	32

WHO, regional average, 2000–2003 (http://www.who.int/whosis/mort/profiles/en/#P).

Top 10 causes of death in all ages in Yemen, Armenia, and Saudi Arabia

	%		
	Yemen	Armenia	Saudi Arabia
Ischemic and hypertensive heart disease	12	35	17
Cerebrovascular disease	4	16	4
Lower respiratory infections	14	NS	6
Diarrheal disease	11	NS	2
Measles	NS	NS	NS
Chronic obstructive lung disease	NS	3	NS
Nephritis and nephrosis	2	NS	2
Diabetes	NS	6	2
Road traffic accidents	4	NS	6
Cancers	NS	8	NS
Inflammatory heart disease	NS	2	NS
Cirrhosis of the liver	2	2	NS

WHO, 2006 (http://www.who.int/whosis/mort/profiles/en/#P).
NS, not stated.

References

1. Memish ZA, Balkhy HH. Brucellosis and international travel. J Travel Med 2004;11(1):49–55.
2. David D, Dveres N, Yakobson BA, Davidson I. Emergence of dog rabies in the northern region of Israel. Epidemiol Infect 2009;137(4):544–8.
3. Seimenis A. The rabies situation in the Middle East. Dev Biol (Basel) 2008;131:43–53.
4. Doganay M, Metan G. Human anthrax in Turkey from 1990 to 2007. Vector Borne Zoonotic Dis 2009;9(2):131–40.
5. El Marsfy YS, Morsy TA. A preliminary study on echinococcosis in Riyadh, Saudi Arabia. J Pak Med Assoc 1975;25:10–11.
6. Al-Tawfiq JA, Abukhamsin A. A 24-year study of the epidemiology of human brucellosis in a health-care system in Eastern Saudi Arabia. J Infect Public Health 2009;2:81–5.
7. Godfroid J, Cloeckaert A, Liautard JP, et al. From the discovery of the Malta fever's agent to the discovery of a marine mammal reservoir, brucellosis has continuously been a re-emerging zoonosis. Vet Res 2005;36:313–26.
8. Pappas G, Papadimitriou P, Akritidis N, Christou L, Tsianos EV. The new global map of human brucellosis. Lancet Infect Dis 2006;6:91–9.
9. Al-Tawfiq JA, Antony A, Abed MS. Antimicrobial resistance rates of Enterobacter spp.: a seven-year surveillance study. Med Princ Pract 2009;18(2):100–4.
10. Al-Tawfiq JA, Antony A. Antimicrobial resistance of Klebsiella pneumoniae in a Saudi Arabian hospital: results of a 6-year surveillance study, 1998–2003. J Infect Chemother 2007; 13(4):230–4.
11. Al-Lawati AM, Crouch ND, Elhag KM. Antibiotic consumption and development of resistance among gram-negative bacilli in intensive care units in Oman. Ann Saudi Med 2000;20:324–7.
12. Al-Dhaheri AS, Al-Niyadi MS, Al-Dhaheri AD, Bastaki SM. Resistance patterns of bacterial isolates to antimicrobials from 3 hospitals in the United Arab Emirates. Saudi Med J 2009;30 (5):618–23.
13. Shibl A, Memish Z, Pelton S. Epidemiology of invasive pneumococcal disease in the Arabian Peninsula and Egypt. Int J Antimicrob Agents 2009;33(5):410.e1–9.
14. Centers for Disease Control and Prevention (CDC). Acinetobacter baumannii infections among patients at military medical facilities treating injured U.S. service members, 2002–2004. MMWR Morb Mortal Wkly Rep 2004;53(45):1063–6.

15. Al-Tawfiq JA, Mohandhas TX. Prevalence of antimicrobial resistance in *Acinetobacter calcoaceticus-baumannii* complex in a Saudi Arabian hospital. Infect Control Hosp Epidemiol 2007;28(7):870–2.

16. Mah MW, Memish ZA, Cunningham G, Bannatyne RM. Outbreak of *Acinetobacter baumannii* in an intensive care unit associated with tracheostomy. Am J Infect Control 2001;29:284–8.

17. Essawi T, Na'was T, Hawwari A, Wadi S, Doudin A, Fattom AI. Molecular, antibiogram and serological typing of Staphylococcus aureus isolates recovered from Al-Makased Hospital in East Jerusalem. Trop Med Int Health. 1998 Jul;3(7):576–83.

18. Al-Tawfiq JA, Clark TA, Memish ZA. Meningococcal disease: the organism, clinical presentation and worldwide epidemiology. J Travel Med 2010; 17(Suppl.): 3–8.

19. Memish ZA. The Hajj: communicable and non-communicable health hazards and current guidance for pilgrims. Euro Surveill 2010; 15(39):19671.

20. Memish ZA, Charrel RN, Zaki AM, Fagbo SF. Alkhurma haemorrhagic fever—a viral haemorrhagic disease unique to the Arabian Peninsula. Int J Antimicrob Agents 2010;36 (Suppl. 1):S53–7.

21. Rashid H, Shafi S, Haworth E, et al. Viral respiratory infections at the Hajj: comparison between UK and Saudi pilgrims. Clin Microbiol Infect 2008;14(6):569–74.

22. Wilder-Smith A, Foo W, Earnest A, Paton NI. High risk of *Mycobacterium tuberculosis* infection during the Hajj pilgrimage. Trop Med Int Health 2005;10(4):336–9.

23. Wilder-Smith A, Earnest A, Ravindran S, Paton NI. High incidence of pertussis among Hajj pilgrims. Clin Infect Dis 2003;37(9): 1270–2.

24. Centers for Disease Control and Prevention. Outbreak of Rift Valley fever—Saudi Arabia, August–October, 2000. MMWR Morb Mortal Wkly Rep 2000;49:905–8.

25. Miller BR, Godsey MS, Crabtee MB, et al. Isolation and genetic characterization of Rift Valley fever virus from *Aedes vexans arabiensis*, Kingdom of Saudi Arabia. Emerg Infect Dis 2002;8:1492–4.

Chapter 16
Eastern Europe

Natalia Pshenichnaya[1] and Malgorzata Paul[2]
[1]Department of Infectious Diseases, Rostov State Medical University, Rostov-on-Don, Russia
[2]Department and Clinic of Tropical and Parasitic Diseases, University of Medical Sciences, Poznan, Poland

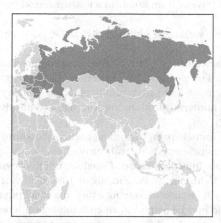

Belarus
Bulgaria
Czech Republic
Hungary
Moldova
Poland
Romania
Russian Federation
Slovakia
Ukraine

Bacteria

An increasing number of *Neisseria meningitidis* serotype C has been isolated from children, adolescents, and young adults (up to 64% of all isolates), including soldiers and military personnel, particularly a hypervirulent clonal complex ST-11/ET-37 of a high invasiveness [3,4]. Resistance in gram-positive and gram-negative bacteria is common including a high frequency of methicillin-resistant *Staphylococcus aureus* (MRSA). Tuberculosis is prevalent with drug-resistant and multi-drug resistant M. tuberculosis being an increasing problem. Infection with *Borrelia* spp. is common in forested areas. Small outbreaks of legionellosis are reported as nosocomial infections.

Viruses

Outbreaks of hepatitis A are recorded regularly and tick-borne encephalitis is seen throughout Russia and the eastern European countries. Eastern Europe (Russia, Ukraine, Bulgaria) Crimean Congo hemorrhagic fever is observed during warm season and Hemorrhagic fever with renal syndrome is registered in Russia, Czech Republic, Slovakia

Infectious Diseases: A Geographic Guide, First Edition.
Edited by Eskild Petersen, Lin H. Chen & Patricia Schlagenhauf.
© 2011 John Wiley & Sons, Ltd. Published 2011 by John Wiley & Sons, Ltd.

and northeast Poland. HIV is increasing among the homeless and intravenous drug abusers.

Parasites

Local transmission of malaria in Russia is low and unstable, and occurs in selected areas at the border with Azerbaijan, recreational lakes for swimming in the Moscow city and Moscow region. Autochthonous *Plasmodium vivax* infections are mostly reported among urban population and constitute up to 47.5% of all imported and domestic malaria cases registered in the Russian Federation every year. Tertian malaria should be considered in a differential diagnosis of a febrile traveler from Russia in a warmer season from late spring to early autumn.

Key symptoms are fever, chills, weakness, sweating, headache, bone and joint pain, anemia, and acute onset.

Infections very typical and characteristic for EE countries. Local outbreaks of trichinosis occurred in the most of eastern Europe territories. Infections caused by raw or under-cooked meat from wild animals (boar, bear) are typically observed in many members of the same family or in groups of hunters. Infections are seasonal, and mostly observed in spring and late autumn.

Key symptoms included fever, muscle pain, periorbital edema, abdominal pain, short-term waterly diarrhea, elevated muscle enzymes, and eosinophilia.

Echinococcus granulosus is a main infectious cause of single or multiple cystic lesions in the liver, mostly located in the right lobe. In Poland, about 10% of all space-occupying lesions in the liver are caused by *E. granulosus*. Having a dog in a small private farm and local slaughtering in a household may be helpful in an epidemiological interview. Cystic echinococcosis in humans from Central and East Europe is caused by "pig" strains of the parasite with genotypes G7 or G9. Infections with a "sheep" strain of *E. granulosus* which dominates in majority countries of the world have not been documented in countries of eastern Europe.

Key symptoms are abdominal discomfort, right upper quadrant pain, and liver cysts usually accidentally diagnosed by ultrasonography.

Due to some culinary traditions and dietary habits, taeniasis is a common intestinal parasitic infection in eastern Europe; *Taenia saginata* is the most prevalent species. Small outbreaks in families are reported. Cysticercosis due to a larval form of *Taenia solium* is sporadically observed in agricultural workers from pigs-raising areas with single, usually calcified, space-occupying lesions of the brain.

Toxocara cati and *canis* responsible for the syndromes of visceral or ocular larva migrans are frequently observed in children and adolescents, similarly from urban agglomerations and agricultural regions. Clinical picture includes hypereosinophilia with leucocytosis, hepatosplenomegaly, nonspecific abdominal pain, weight loss, subretinal or liver granulomas, visual impairment, asthma, chronic urticaria, and other allergic disorders.

CNS infections: meningitis and encephalitis

Acute infections with less than 4 weeks of symptoms

Frequently found microorganisms and conditions	Rare microorganisms	Very rare microorganisms
Viral meningitis (enterovirus group)	*Mycobacterium tuberculosis*	*Treponema pallidum* (neurosyphilis)
Pneumococcus spp. [1]	Human immunodeficiency virus, HIV	Influenza viruses
Arboviruses (tick-borne encephalitis)[a] [2]	*Leptospira* spp.	*Brucella* spp.
N. meningitidis—serogroup B and C [3,4]	Herpes virus (group I and II)	Listeria monocytogenes
Haemophilus influenzae serotype B[b]	*Enterobacteriaceae*	*Yersinia* spp.
	Pseudomonas aeruginosa	*Gnathostoma spinigerum*[c] [5]
	Borrelia burgdorferi genospecies (mostly *Borrelia garinii*)	*Angiostrongylus cantonensis*[c] [5]
	Enterococcus spp.	Lymphocytic choriomeningitis virus (LCMV)
		Lyssavirus (rabies)

[a]Except south of Russia and Ukraine.
[b]In children under 5 years.
[c]In the far-eastern Russia, Kamchatka Peninsula, and Northern Pacific Islands (Kurils).

CNS infections: meningitis and encephalitis with symptoms for more than 4 weeks and in the immunocompromised host

Microorganisms and conditions with symptoms for more than 4 weeks	Microorganisms in the immunocompromised host
HIV	Cytomegalovirus, CMV
Tuberculosis	Epstein–Barr virus, EBV
Neuroborreliosis	Herpes virus
Neurobrucellosis[a]	*Cryptococcus* spp.
T. solium (neurocysticercosis)	*Toxoplasma gondii*
Toxocara canis and *Toxocara cati*	

[a]Very rare.

Ear, nose, and throat infections

Ear, nose, and throat infections with symptoms for less than 4 weeks

Frequently found microorganisms	Rare microorganisms and conditions	Very rare microorganisms
Streptococcal throat infection [6,7]	Peritonsillar abscess[a]	*Corynebacterium diphtheriae*

(Continued)

Frequently found microorganisms	Rare microorganisms and conditions	Very rare microorganisms
EBV [7] Herpes virus (type I and II)	Tuberculosis Necrotizing fasciitis[b] *Yersinia enterocolitica, Yersinia pseudotuberculosis* Fusiform bacteria and spirochetes (Plaut–Vincent angina)	*Francisella tularensis* *L. monocytogenes*

[a]Require acute ENT evaluation.
[b]Require acute surgical evaluation.

Ear, nose, and throat infections with symptoms for more than 4 weeks and in the immunocompromised host

Microorganisms with symptoms for more than 4 weeks	Microorganisms in the immunocompromised host
M. tuberculosis *T. pallidum* (amygdalitis) EBV	*Candida* spp. Herpes virus (type I and II) CMV

Consider noninfectious causes like vasculitis and lymphoma.

Cardiopulmonary infections

Pneumonia with symptoms for less than 4 weeks

Frequently found microorganisms	Rare microorganisms and conditions	Very rare microorganisms
Streptococcus pneumoniae pneumonia [8–10] *Mycoplasma pneumoniae* [8]	*Legionella pneumophila* [8] Influenza *T. canis* and *T. cati*	*Chlamydia psittaci* *Chlamydia pneumoniae*

Endocarditis with symptoms for less than 4 weeks

Frequently found microorganisms	Rare microorganisms and conditions	Very rare microorganisms
Beta-haemolyticus Streptococcus (*Streptococcus viridans*) [11] Nonhemolytic streptococci *Enterococcus* spp. [11] *S. aureus* [11]	*P. aeruginosa* *Beta-haemolyticus Streptococcus* (group A, B, C, D) [11] *S. pneumoniae* Coagulase negative staphylococci (*Staphylococcus epidermidis*)	*Bartonella* spp. *Brucella melitensis* *Neisseria* spp. *Coxiella burnetti*

Frequently found microorganisms	Rare microorganisms and conditions	Very rare microorganisms
	Listeria endocarditis *B. burgdorferi* genospecies (mostly *B. garinii*)[a]	*Salmonella* spp.

[a]*Borrelia* may cause atrioventricular blocade.

Pulmonary symptoms for more than 4 weeks and in the immunocompromised host

Microorganisms and diseases with symptoms for more than 4 weeks	Microorganisms in the immunocompromised host
Tuberculosis *Aspergillus* *P. aeruginosa* *T. canis* and *T. cati* *Paragonimus westermani*[a]	*Pneumocystis jirovecii* CMV Fungi (*Aspergillus, Candida, Actinomyces, Nocardia*) *Strongyloides stercoralis*

Consider noninfectious causes like lung cancer, autoimmune lung fibrosis, Wegener's granulomatosis.
[a]In the Far East Russia.

Endocarditis for more than 4 weeks and in the immunocompromised host

Microorganisms and diseases with symptoms for more than 4 weeks	Microorganisms in the immunocompromised host
Coagulase negative staphylococci (*S. epidermidis*) Nonhemolytic streptococci *P. aeruginosa* HACEK group bacteria	*Aspergillus* *Candida* spp.

Consider noninfectious causes like sarcoidosis.

Gastrointestinal infections

Gastrointestinal infections with symptoms for less than 4 weeks

Frequently found microorganisms	Rare microorganisms and conditions	Very rare microorganisms and conditions
Salmonella (nontyphi) *Escherichia coli* [12] Rotaviruses[a] [13] *Campylobacter*	*Y. enterocolitica* *Clostridium difficile* *Bacillus cereus* toxin *Ascaris lumbricoides*	*M. tuberculosis* Morbus Whipple *Cryptosporidium* spp. *Entamoeba histolytica*

(*Continued*)

Frequently found microorganisms	Rare microorganisms and conditions	Very rare microorganisms and conditions
Enterobius vermicularis	Norovirus, calicivirus, and astravirus [13]	*Diphyllobothrium latum*
Giardia intestinalis	*P. aeruginosa*	*Trichuris trichiura*
Shigella spp.	*Vibrio parahaemolyticus*	*Anisakis simplex*[b]
	HIV-associated gastrointestinal infections	
S. aureus toxin		
Campylobacter spp.		

Consider noninfectious causes like inflammatory bowel disease and intestinal malignancies like colon cancer.
[a]Basically in children.
[b]In the Baltic, Okhotsk, and Bering Seas pericoastal areas.

Diarrhea is often associated with infections with bacteria, virus, and parasites. Repeated negative bacterial cultures and microscopy for parasites should lead to the consideration that the symptoms may not be caused by an infection. Inflammatory bowel diseases like ulcerative colitis and Crohn's disease should be considered in a differential diagnosis, and malabsorption and celiac disease must also be considered.

Gastrointestinal infections with symptoms for more than 4 weeks and in the immunocompromised host

Microorganisms and conditions with symptoms for more than 4 weeks	Microorganisms in the immunocompromised host
Tuberculosis	*Candida* spp.
Morbus Whipple	Herpes virus
Blastocystis hominis[a]	*Cryptosporidium* spp.
Dientamoeba fragilis[a]	*Mycobacterium avium* and *Mycobacterium intracellulare*
E. vermicularis	CMV
E. histolytica	*Isospora belli*
D. latum	Microsporidia
Taenia spp.	*S. stercoralis*
Hymenolepis nana	

Consider noninfectious causes like inflammatory bowel disease, intestinal malignancies like colon cancer, malabsorption, and celiac disease.
[a]Of uncertain pathogenicity in humans.

Infections of liver, spleen, and peritoneum

Acute infections of liver, spleen, and peritoneum with symptoms for less than 4 weeks

Frequently found microorganisms and conditions	Rare microorganisms	Very rare microorganisms
Hepatitis A	Hepatitis E	*Brucella* spp.

Frequently found microorganisms and conditions	Rare microorganisms	Very rare microorganisms
Hepatitis B Hepatitis C	*Leptospira* spp.	

Chronic infections of liver, spleen, and peritoneum with symptoms for more than 4 weeks and in the immunocompromised host

Microorganisms and conditions with symptoms for more than 4 weeks	Microorganisms in the immunocompromised host
Tuberculosis *Fasciola hepatica* and *Fasciola gigantica* *E. histolytica* *Opisthorchis felineus*[a] *Clonorchis sinensis*[b] *Echinococcus granulosus* and *Echinococcus multilocularis*[c] [28,29]	Herpes virus *M. avium* and *M. intracellulare* CMV

[a]In the basins of rivers of Russia (predominantly Ob, Irtysh, Kama, Volga, and also Don, Donets, Severnaya Dvina, Neman) and Ukraine (Dnepr).
[b]In Far East Russia.
[c]In the forests of northern Poland and the Carpathian Mountains.

Alveolar echinococcosis. *E. multilocularis* has become an emerging infection in majority of EE region; a number of new human cases are constantly increasing in Poland, Slovakia, and Czech Republic. Irregular space-occupying lesions of the liver with necrosis, fibrosis, calcifications, and a tendency to infiltration of adjacent tissues and organs, as well as a formation of distant metastases in CNS and lungs make a differential diagnosis difficult because of its clinical similarity to an advanced stage of liver malignancy. Living in forested areas of EE or working in forestry occupations, hunting, picking-up dry twigs, mushrooms, or blueberries are the main risk factors. So far, the infection has not been documented in children and young people.

Genitourinary infections

Cystitis, pyelonephritis, and nephritis with symptoms for less than 4 weeks

Frequently found microorganisms	Rare microorganisms and conditions	Very rare microorganisms
E. coli *Klebsiella pneumoniae* *Proteus mirabilis* [14] *P. aeruginosa* *S. aureus* *S. epidermidis* *Staphylococcus saprophyticus*	Perirenal abscess *Enterobacter* spp. [14] *P. aeruginosa* *Acinetobacter* spp. *Serratia marcescens* *Citrobacter* spp. *Candida albicans*	*M. tuberculosis* *Providencia, Morganella* spp. *H. influenzae, Haemophilus parainfluenzae* *Mycoplasma hominis* *Bordetella bronchiseptica* *Pasteurella* spp.

(Continued)

Frequently found microorganisms	Rare microorganisms and conditions	Very rare microorganisms
Enterococcus faecalis *Chlamydia trachomatis*	*Serratia* spp. *Klebsiella* spp. Hantavirus[a] [15] *Leptospira* spp.	

Consider noninfectious causes, especially malignancies like renal cell carcinoma.
[a]Except south of Russia and Ukraine.

Sexually transmitted infections with symptoms for less than 4 weeks

Frequently found microorganisms	Rare microorganisms and conditions	Very rare microorganisms
Chlamydia spp. *Neisseria gonorrhoeae* *Trichomonas vaginalis* *Ureaplasma urealyticum*	*Lymphogranuloma venerum* HIV *Mycobacterium genitalium,* *Mycobacterium hominis*	*Haemophilus ducreyi* *Calymmatobacterium granulomatis*

Cystitis, pyelonephritis, and nephritis with symptoms for more than 4 weeks and in the immunocompromised host

Microorganisms with symptoms for more than 4 weeks	Microorganisms in the immunocompromised host
Bacterial infections in patients with long-term catheters and renal stones *M. tuberculosis* *B. melitensis*	*Candida* spp. Herpes viruses type I, II

Consider noninfectious causes, especially malignancies like renal cell carcinoma.

Sexually transmitted infections with symptoms for more than 4 weeks and in the immunocompromised host

HIV should always be considered. The most common infections with a long incubation period are syphilis, herpes virus, and papillomavirus. In the immunocompromised host, diagnosis can be difficult as the antibody response may be false negative.

Joint, muscle, and soft tissue infections

Joint, muscle, and soft tissue infections with symptoms for less than 4 weeks

Frequently found microorganisms	Rare microorganisms and conditions	Very rare microorganisms and conditions
S. aureus *S. pneumoniae*	Necrotizing fasciitis (*Streptococcus pyogenes*) [16]	Fourniers gangrene (perineum and urogenital) [17]

Frequently found microorganisms	Rare microorganisms and conditions	Very rare microorganisms and conditions
Streptococcus agalactiae	Group C and G streptococci	
S. pyogenes	*S. epidermidis*	
Enterobacter spp.	*E. faecalis*	
Y. pseudotuberculosis,	*E. coli*	
Y. enterocolitica	*P. aeruginosa*	

Joint, muscle, and soft tissue infections with symptoms for more than 4 weeks and in the immunocompromised host

Microorganisms with symptoms for more than 4 weeks	Microorganisms in the immunocompromised host
B. burgdorferi and other species (mostly *B. garinii*) [18]	*Candida* spp.
M. tuberculosis	*Dirofilaria repens* [19]
Brucella spp.	

Skin infections

Skin infections with symptoms for less than 4 weeks

Frequently found microorganisms	Rare microorganisms and conditions	Very rare microorganisms and conditions
Erysipelas (*Streptococcus pyogenes*) [16], *S. pneumoniae*	*Erysipelothrix rhusiopathiae* [16]	Mycoses (*Candida, Trichophyton rubrum, Epidermophyton floccosum,* etc.)
S. aureus [16]	*H. influenzae* type B (HIB)	*Pasteurella multocida*
B. burgdorferi genospecies (mostly *B. garinii*) [18]	*Corynebacterium minutissimum*	*Mycobacterium leprae*[a] [20]
Herpes virus type I, II, III (VZV)	*Propionibacterium acnes*	Scabies
		Pediculus capitis, P. humanus Ancylostoma caninum Bacillus anthracis

[a]Very rare sporadic cases.

We have not listed a rash due to viral infections as this is not considered as an infection limited to the skin.

Skin infections with symptoms for more than 4 weeks and in the immunocompromised host

Microorganisms with symptoms for more than 4 weeks	Microorganisms in the immunocompromised host
T. pallidum	Mycoses (*Candida, Trichophyton, Epidermophyton*)
M. tuberculosis	*Strongyloides stercoralis*
M. leprae [20]	Atypical mycobacteria
Demodex folliculorum	
G. spinigerum[a]	

[a]In the far-eastern Russia, Kamchatka Peninsula, and Northern Pacific Islands.

Adenopathy

Adenopathy of less than 4 weeks' duration

Frequently found microorganisms	Rare microorganisms and conditions	Very rare microorganisms and conditions
EBV [21] CMV [21] *T. gondii* [21] HIV Adenovirus[a]	*F. tularensis* *Bartonella henselae* *M. tuberculosis* *Toxocara* spp.[a]	*Ehrlichia chaffensis* *Anaplasma phagocytophilum* *Babesia divergens* and *Babesia microti* Parvovirus B19 *Brucella* spp. *Rickettsia slovaca*[b]

[a]Basically in children.
[b]Formerly TIBOLA (tick-borne lymphadenopathy).

Adenopathy of more than 4 weeks' duration and in the immunocompromised host

Microorganisms with symptoms for more than 4 weeks	Microorganisms in the immunocompromised host
T. gondii *M. tuberculosis* *B. melitensis*	Adenovirus CMV *M. avium*

If the diagnosis is not made within a few days, biopsies should be performed to exclude malignancies like lymphoma and carcinomas.

Fever without focal symptoms

Fever less than 4 weeks without focal symptoms

Frequently found microorganisms and conditions	Rare microorganisms and conditions	Very rare microorganisms and conditions
Endocarditis EBV CMV *T. gondii* HIV *Trichinella* spp.	Tuberculosis *C. burnetti* *Leptospira* spp. *Yersinia* spp. *Borrelia* spp. (Lyme disease) Viral hepatitis viruses (HAV, HBV, HCV) CCHF virus[a], CFRS virus *P. vivax*[b] [22]	*Salmonella enterica* typhi, paratyphi A, B *Brucella* spp. Parvovirus B19 *E. chaffensis* [23] *A. phagocytophilum* [23] *B. divergens* and *B. microti* [24] *F. tularensis*

Frequently found microorganisms and conditions	Rare microorganisms and conditions	Very rare microorganisms and conditions
		Rickettsia prowazekii, *R. slovaca* [25] Hantaviruses [15]

[a]In the south of Russia.

[b]In the south of Russia, there is a rare domestic transmission of *P. vivax* malaria by a border with Azerbaijan. Also sporadic cases are rarely registered in the basins of rivers Don and Volga. In Moscow city and Moscow region, 30–47.5% of reported malaria infections are locally acquired every year, and actually a number of new *P. vivax* cases are significantly diminishing. Russian travelers infected abroad and local *Anopheles* mosquitoes multiplying in recreational lakes for swimming are the source of introduced malaria infection. All the strains of *P. vivax* are sensitive to chloroquine [22].

Fever for more than 4 weeks without focal symptoms and in the immunocompromised host

Microorganisms with symptoms for more than 4 weeks	Microorganisms in the immunocompromised host
T. gondii *M. tuberculosis* *B. melitensis*	CMV Adenovirus *E. chaffensis* *A. phagocytophilum*

Noninfectious causes should be considered from the beginning including malignancies like lymphoma and autoimmune diseases.

Eosinophilia and elevated IgE

Eosinophilia and elevated IgE for less than 4 weeks

Frequently found microorganisms	Rare microorganisms and conditions	Very rare microorganisms and conditions
A. lumbricoides and *Ascaris suum* *Trichinella spiralis*, *Trichinella britovi*, and *Trichinella pseudospiralis*[b], [26] *T. canis* and *T. cati* *T. saginata* *O. felineus*[d], *C. sinensis*[a] *E. vermicularis*	*S. stercoralis* *Ancylostoma* spp. *D. repens* *T. solium* *F. hepatica*, *F. gigantica* *E. granulosus* and *E. multilocularis*[c] [28,29]	*P. westermani*[a] [27] *A. cantonensis*[d] *H. nana*

[a]In Far East Russia.

[b]Outbreaks related to eating of raw meat from wild boars and domestic pigs.

[c]In the forests of northern Poland and the Carpathian Mountains.

[d]In the basins of rivers of Russia (predominantly Ob, Irtysh, Kama, Volga, and also Don, Donets, Severnaya Dvina, Neman) and Ukraine (Dnepr).

Eosinophilia and elevated IgE for more than 4 weeks and in the immunocompromised host

Microorganisms with symptoms for more than 4 weeks	Microorganisms in the immunocompromised host
A. lumbricoides and *A. suum* *E. granulosus* and *E. multilocularis* *T. canis* and *T. cati* *F. hepatica* and *F. gigantica* *H. nana*	*D. repens* *S. stercoralis*

Antibiotic resistance

Up to 12% of *S. pneumoniae* have resistance to first- and second-generation cefalosporines and macrolides, and more than 50% are resistant to co-trimoxazole and tetracyclines, and resistance to fluoroquinolones is increasing [10].

Ten to twenty percent of *Streptococcus pyogenes* are resistant to macrolides, and more than 50% to tetracyclines. Ten percent of *H. influenzae* are resistant to co-trimoxazole (sulfamethoxazole plus trimethoprim) and 15% to ampicillin [8,9,16].

Up to 20% of *S. aureus* are resistant to methicillin (MRSA), and resistance to macrolides and tetracyclines is also common. Hospital isolated *S. aureus* show a high frequency of resistance to lincosamides and aminoglycosides, and the number of ciprofloxacin-resistant strains approaches 40%. Over 60% of strains produce β-lactamase. MRSA is recorded in approximately 30% of hospital isolated strains [6,8,9]. Resistance to benzylpenicillin and oxacillin is almost universal.

In recent years in Russia, the high frequency resistance to ampicillin in community-acquired strains of *E. coli* has been found—uncomplicated infections, 37% and complicated, 46%, and for co-trimoxazole—uncomplicated infections, 21% and complicated, 30% [12,14].

The levels of primary drug-resistant *M. tuberculosis* vary from 12% to 18%. Levels of secondary drug resistance are in frames of 56–68%. Multi-drug resistance *M. tuberculosis* is detected in 4–5% of newly diagnosed patients and in 40–72% of previously treated patients. In newly diagnosed patients, resistance to streptomycin, rifampicin, and their combinations is common, whereas among treated patients, resistance to isoniazid, rifampicin, and streptomycin is seen in up to 30% of cases [30].

More than 60% of *P. aeruginosa* isolates are resistant to third-generation cephalosporins usually active against *Pseudomonas*, ciprofloxacin, gentamicin, netilmicin, and about 40% to piperacillin, ceftazidime, and amikacin. Resistance of *P. aeruginosa* to imipenem and meropenem has been found in up to 30% of isolates [16].

From 47% to 74% of strains in certain years were resistant to chloramphenicol, ampicillin, ceporin, neomycin, carbenicillin, and nalidixic acid [12].

N. meningitidis strains responsible for recent outbreaks of severe meningococcal sepsis in Poland were mostly susceptible to penicillin; and reduced susceptibility to benzylpenicillin was found in 10.1–32.1% of isolates [3].

Vaccine preventable diseases in children

The childhood vaccination programs have a high adherence in the republics of former Soviet Union (Russia, Belarus, Ukraine, Moldova). Among people who due to different reasons have not been vaccinated (migrants, homeless, peoples who refuse vaccinations for different reasons) or have low level of protecting antibodies, sporadic cases of diphtheria, mumps, rubella, small outbreaks of measles, and hepatitis A are seen. Vaccination against hepatitis A is not mandatory. Free of charge immunization program for children in Russia includes vaccination against tuberculosis, poliomyelitis, measles, mumps, rubella, diphtheria, whooping cough, tetanus, and hepatitis B. Also vaccination against HIB is available on a commercial basis. Seasonal vaccination against influenza is provided to children and groups of risks. In endemic areas, vaccination against tick-borne encephalitis is recommended.

In Poland, more than 95% of population are included into the national mandatory and free of charge immunization program for children and young people. Vaccinations against pneumococci, varicella, rotavirus, hepatitis A, influenza, and human papillomavirus are not implemented into the routine immunization schedule. A small number of local outbreaks of chickenpox, hepatitis A, mumps, and rubella are reported every year, but their incidence is decreasing. Congenital rubella is reported sporadically. Diphtheria has been successfully eliminated in the 1970s, and measles is in the process of eradication. The number of pertussis cases tends to fluctuations, but its actual occurrence is rapidly declining in teenagers after the mass introduction of the additional dose of vaccine at age of 6 years.

Meningococcal vaccine is not included into the mandatory vaccinations program. However, since 2003, vaccination against serogroup C meningococci is recommended for children above 2 years of age and for asplenic patients. In recent years, emerging outbreaks of severe invasive meningococcal disease associated with a high percentage of cases with fulminant septicemia (up to 62%) and a high case fatality rate of 42.9% have been seen. An increasing number of N. *meningitidis* serotype C have been isolated from children, adolescents, and young adults (up to 64% of all isolates), including soldiers and military personnel, particularly a hypervirulent clonal complex ST-11/ET-37 of a high invasiveness [3,4]. Because of the emerging epidemiological situation of severe meningococcal sepsis in the Polish army, a mass introduction of conjugated vaccine against meningococci group C in military recruits is actually considering.

For people staying in rural wooded areas of the northern part of the country or seasonally working in forestry occupations, especially young people involved in recreational outdoor activities from March to November, vaccination against tick-borne encephalitis (central European encephalitis virus) is strongly recommended.

Basic economic and demographic data

Basic demographics*	GNI[a] per capita (USD)	Life expectancy at birth (total, years)	School enrollment, primary (% net)
Belarus	5,380	70	90
Bulgaria	5,490	73	95
Czech Republic	16,600	77	93
Hungary	12,810	73	87
Moldova	1,470	69	88
Poland	11,880	75	96
Romania	7,930	73	94
Russian Federation	9,620	68	NS
Slovakia	14,540	74	92
Ukraine	3,210	68	89

*World Bank, 2008.
NS, not stated.
[a]Gross national income per capita.

Causes of death in children under 5 years—regional average

	%
Neonatal causes	44
Pneumonia	13
Diarrheal diseases	10
HIV/AIDS	0
Measles	0
Injuries	6
Others	25

WHO, 2000–2003 data.

Most common causes of deaths in all ages in Moldova, Russian Federation, and Czech Republic

	%		
	Moldova	Russian Federation	Czech Republic
Ischemic and hypertensive heart disease	39	30	25
Cerebrovascular disease	16	22	15
Cancers	1	6	13
Liver cirrhosis	8	2	2
Lower respiratory infections	2	NS	2
Tuberculosis	1		NS
Poisoning	NS	3	NS
Chronic obstructive pulmonary disease	4	NS	2
Falls	NS	NS	2
Road and traffic accidents	1	2	NS
Self-inflicted injuries	2	3	2
Violence	NS	2	NS

WHO, 2006.
NS, not stated.

References

1. Yakovlev SV. [Bacterial meningitis in the intensive care unit]. Consilium Medicum 2001;3:23–7 (Russian).
2. Donoso MO, Schädler R, Niedrig M. A survey on cases of tick-borne encephalitis in European countries. Euro Surveill 2008;13(17): pii:18848.
3. Skoczyńska A, Kadłubowski M, Knap J, et al. Invasive meningococcal disease associated with a very high case fatality rate in the North-West of Poland. FEMS Immunol Med Microbiol 2006;46:230–5.
4. Gryniewicz O, Kolbusz J, Rosinska M, et al. Epidemiology of meningococcal meningitis and changes in the surveillance system in Poland, 1970–2006. Euro Surveill 2007;12(5). Available online at http://www.eurosurveillance.org/ViewArticle.aspx?ArticleId=19786.
5. Ramirez-Avila L, Slome S, Schuster FL, et al. Eosinophilic meningitis due to *Angiostrongylus* and *Gnathostoma* species. Clin Infect Dis 2009;48:322–7.

6. Dvoretsky LI, Yakovlev SV. [Errors in antibiotic therapy respiratory tract infections in ambulatory practice]. Attend Phys 2003;8:1–8 (Russian).

7. Modestov AA, Sokovich OG, Terletska RN. [Current tendencies of respiratory diseases morbidity in the child population of the Russian Federation]. Siberian Med Rev 2008;6:3–8 (Russian).

8. Chuchalin AG, Synopalnikov AI, Strachunskiy LS, Kozlov RS, Rachina SA, Yakovlev SV [Community-acquired pneumonia in adults: practical recommendations for diagnosis, treatment and prevention]. Clin. Microbiol Antimicrob Chemother 2006;8(1):54–86 (Russian).

9. Tatochenko VK. Antibacterial therapy of pneumonia in children. Farmateka 2002;11:24–6.

10. Kozlov RS, Krechikova OI, Sivaya OV, et al. Antimicrobial resistance of *Streptococcus pneumoniae* in Russia: results of a prospective multicenter study. Clin Microbiol Antimicrob Chemother 2002;3:267–77.

11. Gurevich MA, Tazin SJ. [Features of modern infective endocarditis]. Russ Med J 1999;8: 27–32 (Russian).

12. Brodov LE, Yushchuk ND. [Infectious diarrhea]. Russ Med J 2001;9:679–83 (Russian).

13. Podkolzin AT, Fenske EB, Abramycheva EY, et al. [Seasonality and age structure of the morbidity by acute intestinal infections on the territory of the Russian Federation]. Ther Arch 2007;11:10–16 (Russian).

14. Moiseev SV. [Practical recommendations for antimicrobial therapy and prevention of urinary tract infections from the standpoint of evidence based medicine]. Infect Antimicrob Ther 2003;5:89–92 (Russian).

15. Sadkowska-Todys M, Gut W, Baumann, A, et al. [Occurrence of human *Hantavirus* infections in Poland]. Przegl Epidemiol 2007;61 (3):497–503 (Polish).

16. Zubkov MN. [Etiology and antimicrobial therapy of superficial and deep infections of skin]. Consilium Medicum 2002;4:6–9 (Russian).

17. Efimenko NA, Privolnev VV. [Fourniers gangrene]. Clin Microbiol Antimicrob Chemother 2008;10:34–42 (Russian).

18. Lencakova D, Hizo-Teufel C, Petko B, et al. Prevalence of *Borrelia burgdorferi* s.l. OspA types in *Ixodes ricinus* ticks from selected localities in Slovakia and Poland. Int J Med Microbiol 2006; S1:108–18.

19. Zarnowska-Prymek H, Cielecka D, Salamatin R. [Dirofilariasis—*Dirofilaria repens*—first time described in Polish patients]. Przegl Epidemiol 2008;62:547–51 (Polish).

20. Duyko VV, Gross OG, Riabukha MG. [Leprosy in the south of Russia]. Chief Doctor of Southern Russia 2007;3:21–5 (Russian).

21. Dvoretsky LI. [Differential diagnosis of lymphadenopathy. Manual of outpatient physician]. 2005;3(2). Available online at http://old.consilium-medicum.com/media/refer/05_02/3.shtml (Russian).

22. Leksikova LV, Savinkin VA. [Malaria situation in the Moscow region]. Med Parazitol (Mosk) 2009;1:19–21 (Russian).

23. Grzeszczuk A, Stanczak J, Kubica-Biernat B. Serological and molecular evidence of human granulocytic ehrlichiosis focus in the Bialowieza Primeval Forest (Puszcza Bialowieska), northeastern Poland. Eur J Clin Microbiol Infect Dis 2002;21:6–11.

24. Sinski E, Welc-Faleciak R. [*Babesia* spp. in Poland: the identity and epidemic reality]. Post Microbiol 2008;47(3):299–305 (Polish).

25. Chmielewski T, Tylewska-Wierzbanowska S. [New rickettsioses in Europe]. Post Microbiol 2008;47(3):307–311 (Polish).

26. Cabaj W. Wild and domestic animals as permanent *Trichinella* reservoir in Poland. Wiad Parazytol 2006;52(3):175–9.

27. Kaminsky YB, Sukhanov GI. [Lung fluke disease]. Med Newspaper 2002;37. Available online at http://medgazeta.rusmedserv.com/2002/37/article_782.html (Russian).

28. Dubinsky P, Malczewski A, Miterpakova M, Gawor J, Reiterova K, Girardoux P. *Echinococcus multilocularis* in the Carpathian regions of Poland and Slovakia. Helminthol J 2006;80: 243–7.

29. Gawor J, Malczewski A, Stefaniak J, et al. [Risk of alveococcosis for humans in Poland]. Przegl Epidemiol 2004;58(3):459–65 (Polish).

30. Vasilenko NV. [Monitoring drug resistance *Mycobacterium tuberculosis* in the Republic of Belarus]. Clin Microbiol Antimicrob Chemother 2005;7(2):17–21 (Russian).

Chapter 17
Northern Europe

Birgitta Evengård,[1] Audrone Marcinkute[2] and Eskild Petersen[3]
[1]Division of Infectious Diseases, Department of Clinical Microbiology, Umeå University, Umeå, Sweden
[2]University Hospital of Tuberculosis and Infectious Diseases, Vilnius, Lithuania
[3]Department of Infectious Diseases, Aarhus University Hospital, Skejby, Aarhus, Denmark

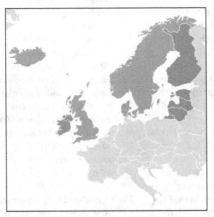

Denmark
Estonia
Finland
Iceland
Ireland
Latvia
Lithuania
Norway
Sweden
United Kingdom

The most common community-acquired infectious diseases are upper and lower respiratory tract infections, gastroenteritis, and urinary tract infections. Among vector-borne infections, *Borrelia* dominate but tick-borne encephalitis is found in the Baltic countries and parts of Sweden and a few cases have been reported from Denmark. The most common cause of viral meningitis is enterovirus, and herpes virus is the most common cause of encephalitis. Bacterial meningitis is rare and the most common causes are pneumococci and meningococci type B. Hepatitis A is very rare but local outbreaks are described from single imported cases. Hepatitis B is often sexually transmitted and B and C are usually related to intravenous drug abuse. Gastroenteritis due to virus is seen and food-borne outbreaks are rare but seen regularly due to virus and especially *Campylobacter* and *Salmonella* spp. (*Campylobacter*, the most reported in Sweden.) The prevalence of HIV is below 1% in the population and all patients are offered free antiretroviral treatment. Infections related to immunosuppressed patients like transplant recipients and patients for other reasons receiving immunosuppressive treatment are increasing primarily due to an increasingly aging population. Tuberculosis is still common in the Baltic countries where MDR is also a problem. Parasitic infections are rare, but waterborne outbreaks of *Giardia* have been described from Norway and Sweden. In the Baltic countries *Echinococcus multilocularis* seems to be spreading and *Trichinella* infections from consumption of infected meat has been described.

Infectious Diseases: A Geographic Guide, First Edition.
Edited by Eskild Petersen, Lin H. Chen & Patricia Schlagenhauf.
© 2011 John Wiley & Sons, Ltd. Published 2011 by John Wiley & Sons, Ltd.

CNS infections: meningitis and encephalitis

Acute infections with less than 4 weeks of symptoms

Frequently found microorganisms	Rare microorganisms	Very rare microorganisms
Viral meningitis (enterovirus group)	*Listeria monocytogenes*	Influenza
Pneumococcal meningitis	Neurosyphilis	*Naegleria* and other free-living
Herpes virus (group I and II) [1]	Human immunodeficiency virus (HIV)	ameba
Borrelia spp.	Tick-borne encephalitis (TBE)[a]	*Brucella*
Neisseria meningitidis	Tuberculosis	Rabies[b]
	Haemophilus influenzae[c]	

[a]Especially common in the Baltic countries and parts of Sweden. One case has been reported from Northern Sealand, Denmark.
[b]Rabies is found in bats, and persons exposed to bat bites should receive rabies postexposure immunization.
[c]Vaccination against *H. influenzae* has almost eradicated meningitis due to *H. influenzae* in Northern Europe.

CNS infections: meningitis and encephalitis with symptoms for more than 4 weeks and in the immunocompromised host

Microorganisms and conditions with symptoms for more than 4 weeks	Microorganisms in the immunocompromised host
HIV	CMV
Tuberculosis	Polyomavirus
Borreliosis	*Cryptococcus* spp.
Brucellosis	JC, BK virus or papovavirus
	Adenovirus
	Toxoplasma gondii
	Nocardia

Consider noninfectious causes like vasculitis and lymphoma.

Ear, nose, and throat infections

Ear, nose, and throat infections with less than 4 weeks of symptoms

Frequently found microorganisms	Rare microorganisms and conditions	Very rare microorganisms
Streptococcal throat infection	Peritonsillar abscess[a]	Diphtheria
Epstein–Barr virus (EBV)	Tuberculosis	*Fusobacterium necrophorum*
Herpes virus (type I and II)	Necrotizing fasciitis[a]	
Adenovirus	*Francisella tularensis*	

[a]Require acute ENT evaluation.

Ear, nose, and throat infections with symptoms for more than 4 weeks and in the immunocompromised host

Microorganisms with symptoms for more than 4 weeks	Microorganisms in the immunocompromised host
Tuberculosis *Actinomyces*	*Candida* Herpes virus Adenovirus *Aspergillus* Coxsackievirus

Consider noninfectious causes like vasculitis and lymphoma.

Cardiopulmonary infections

Pneumonia with less than 4 weeks of symptoms

Frequently found microorganisms	Rare microorganisms and conditions	Very rare microorganisms
Streptococcus pneumoniae [2] *Mycoplasma pneumoniae* [3] *Chlamydia pneumoniae* *H. influenzae* *Moraxella catarrhalis* *Staphylococcus aureus* Influenza	*Legionella* *Chlamydia psittaci* *Klebsiella pneumoniae* Puumala virus[b] *F. tularensis*	Diphtheria *Simkania negevensis* [4][a] Q fever *Ehrlichia* Anaplasma

[a]*S. negevensis* is an atypical bacteria like *Chlamydia* and *Mycoplasma*.
[b]Puumala virus belong to the Hantavirus group (Bunyaviridae). It is common in Northern Sweden, Finland, and the Baltic countries, especially in Estonia, but very rare in Denmark and has not been reported from the United Kingdom, Ireland, and Iceland.

Endocarditis with less than 4 weeks of symptoms

Frequently found microorganisms	Rare microorganisms and conditions	Very rare microorganisms
S. aureus [5] Nonhemolytic streptococci Coagulase-negative staphylococci (*Staphylococcus epidermidis*) *S. pneumoniae* *Enterococcus*	*Neisseria gonorrhoeae* *Coxiella burnetii* *Propionibacterium* HACEK group[a] *Salmonella*	*Bartonella* spp. *Brucella*

[a]*Haemophilus aphrophilus, Haemophilus paraphrophilus, Actinobacillus actinomycetemcomitans, Cardiobacterium hominis, Eikenella corrodens, Kingella kingae.*

Pulmonary symptoms for more than 4 weeks and in the immunocompromised host

Microorganisms and diseases with symptoms for more than 4 weeks	Microorganisms in the immunocompromised host
Chronic obstructive pulmonary disease (COPD)	*Pneumocystis jirovecii*
Tuberculosis	CMV
Aspergillus	*Aspergillus, Candida*
Adenovirus	*Pseudomonas aeruginosa*
C. pneumoniae, C. psittaci	*T. gondii*
	Influenza
	Herpes simplex

Consider noninfectious causes like lung cancer, autoimmune lung fibrosis, Wegener's granulomatosis.

Endocarditis for more than 4 weeks and in the immunocompromised host

Microorganisms and diseases with symptoms for more than 4 weeks	Microorganisms in the immunocompromised host
Coagulase-negative staphylococci (*S. epidermidis*)	*Aspergillus*
C. burnetii	*C. burnetii*
Nonhemolytic streptococci	

Consider noninfectious causes like sarcoidosis.

Gastrointestinal infections

Gastrointestinal infections with less than 4 weeks of symptoms

Frequently found microorganisms	Rare microorganisms and conditions	Very rare microorganisms
Norovirus and calicivirus	*Cryptosporidium* spp.	Tuberculosis
Campylobacter	*S. aureus* toxin	Morbus Whipple
VTEC	*Bacillus cereus* toxin	
Giardia intestinalis	*Ascaris lumbricoides*	
Salmonella (nontyphi)	*Entamoeba histolytica/Entamoeba dispar*[a]	
Enterobius vermicularis		
Adenovirus		
Rotavirus		

Consider noninfectious causes like inflammatory bowel disease and intestinal malignancies like colon cancer. Colitis ulcerosa and Mb Crohn are differential diagnosis and malabsorption and celiac disease must also be considered. Some parasites generally considered apathogenic might in some individuals cause symptoms and an ex juvantibus therapy can be indicated.

[a]Autochthonous intestinal and liver amebiasis is very rare in the Baltic countries, only *Entamoeba coli* is very prevalent. Diarrhea is often associated with infections with bacteria, virus, and parasites. Repeated negative bacterial cultures and microscopy for parasites should lead to the consideration that the symptoms may not be caused by an infection.

Gastrointestinal infections with symptoms for more than 4 weeks and in the immunocompromised host

Microorganisms with symptoms for more than 4 weeks	Microorganisms in the immunocompromised host
Giardia and *Cryptosporidium*	*Cryptosporidium*
Tuberculosis	CMV
Morbus Whipple	*Candida*
Blastocystis[a]	Herpes virus
Dientamoeba fragilis[a]	

Consider noninfectious causes like inflammatory bowel disease, intestinal malignancies like colon cancer, malabsorption, intestinal lymphoma, and celiac disease.

[a]Of uncertain pathogenicity in humans.

Hepatobiliary infections

Hepatitis with less than 4 weeks of symptoms

Frequently found microorganisms	Rare microorganisms and conditions	Very rare microorganisms
Hepatitis B	Hepatitis A	Tuberculosis
CMV	Hepatitis E	*T. gondii*
EBV	Hepatitis C	

Hepatitis with symptoms for more than 4 weeks and in the immunocompromised host

Microorganisms with symptoms for more than 4 weeks	Microorganisms in the immunocompromised host
Hepatitis B	Herpes virus
Hepatitis C	
Opisthorchis felineus[a]	

Consider noninfectious causes like autoimmune hepatitis, sarcoidosis, toxic reaction to drugs or other substances.

[a]Consider rare eosinophilic hepatitis cases.

Echinococcus multilocularis is found in wildlife in Svalbard islands, but no human cases has been reported [6]. A single case in a fox has been found in Denmark and in Sweden. Recently, the occurrence of *E. multilocularis* has been reported in the Baltics and in Sweden. In Lithuania, *E. multilocularis* was detected in 58.7% of red foxes and 8.2% of raccoon dogs. 0.8% dogs from rural areas in the southwestern parts of Lithuania were found infected with *E. multilocularis*. Necrotic lesions in pig livers in 0.4% of cases were identified as *E. multilocularis* by PCR. From 1997 to 2010, 127 human cases of *E. multilocularis* have been diagnosed in Vilnius, Lithuania.

Genitourinary infections

Cystitis, pyelonephritis, and nephritis with less than 4 weeks of symptoms

Frequently found microorganisms	Rare microorganisms and conditions	Very rare microorganisms
E. coli *K. pneumoniae* *Staphylococcus saprophyticus* *Proteus mirabilis* *Enterococcus faecalis*	Perirenal abscess Puumala virus[a] *P. aeruginosa* *Chlamydia trachomatis*	Tuberculosis

Consider noninfectious causes especially malignancies like renal cell carcinoma.

[a]Endemic in northern parts of Scandinavia and the Baltic countries where it causes epidemic nephrotic syndrome.

Sexually transmitted infections with less than 4 weeks of symptoms

Frequently found microorganisms	Rare microorganisms and conditions	Very rare microorganisms
Chlamydia spp. *N. gonorrhoeae* *Trichomonas vaginalis*	Lymphogranuloma venereum *E. dispar* and *E. histolytica* Syphilis	

Cystitis, pyelonephritis, and nephritis with symptoms for more than 4 weeks and in the immunocompromised host

Microorganisms with symptoms for more than 4 weeks	Microorganisms in the immunocompromised host
Bacterial infections in patients with long-term catheters and renal stones Tuberculosis	*Candida*

Consider noninfectious causes especially malignancies like renal cell carcinoma.

Sexually transmitted infections with symptoms for more than 4 weeks and in the immunocompromised host

Microorganisms with symptoms for more than 4 weeks	Microorganisms in the immunocompromised host
HIV Herpes virus type I,II Papillomavirus *T. pallidum*	HIV *Treponema pallidum*

Joint, muscle, and soft tissue infections

Joint, muscle, and soft tissue infections with less than 4 weeks of symptoms

Frequently found microorganisms	Rare microorganisms and conditions	Very rare microorganisms and conditions
S. aureus S. pneumoniae	Necrotizing fasciitis (group G streptococci)	Fournier's gangrene (perineum and urogenital) Sindbis virus

Joint, muscle, and soft tissue infections with more than 4 weeks of symptoms and in the immunocompromised host

Microorganisms with symptoms for more than 4 weeks	Microorganisms in the immunocompromised host
Borreliosis (Lyme disease) Tuberculosis	*Candida*

Reactive arthritis is common.

Skin infections

Skin infections with less than 4 weeks of symptoms

Frequently found microorganisms	Rare microorganisms and conditions	Very rare microorganisms and conditions
Erysipelas, *S. pneumoniae* S. aureus *Borrelia* spp. *Malassezia furfur*	Scabies Fungi	Rat-bite fever (*Spirillum minus*)

Rash due to viral infections has not been listed.

Skin infections with more than 4 weeks of symptoms and in the immunocompromised host

Microorganisms with symptoms for more than 4 weeks	Microorganisms in the immunocompromised host
Syphilis Tuberculosis	*Candida*

Rash due to viral infections has not been listed.

Infections due to streptococci (erysipelas) are common which may be complicated by staphylococci infection. Erythema migrans caused by *Borrelia* spp. is common. Scabies caused by the mite, *Sarcoptes scabiei*, is rare but seen also in outbreaks and in any skin disease with itching scabies should be considered.

Consider noninfectious causes like psoriasis. Consult a dermatologist if the condition is unclear.

Adenopathy

Adenopathy of less than 4 weeks' duration

Frequently found microorganisms	Rare microorganisms and conditions	Very rare microorganisms and conditions
EBV	Tularemia	*Ehrlichia*
Cytomegalovirus (CMV)	*Bartonella* spp.	*Babesia microti*
Parvovirus B19		
T. gondii		
HIV		

Adenopathy of more than 4 weeks' duration and in the immunocompromised host

Microorganisms with symptoms for more than 4 weeks	Microorganisms in the immunocompromised host
T. gondii	Adenovirus
Tuberculosis	CMV

If the diagnosis is not made within a few days, biopsies should be performed to exclude malignancies like lymphoma and carcinomas.

Fever without focal symptoms

Fever for less than 4 weeks without focal symptoms

Frequently found microorganisms and conditions	Rare microorganisms and conditions	Very rare microorganisms and conditions
Endocarditis	Tuberculosis	Tularemia
EBV	*C. burnetii*	*Ehrlichia*

(Continued)

Frequently found microorganisms and conditions	Rare microorganisms and conditions	Very rare microorganisms and conditions
CMV Parvovirus B19 *T. gondii* HIV	Puumala virus (epidemic nephrotic syndrome)	*Babesia* Sindbis virus (Ockelbo disease) Anthrax[a]

[a]Anthrax from contaminated heroin has been reported in heroin users in the United Kingdom.

Fever for more than 4 weeks without focal symptoms and in the immunocompromised host

Microorganisms with symptoms for more than 4 weeks	Microorganisms in the immunocompromised host
T. gondii Tuberculosis HIV	CMV Adenovirus Herpes virus

Noninfectious causes should be considered from the beginning including malignancies like lymphoma and autoimmune diseases.

Eosinophilia and elevated IgE

Eosinophilia and elevated IgE for less than 4 weeks

Frequently found microorganisms	Rare microorganisms and conditions	Very rare microorganisms and conditions
A. lumbricoides and *Ascaris suum* *Schistosoma* spp.[b]	*Toxocara* spp. [7] *Trichinella spiralis*[c]	*Strongyloides stercoralis*[a]

[a]Very rare in Baltic countries, but has been described.
[b]Free-living cercaria cause swimmer's itch.
[c]*T. spiralis* in humans have been reported from the Baltic countries.

Eosinophilia and elevated IgE for more than 4 weeks and in the immunocompromised host

Microorganisms with symptoms for more than 4 weeks	Microorganisms in the immunocompromised host
A. *lumbricoides* and A. *suum* *Schistosoma* spp.[a] *T. spiralis*[b] *Echinococcus granulosus*[c] and E. *multilocularis* Northern Sweden, Norway, and Finland?	*Toxocara* spp. S. *stercoralis*

[a]Free-living cercaria cause swimmer's itch.

[b]*T. spiralis* in humans have been reported from the Baltic countries. Between 1999 and 2008, a total of 359 cases were registered, including 66 sporadic cases and 42 outbreaks. An outbreak of trichinellosis, with affected 107 people, due to wild boar meat was detected in Lithuania in June 2009. During these 10 years, the incidence of trichinellosis decreased from 1.7 to 1.2 cases per 100,000 population. Fifty-eight percent of the cases were due to consumption of meat from home-raised pigs, 10% due to infected wild boar meat, and 8% due to illegal sale of meat.

[c]*E. granulosus* is endemic in reindeers and wolves in Finland, but human cases have not been reported [8]. The last human autochthonous case in Sweden was in 1984 [9]. Human infections with E. *granulosus* is of increasing concern in Lithuania. 13.7% of rural dogs and pigs were found to be infected with E. *granulosus* in South West Lithuania.

Antibiotic resistance

Methicillin-resistant *Staphylococcus aureus* (MRSA) is common in the United Kingdom, but is still rare in Scandinavia and increasing especially in Finland [10]; however, the problem with community-acquired MRSA is increasing as in other parts of Europe [11]. In Scotland 7.5% of patients were colonized with MRSA on admission to hospital [12]. In Lithuania 11.4–12% of S. *aureus* seems to be methicillin resistant. Vancomycin-resistant *Enterococcus faecalis* is rare in Baltic countries, but increasing in vancomycin-resistant *Enterococcus faecium* (10.5% cultures of E. *faecium* were resistant in 2009).

In Lithuania penicillin-resistant pneumococci were identified in 6.5% of cases in 2009. Ampicillin- and trimethoprim/sulfamethoxazole-resistant *Salmonella* are very common in Lithuania. E. *coli* ciprofloxacin resistant in 14.6% of culture cases. Ciprofloxacin-resistant *Campylobacter jejuni* was in 21.1% of isolates.

Vaccine-preventable diseases in children

The childhood vaccination programs have a high adherence in the Scandinavian countries and in Baltic countries, but small outbreaks due to imported cases are seen in the age groups which are not yet immunized [13]. Measles is increasing in Ireland with substantial transmission [14]. Two cases of measles among adults, imported from United Kingdom and Italy, were registered in Lithuania in 2010. Mumps has been reported in the United Kingdom in 2010 and occasional outbreaks of pertussis are also seen.

Basic economic and demographic data

	GNI per capita (USD)	Life expectancy at birth (total, years)	School enrollment, primary (% net)
Denmark	59,130	78	96
Estonia	14,270	73	95
Finland	48,120	79	96
Iceland	40,070	81	97
Ireland	49,590	79	96
Latvia	11,860	71	90
Lithuania	11,870	71	91
Norway	87,070	80	99
Sweden	50,940	81	94
United Kingdom	45,390	79	97

GNI, gross national income.
World Bank, 2008.

Causes of death in children under 5 years—regional average

	%
Neonatal causes	44
Pneumonia	13
Diarrheal diseases	10
HIV/AIDS	0
Measles	0
Injuries	6
Others	25

WHO, 2000–2003 data.

Ten most common causes of death in all ages in three countries selected for a regional low (Latvia), middle (Iceland), and high (Norway) BNI per capita

	%		
	Latvia	Iceland	Norway
Ischemic and hypertensive heart disease	30	22	20
Cerebrovascular disease	22	10	11
Lower respiratory infections	NS	5	6
Inflammatory heart disease	2	NS	NS
Alzheimer and other dementias	NS	5	3

	%		
	Latvia	Iceland	Norway
COPD	NS	4	4
Road traffic accidents	2	NS	NS
Cancers	8	16	13
Falls	NS	1	2
Self-inflicted injuries	2	NS	NS

WHO, 2002.
NS, not stated.

References

1. Aurelius E, Forsgren M, Gille E, Sköldenberg B. Neurologic morbidity after herpes simplex virus type 2 meningitis: a retrospective study of 40 patients. Scand J Infect Dis 2002;34:278–83.
2. Korsgaard J, Møller JK, Kilian M. Antibiotic treatment and the diagnosis of *Streptococcus pneumoniae* in lower respiratory tract infections in adults. Int J Infect Dis 2005;9(5):274–9.
3. Ragnar Norrby S. Atypical pneumonia in the Nordic countries: aetiology and clinical results of a trial comparing fleroxacin and doxycycline. Nordic Atypical Pneumonia Study Group. J Antimicrob Chemother 1997;39:499–508.
4. Heiskanen-Kosma T, Paldanius M, Korppi M. *Simkania negevensis* may be a true cause of community acquired pneumonia in children. Scand J Infect Dis 2008;40:127–30.
5. Knudsen JB, Fuursted K, Petersen E, et al. Infective endocarditis: a continuous challenge. The recent experience of a European tertiary center. J Heart Valve Dis 2009;18:386–94.
6. Fuglei E, Stien A, Yoccoz NG, et al. Spatial distribution of *Echinococcus multilocularis*, Svalbard, Norway. Emerg Infect Dis 2008;14:73–5.
7. Stensvold CR, Skov J, Møller LN, et al. Seroprevalence of human toxocariasis in Denmark. Clin Vaccine Immunol 2009;16:1372–3.
8. Hirvelä-Koski V, Haukisalmi V, Kilpelä SS, Nylund M, Koski P. *Echinococcus granulosus* in Finland. Vet Parasitol 2003;111:175–92.
9. Akuffo H (ed). Parasites of the Colder Climates. London, UK: Taylor and Francis, 2003.
10. Skov R, SSAC MRSA Working Party. MRSA infections increasing in the Nordic countries Denmark, Finland, Iceland, Norway, Sweden. Euro Surveill 2005;10:pii2765.
11. Skov RL, Jensen KS. Community-associated methicillin-resistant *Staphylococcus aureus* as a cause of hospital-acquired infections. J Hosp Infect 2009;73:364–70.
12. Reilly JS, Stewart S, Christie P, et al. Universal screening for methicillin-resistant *Staphylococcus aureus*: interim results from the NHS Scotland pathfinder project. J Hosp Infect 2010;74:35–41.
13. Groth C, Bottiger B, Plesner A, Christiansen A, Glismann S, Hogh B. Nosocomial measles cluster in Denmark following an imported case, December 2008–January 2009. Euro Surveill 2009;14:19126.
14. Gee S, Cotter S, O'Flanagan D; National Incident Management Team. Spotlight on measles 2010: measles outbreak in Ireland 2009–2010. Euro Surveill 2010;15:19500.

Chapter 18
Southern Europe

Francesco Castelli, Fabio Buelli and Pier Francesco Giorgetti
Institute for Infectious and Tropical Diseases, University of Brescia, Brescia, Italy

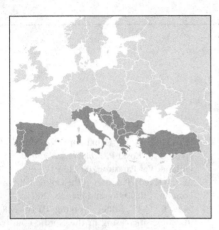

Albania	Portugal
Andorra	San Marino
Bosnia and	Serbia
Herzegovina	Slovenia
Croatia	Spain
Cyprus	The Former Yugoslav Republic of
Gibraltar	Macedonia (FYROM in the text)
Greece	Turkey
Holy See	
Italy	
Malta	
Montenegro	

In this chapter, the following countries will be considered as part of Southern Europe (http://www.nationsonline.org/oneworld/index.html) as they share common character-istics from the epidemiological standpoint: countries of the Iberian and Italian penin-sulas, most of the Balkan countries, Cyprus, Malta, and Turkey. The total population of the region is 220 million of inhabitants and the average number of tourists per year is 180 millions.

Southern Europe is a temperate climate region acting as a bridge between the South and the North, located at the crossroad of migration. Apart from pandemic infections, such as infections with Human Immunodeficiency Virus (HIV), Hepatitis B Virus (HBV) and Hepatitis C Virus (HCV), Southern Europe offers peculiar epidemiological features that may be considered. This is mainly due to the presence of specific possible vectors of viral (Tuscany virus, etc.) and protozoan (*Leishmania*, potentially *Plasmodium vivax* malaria) infections. These features make Southern Europe at risk for vector-borne emerging dis-eases, such as Chikungunya, dengue, and West Nile, as recently demonstrated although sporadically. Due to its warm climate and long seashores, Southern Europe may also be potentially considered a suitable place for the transmission of fecal-oral pathogens (hepatitis A, typhoid fever, traveler's diarrhea, etc.) although the dramatic improvement of hygienic conditions during the last decades has substantially decreased this risk.

Infectious Diseases: A Geographic Guide, First Edition.
Edited by Eskild Petersen, Lin H. Chen & Patricia Schlagenhauf.
© 2011 John Wiley & Sons, Ltd. Published 2011 by John Wiley & Sons, Ltd.

The high antibiotic pressure exerted on in the past decades on many bacterial species has given rise to the worrying phenomenon of bacterial drug resistance in the region, particularly in those countries with higher living standards. Unfortunately epidemiological data on many infectious diseases are limited (*Bartonella*, *Borrelia*), with uncertain prevalence and incidence values.

Infectious diseases in travelers

To assess an ill returning traveler, the knowledge of the incubation periods of the suspected infectious diseases is of great support.

Infectious diseases with incubation periods shorter than 4 weeks

Infectious diseases with short incubation periods are more easily related to the recent travel.

Possible etiologic agents by clinical presentation

Undifferentiated fever:
  Malaria[a]
  Rickettsial infections[a]
  Typhoid and paratyphoid fevers[a]
  Brucellosis[a]
  Leptospirosis
  Acute HIV infection
  Toxoplasmosis
  Relapsing fevers

Fever associated with respiratory findings:
  Pneumonia due to common bacterial and viral agents
  Influenza
  Legionellosis
  Q fever

Fever associated with hemorrhage:
  Viral hemorrhagic fevers (Crimean–Congo)[a]
  Leptospirosis and other acute bacterial infections

Fever associated with the involvement of the central nervous system:
  Arbovirus encephalitis (tick-borne encephalitis, West-Nile virus infection, Chikungunya virus infection, viral infection transmitted by sandfly)[a]
  Rabies[a]
  Meningococcal meningitis
  Other viral or bacterial causes of meningitis or encephalitis

Gastrointestinal infections:
  Infectious diarrhea (infections due to *Campylobacter*, *Salmonella*, *Shigella* and other bacterias, viral infections)[a]
  Hepatitis A

Fever associated with genitourinary findings:
  Urinary tract infections
  Sexually transmitted diseases

[a]Description of the disease follows in the text.

Epidemiological details of some infections that may be encountered by travelers to South Europe are provided below.

Malaria   Risk of contracting malaria is present only in the south-eastern part of Turkey from May to October and the infection is exclusively due to *P. vivax*. For those who travel in this region, the following measures are recommended: (i) mosquito bite prevention and (ii) chloroquine chemoprophylaxis [1]. Turkish provinces with low risk of malaria infection are: Adana, Adiyaman, Batman, Bingöl, Bitlis, Diyarbakir, Elazig, Gaziantep, Hakkâri, Hatai, K. Maras, Kilis, Mardin, Mus, Osmaniye, Sanliurfa, Sirnak, Siirt, and Van [2]. After nearly 50 years, an autochthonous case of *P. vivax* malaria has recently been reported in the Aragon region of Spain in October 2010. The presence of a potential malaria vector (*Anopheles atroparvus*) in Southern Europe (i.e., Italy and Greece) requires careful surveillance.

Rickettsial infections   The most common rickettsial infection in Southern Europe is *Mediterranean spotted fever* due to *Rickettsia conorii*, transmitted to humans by tick bite. The disease is present in Albania, Andorra, Bosnia and Herzegovina, the coastal region of Croatia, in Cyprus and Greece, in the southern regions and islands of Italy, in the former Yugoslav Republic of Macedonia (FYROM), Malta, Montenegro, and Portugal, in the south of Spain, Serbia, Slovenia, and Turkey. In rural areas of certain countries, the seroprevalence of the infection in humans can be as high as 44% [3]. The murine typhus (*Rickettsia typhi*) is sporadically observed. Travelers who have been camping or hiking are to be considered at higher risk of contracting the infection.

Typhoid and paratyphoid fevers   Typhoid fever (due to *Salmonella enterica* serotype typhi) and paratyphoid fever are two of the most important infectious diseases in developing countries, whereas in Southern Europe they have a low incidence rate. However, the global diffusion of enteric fevers urges the medical practitioner to consider this differential diagnosis while approaching to a traveler coming back from this region and clinical findings suggestive for the disease. As to countries of Southern Europe, those of the Iberian and Italian peninsulas have an incidence rate lower than 10 cases per 100,000 population/year, whereas those of the Balkan peninsula, Cyprus, Malta, and Turkey show an incidence rate between 10 and 100 per 100,000 population/year. However, more than 50% of the notified cases are imported cases contracted abroad [4].

Brucellosis   Brucellosis is present in every country of the region and is due to *Brucella melitensis*, *Brucella abortus*, and *Brucella suis*. It is mainly a professional disease and those who work in contact with animals show a seroprevalence of about 3%, as reported in Spain [5]. Among the animals responsible for the transmission of disease (ovine, bovine, swine), the proportion of the affected cattle has been reported to be around 20–30% [6]. The disease is spread in Albania, Bosnia, Croatia, in north-western and central regions of Greece, in the south of Italy, in the FYROM, Montenegro, Portugal, Slovenia, Spain, and Turkey; the highest annual incidence rates, despite still very low, are reported in Greece, Italy, Portugal, and Spain (from 0.3 to 0.9 per 100,000 population/year) [7]. In Andorra and Malta no cases have been notified in recent years, whereas in Cyprus, previously declared brucellosis-free, the disease reemerged during last decade, even if with very low incidence rates.

Crimean–Congo hemorrhagic fever Crimean–Congo hemorrhagic fever (CCHF) virus has been reported in more than 30 countries in Africa, Asia, south-eastern Europe, and the Middle East. As for Southern Europe, the virus is present in the Balkan region (sporadic cases are reported every year and during 2003 and 2004 two outbreaks occurred in this area, respectively, in Albania and Kosovo) [8,9] and in Turkey, especially in the middle and eastern Anatolia region where the number of cases has been increasing over the years since 2002 [10]. During 2008, the first CCHF case was notified in the north of Greece [11].

Tick-borne encephalitis Tick-borne encephalitis (TBE) is the most common encephalitis due to a Flavivirus in Europe. The main subtype is the European one, responsible for less severe diseases than those due to the Siberian or Far Eastern viruses. The disease starts with an uncharacteristic influenza-like illness. After a symptom-free interval, the neurological involvement appears (meningitis, meningoencephalitis, meningoencephalomyelitis, or meningoencephalo-radicu-litis). The disease is spread in the south of Albania, in the northern regions of Bosnia and Herzegovina, in Croatia, in the north of Greece, in the north-east of Italy, in the FYROM, Serbia and Montenegro, and Slovenia. Countries of Balkan Peninsula show the highest prevalence rates [12]. In Slovenia, the disease accounts for 28.8% of encephalitis in children [13]. In Spain and Portugal, TBE is not indigenous. In Turkey, there are no confirmed cases of the disease [14]. TBE vaccine should be considered for all persons living in TBE-endemic areas, for those at occupational risk in endemic areas (e.g., farmers, forestry workers, and soldiers) and for travelers to rural endemic areas during late spring and summer [15].

West Nile virus West Nile virus is transmitted by infected *Culex* mosquitoes and is present in all countries of Southern Europe. The infection can be asymptomatic or associated with an influenza-like illness (fever, headache, vomiting, conjunctivitis, eye pain, and anorexia). In some cases patients can develop neurological signs due to the presence of encephalitis. It is present in the coastal region of Albania, in Andorra, Bosnia and Herzegovina, Cyprus, Croatia, Greece, in north-eastern regions of Italy (during 2009 16 cases were reported in Veneto, Emilia–Romagna, and Lombardia) [16], in the FYROM, Malta, Serbia and Montenegro, in southern regions of Portugal, in Slovenia, Spain and in the central regions of Turkey. Recently, in August 2010, an outbreak occurred in Greece and Turkey, with 14 deaths and more than 100 confirmed cases of the disease.

Chikungunya virus The Chikungunya virus is present in more than 40 countries (mainly in Africa and Asia) and is transmitted by infectious mosquitoes (*Aedes albopictus* also known as the "tiger mosquito"). In Southern Europe the disease has been identified only in Italy, where an outbreak occurred in Emilia–Romagna during 2007, introduced by a man coming from the Indian state of Kerala [17]. In the following years no other new cases were notified, but this episode suggests the chance of a stable introduction of the virus in the region in the future.

Diseases transmitted by sand flies Sand flies may be responsible for the transmission of many viral, bacterial (bartonellosis), and protozoan (leishmaniasis) diseases. Among viruses responsible for human diseases, in Southern Europe the Tuscany virus, the Sicily and Naples viruses can be encountered. Other viruses have been isolated from asymptomatic carriers, even if currently no data are available on their pathogenicity for human host: the Corfu virus (identified in Greece and closely related to the Sicily virus), Arbia virus, Punta Toro virus, Chandipura virus, and Changuinola virus.

These viruses are endemic in Europe and, although a limited number of cases have been reported in few states, their presence might extend to all areas where carriers are present [18].

Tuscany virus　Tuscany virus is generally responsible for asymptomatic infections. However, in some cases a flu-like syndrome occurs and, due to its neurotropism, meningitis and/or encephalitis are also reported. Cases of neurological involvement were reported in Cyprus, Greece, Italy, Portugal, Spain, and Turkey. In Italy, particularly in spring and summer, Tuscany virus is one of the three most frequent causes of viral meningitis. Tuscany virus infections should always be investigated should a traveler with signs and symptoms of meningoencephalitis return from Southern Europe [18].

Sicily and Naples viruses　The illness caused by Sicily or Naples viruses is a flu-like syndrome consisting of fever, eyes' pain, bone pain, and fatigue, which usually resolves in about a week. Cases of human disease and isolation of vectors are reported in Cyprus, Italy, Portugal, states of former Yugoslavia (especially Serbia), and Turkey [18].

Rabies　In Southern European countries, rabies infection usually affects wild animals (foxes, bats, and raccoons in particular) rather than domestic ones. The virus affects the central nervous system causing progressive paralysis, encephalitis, and coma. Based on the WHO assessment of risk of infection, Southern European countries can be divided into low-risk (Andorra, Cyprus, Greece, Italy, Malta, Portugal, and Spain), medium-risk (Slovenia), and high-risk (Albania, Bosnia and Herzegovina, Croatia, Macedonia, Serbia, Montenegro, and Turkey) countries [19]. Recently, an outbreak of animal rabies in northern Italy has been documented after many years of absence of the diseases in the country: since October 2008 more than 100 confirmed cases of rabies were reported in wild and domestic animals in two regions of northern Italy, Friuli Venezia Giulia and Veneto [20].

In cases of exposure to a suspected infected animal, postexposure prophylaxis is mandatory. Pretravel vaccination is to be considered according to the estimated risk of the travel.

Infectious diarrhea　Diarrheal diseases are directly related to hygienic environmental condition and alimentary practices. The etiological spectrum of traveler's diarrhea is composed principally by bacterial agents (*Escherichia coli*, *Salmonella* spp., *Campylobacter* spp., *Shigella* spp., etc.), but also by enteropathogenic viruses (more than 70% of diarrheal cases in children in Albania) [21] and, especially in immunocompromised patients, protozoa such as *Entamoeba histolytica* and/or *Giardia lamblia* (4–5% of all cases). Diarrhea episodes that are bacterial or viral in nature usually have a short incubation period (less than 2 weeks) with acute course, while protozoan forms normally follow a more chronic course (see chapter "Infectious diseases with incubation periods longer than 4 weeks").

Infectious diseases with incubation periods longer than 4 weeks

Infectious diseases with long incubation periods may be more difficult to approach from an epidemiological standpoint. The most important etiological entities by clinical presentations are listed below.

Possible etiologic agents by clinical presentation

Undifferentiated fever:
  Leishmaniasis[a]
  HIV/AIDS infection
  HBV and/or HCV infection

Fever and respiratory symptoms:
  Tuberculosis[a]

Fever and gastrointestinal symptoms:
  Protozoan diarrhea

---

[a]Description of the disease follows in the text.

Leishmaniasis In Southern Europe, leishmaniasis is mainly caused by *Leishmania donovani* and *Leishmania infantum*, even *Leishmania tropica* has been detected in some cases. The two main clinical forms of leishmaniasis are (i) cutaneous leishmaniasis, the most common form limited to skin involvement, and (ii) visceral leishmaniasis, the most serious and potentially lethal form with systemic spread of pathogens. In Southern Europe, visceral leishmaniasis also commonly affects HIV-infected patients. In these patients, the less pathogenic strains of *Leishmania* spp. can also spread and cause serious systemic disease [22]. The disease is common in the coastal regions of Albania, Serbia, and Slovenia (including islands), in Andorra, Bosnia and Herzegovina, Croatia, and Cyprus. It may also be encountered in some regions of Greece, Italy, and Spain, in Malta, Portugal, and in the south-east of Turkey.

Tuberculosis All countries of Southern Europe region normally report cases of tuberculosis, but substantial differences among countries exist. Tuberculosis epidemiological data (cases/ 100,000 inhabitants per year) permit to distinguish three different group of countries: (i) incidence rate less than 10 cases/100,000 (Cyprus, Italy, and Malta), (ii) from 10 to 25 cases/ 100,000 (Albania, Andorra, Gibraltar, Greece, and Slovenia), and (iii) more than 30 cases/ 100,000 (Portugal, Spain, Turkey, and ex-Yugoslavian countries, except Slovenia where tuberculosis vaccination is routinely administered within normal infant vaccination schedule) [23]. The possibility of active tuberculosis has to be taken into account when subjects with typical symptoms (persistence of cough, fever and loss of weight) report previous travels to high prevalence rate countries of the region.

Drug resistance

Although it is very difficult to compare countries with significantly different health expenditures, the drug resistance phenomenon toward the most common pathogens, such as *Streptococcus pneumoniae* and *E. coli*, is almost universally present due to the high and often inappropriate use of antibiotics in recent years (in Spain about 25% of pneumococcal strains is resistant to penicillin) [7]. Drug resistance to tuberculosis is different among states in the region: in Italy 17/4137 (0.41%) strains showed multidrug resistance (MDR strains) and eight cases of XDR (extensively drug-resistant tuberculosis) were reported from 2003 to 2005 [23]. The FYROM reported 6/698 (0.85%) cases of MDR strains in the same years with a double incidence than the Italian one. It is important to underline that differences in the disease reporting exist from country to country, also as a consequence of differences in diagnostic capacities, despite the intense efforts that have been made to enhance the level of monitoring and reporting. In Southern Europe, since the early 1990s after highly active antiretroviral therapy (HAART) has been made available, many HIV strains have become resistant to different classes of drugs, namely, nucleoside reverse transcriptase inhibitors (NRTIs), nonnucleoside reverse transcriptase inhibitors (NNRTIs), and protease inhibitors (PIs).

Recent studies show that as many as 5–20% of new HIV infections in Southern Europe are caused by HIV-resistant strains, requiring resistance testing to be performed before starting therapy in a naïve patient [24,25].

Vaccines

Infants' immunization schedule is substantially comparable among the different countries of Southern Europe. Vaccine for tetanus, diphtheria, and whooping cough (usually administered in combination) and polio and hepatitis B vaccine are compulsory in all the states in the region, although different coverage rates are recorded from state to state. BCG (Bacillus Calmette-Guerin) vaccine against tuberculosis is required only by some states in the region.

Vaccination coverage of the main vaccine-preventable diseases by country, according to WHO-UNICEF estimates [26]

	AL	AND	BiH	CY	E	GR	HR	I	M	MK	MNE	P	SLO	SRB	TR
BCG	97	/	95	/	/	91	99	/	/	98	95	98	/	98	96
DTP3	98	99	90	99	96	99	96	96	73	96	92	96	96	95	96
HepB3	98	96	90	96	96	95	97	96	86	95	87	96	/	93	92
MCV	97	98	93	87	98	99	98	91	82	96	86	95	95	95	97
Pol3	98	99	90	99	96	99	96	97	73	96	91	96	96	97	96
Hib3	98	97	80	96	96	83	96	96	73	82	87	96	95	94	96

International countries codes: AL, Albania; AND, Andorra; BiH, Bosnia and Herzegovina; CY, Cyprus; E, Spain; GR, Greece; HR, Croatia; I, Italy; M, Malta; MK, The former Yugoslav Republic of Macedonia; MNE, Montenegro; P, Portugal; SLO, Slovenia; SRB, Serbia; TR, Turkey.

Vaccine abbreviations: BCG, Bacillus Calmette-Guérin vaccine; DTP3, three doses Diphtheria-Tetanus-Pertussis vaccine; HepB3, three doses Hepatitis B vaccine; MCV, Measles-Containing vaccine; Pol3, three doses Polio vaccine; HiB3, three doses Haemophilus influenzae type B vaccine.

Travelers to Southern Europe may be willing to consider the following specific vaccination should condition of risk exist: hepatitis A, cholera, typhoid fever, *Haemophilus influenzae* B, rabies, human papilloma virus (HPV), measles and rubella, *S. pneumoniae*, rotavirus, TBE, and tuberculosis. Each traveler should check his/her own immunization coverage and update his/her vaccination schedule. At present, no Southern European country requires yellow fever vaccination for those entering the national territory with the notable exception of Albania that requires yellow fever vaccination certificate from travelers coming from yellow fever-endemic regions.

References

1. WHO. International travel and health. Situation as on January 1, 2010. WHO Library Cataloguing-in-Publication Data 2010:198–225.

2. International Association for Medical Assistance to Travelers. Available at http://www.iamat.org/country_profile.cfm?id=100.

3. Punda-Polic V, Klismanic Z, Capkun V. Prevalence of antibodies to spotted fever group rickettsiae in the region of Split (southern Croatia). Eur J Epidemiol 2003;18:451–5.

4. Crump JA, Luby SP, Mintz ED. The global burden of typhoid fever. Bull World Health Organ 2004;82:346–53.

5. Villamarin-Vazquez JL, Chva-Nebot F, Arnedo-Pena A. Seroprevalencia de brucelosis en trabajadores agrícolas de las comarcas costeras de Castellón, España. Salud Pública Méx 2002;44: 137–9.

6. Reviriego FL, Moreno MA, Doninguez L. Risk factors for brucellosis seroprevalence of sheep and goat flocks in Spain. Prev Vet Med 2000;44:167–73.

7. ECDC. Annual Epidemiological Report on Communicable Diseases in Europe 2009. Available from http://www.ecdc.europa.eu/en/publications/Publications/0910_SUR_Annual_Epidemiological_Report_on_Communicable_Diseases_in_Europe.pdf.

8. Maltezou HC, Andonova L, Andraghetti R, et al. Crimean-Congo hemorrhagic fever in Europe: current situation calls for preparedness. Euro Surveill 2010;15(10):19504. Available from http://www.eurosurveillance.org/ViewArticle.aspx?ArticleId=19504.

9. Ahmeti S, Raka L. Crimean-Congo haemorrhagic fever in Kosova: a fatal case report. Virol J 2006;3:85.

10. Yilmaz GR, Buzgan T, Irmak H, et al. The epidemiology of Crimean-Congo hemorrhagic fever in Turkey, 2002–2007. Int J Infect Dis 2009;13(3):380–6.

11. Papa A, Maltezou HC, Tsiodras S, et al. A case of Crimean-Congo haemorrhagic fever in Greece, June 2008. Euro Surveill 2008;13(33):18952. Available from http://www.eurosurveillance.org/ViewArticle.aspx?ArticleId=18952.

12. Süss J. Tick-borne encephalitis in Europe and beyond—the epidemiological situation as of 2007. Euro Surveill 2008;13(26):18916. Available from http://www.eurosurveillance.org/ViewArticle.aspx?ArticleId=18916.

13. Ckižman M, Jazbec J. Etiology of acute encephalitis in childhood in Slovenia. Pediatr Infect Dis J 1993;12(11):903–8.

14. Esen B, Gozalan A, Coplu N, et al. The presence of tick-borne encephalitis in an endemic area for tick-borne diseases, Turkey. Trop Doct 2008;38(1):27–8.

15. Hayasaka D, Goto A, Yoshii K, Mizutani T, Kariwa H, Takashima I. Evaluation of European tick-borne encephalitis virus vaccine against recent Siberian and far-eastern subtype strains. Vaccines 2001;19(32):4774–9.

16. Rizzo C, Vescio F, Declich S, et al. West Nile virus transmission with human cases in Italy, August—September 2009. Euro Surveill 2009;14(40):19353. Available from http://www.eurosurveillance.org/ViewArticle.aspx?ArticleId=19353.

17. Rezza G, Nicoletti L, Angelini R, et al. Infection with Chikungunya virus in Italy: an out break in a temperate region. Lancet 2007;370:1–7.

18. Depaquit J, Grandadam M, Fouque F, Andry P, Peyrefitte C. Arthropod-borne viruses transmitted by Phlebotomine sandflies in Europe: a review. Euro Surveill 2010;15(10):19507. Available from http://www.eurosurveillance.org/ViewArticle.aspx?ArticleId=19507.

19. Rabies Information System of the WHO Collab Centre for Rabies Surveillance and Research. Available from http://www.who-rabies-bulletin.org/Travel/Recommendations.aspx.

20. OIE-WAHID. Disease Summary. Available from http://www.oie.int/wahis/public.php?page=event_summary&reportid=7444.

21. Fabiana A, Donia D, Gabrieli R, et al. Influence of enteric viruses on gastroenteritis in Albania: epidemiological and molecular analysis. J Med Virol 2007;79(12):1844–9.

22. Alvar J, Cañavate C, Gutiérrez-Solar B, et al. Leishmania and human immunodeficiency virus coinfection: the first 10 years. Clin Microbiol Rev 1997;10:298–319.

23. WHO. TB countries profiles 2007. Available from http://www.euro.who.int/en/what-we-do/health-topics/diseases-and-conditions/tuberculosis/country/work.

24. Ceccherini-Silberstein F, Cento V, Calvez V, Perno CF. The use of HIV resistance tests in clinical practice. Clin Microbiol Infect 2010;16 (10):1511–7.

25. Deenan P. Current patterns in the epidemiology of primary HIV drug resistance in North America and Europe. Antivir Ther 2004;9:695–702.

26. WHO-UNICEF. Estimates of immunization coverage for single countries. Available from http://apps.who.int/immunization_monitoring/en/globalsummary/countryprofileselect.cfm.

Chapter 19
Western Europe

Peter J. de Vries
Division of Infectious Diseases, Tropical Medicine and AIDS, Academic Medical Center, Amsterdam, the Netherlands

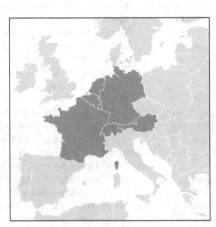

Austria
Belgium
France
Germany
Liechtenstein
Luxembourg Monaco
the Netherlands
Switzerland

The epidemiology of infectious disease in Western Europe is dominated by infections typical of industrialized, urbanized regions in the temperate climate zones. Public health policies, including mass vaccination, has reduced the incidence of community-acquired infections. Most infections are airborne respiratory tract infections. Food-borne gastro-intestinal infections are relatively rare. Zoonotic and parasitic infections are rare. Their distribution varies with changing landscape and climate. Vector-borne infections are mainly tick borne. Leishmaniasis and *Aedes albopictus*-transmitted dengue and Chikungunya have been reported in Southern France. STIs have become rare. Prevalence of antibiotic resistance varies and is partly associated with extensive use of antibiotics in the bioindustry.

Infectious Diseases: A Geographic Guide, First Edition.
Edited by Eskild Petersen, Lin H. Chen & Patricia Schlagenhauf.
© 2011 John Wiley & Sons, Ltd. Published 2011 by John Wiley & Sons, Ltd.

Introduction

The region defined as Western Europe encompasses different ecological regions: the river delta region of the Netherlands and Belgium (Flanders) and the almost similar northwestern parts of France flanking the North Sea; the Pyrenees and Alpine region in Germany, France, Switzerland, Liechtenstein, and Austria; the Mediterranean zone of France and Monaco and the midland that connects the previous three.

The human infections in this region are dominated by diseases of crowding and not so much by zoonotic infections or vector-borne diseases. This is especially true for the lowlands that are characterized by a temperate sea climate, high population densities, intensive bioindustry, and little natural vegetation. The Alpine region with its highest peak reaching to 4.8 km above sea level, and the Pyrenees in France are far less densely populated and include large forested areas and parks that are frequented by tourists from all over Europe. In the winter season these regions are cold and covered with snow. The Mediterranean region has a dry subtropical climate which is suitable for vector-borne diseases, has variable population densities with large urbanized areas along the coast that attract large flocks of tourists in the summer. The midland is of variable nature but typically a mixture of agricultural land and coniferous and deciduous forests, the habitat for the European fauna that may serve as a zoonotic reservoir of particular diseases. Overall, the climate in Western Europe shows a seasonal pattern that affects the transmission patterns of infectious diseases. The effects of global warming are not yet clearly visible on disease transmission with perhaps the exception of bluetongue, a vector-borne viral infection of ruminants, that recently showed up in Northwestern Europe [1].

Endemic communicable infections will be discussed in the following with frequent reference to European (EU) Surveillance data [2]. The large group of ubiquitous, opportunistic, or nosocomial infections will only be mentioned if there is a particular condition such as antibiotic nonsusceptibility that deserves mentioning.

CNS infections: meningitis, encephalitis, and other infections with neurological symptoms

Acute infections with less than 4 weeks of symptoms

Frequently found microorganisms and conditions	Rare microorganisms and conditions	Very rare microorganisms and conditions
Viral meningitis (enterovirus group)	*Listeria monocytogenes*	*Naegleria* and other free-living ameba
Meningococcal meningitis	Neurosyphilis	Influenza
Pneumococcal meningitis		
Herpes virus (group I and II)	Human immunodeficiency virus (HIV)	*Brucella*
Borrelia	Tick-borne encephalitis	

CNS infections: meningitis and encephalitis with symptoms for more than 4 weeks and in the immunocompromised host

Microorganisms with symptoms for more than 4 weeks	Microorganisms in the immunocompromised host
HIV	*Nocardia*
Tuberculosis	Polyomavirus
Neuroborreliosis	*Cryptococcus*
	Adenovirus

Enterovirus infections   Enterovirus infections are the most common cause of viral meningitis, especially in children. Nonpolio enterovirus infections show a seasonal pattern with peaks in the summer and early fall extending into the cold season [3,4].

Meningococcal meningitis   *Neisseria meningitidis* serotypes B and C are the most frequent cause of bacterial meningitis, especially in the younger age group in Western Europe. The introduction of the conjugated meningococcal serogroup C vaccine caused a significant decrease in serogroup C infections.

Pneumococcal meningitis   The notification rate of invasive pneumococcal disease in the EU zone is approximately 6 per 100,000, with the highest incidence in winter time [2]. Pneumococcal meningitis is not counted separately. Elderly and under fives are the most affected groups.

Viral meningoencephalitis   Severe viral CNS infections are predominantly caused by herpes simplex virus (HSV) followed by varicella zoster virus infections [5].

Neuroborreliosis   The causative agents of borreliosis, *Borrelia burgdorferi* sensu stricto, *Borrelia garinii* and *Borrelia afzelii* and other species in the *B. burgdorferi* sensu lato complex, have been isolated from castor bean ticks (*Ixodes ricinus*) and vertebrate hosts from all over Europe, except the Mediterranean coast and the altitudes above 1,500 m [6–9]. Tick infestation rates are on average 7%, low in the low countries and high in the Alpine area.

Listeriosis   *Listeria monocytogenes* infection may present as a febrile gastroenteritis, associated with consumption of food products such as soft cheese or meat/pork/chicken products. Elderly and immunocompromised individuals are at risk for septicemia and meningoencephalitis [10]. The EU zone average notification rate is 0.34 per 100,000, with a small increase over the last years [2,11].

Tuberculosis   Notification rates of tuberculosis are very low in Western Europe and one- to two-thirds of all cases have a foreign origin.

Syphilis   Syphilis is rare in Western Europe although the incidence increased over the last decade, mainly among men having sex with men (MSM) [12]. Syphilis of the central nervous system is a very rare complication and is often associated with HIV infection.

HIV   CNS manifestations of acute and chronic HIV-1 infections (meningitis, cranial nerve involvement, major cognitive or motor disorder, dementia, and encephalopathy) are rare.

Tick-borne encephalitis The European subtype of tick-borne encephalitis virus (TBEV-Eu) is transmitted by *I. ricinus* and endemic in parts of Austria, Switzerland, and Germany. Sporadic cases have been reported from France [13]. There is no TBEV in the Benelux. Transmission to humans is associated with leisure activities and collecting forest products and is highest during the summer months.

Two TBEV-Eu strain-based vaccines are marketed in Western Europe. In Austria, people in risk areas, are routinely being vaccinated.

Free-living ameba The chronic granulomatous amebic encephalitis (GAE) caused by *Acantha-moeba* spp. and *Balamuthia mandrillaris* particularly affects immunocompromised individuals. *Naegleria fowleri* may cause an acute, more fulminant, necrotizing, hemorrhagic meningoen-cephalitis in children and young adults [14].

Acanthamoeba spp. are ubiquitous and have been isolated from soil, fresh and brackish waters, and a range of water-containing appliances. *B. mandrillaris* has not been reported from Western Europe. *N. fowleri* proliferates in water at ambient temperatures above 30°C. Swimming in unchlorinated pools or thermal effluents from nuclear power plants is a risk factor, notably during summer.

Influenza Neurological complications of influenza are rare and follow the epidemiology of respiratory influenza, i.e., almost exclusively during the cold season (the months with an "R").

Capnocytophaga canimorsus *Capnocytophaga canimorsus* infection is sporadic and occurs after a dog or cat bite. Sepsis occurs more frequently than meningitis. Male sex, asplenia, and alcohol abuse are risk factors [15].

Brucellosis Brucellosis is extremely rare in Western Europe. Sporadic cases are often imported from endemic areas or associated with imported food products that bypassed the routine food control systems.

CNS infections in the immunocompromised host

Nocardiosis Nocardiosis is ubiquitous. Inhalation, but also ingestion, intravenous inoculation by IV drug users, and direct skin inoculation are means of infection. The incidence is very low in Western Europe.

Polyomaviruses JC virus causes progressive multifocal leukoencephalopathy and is probably transmitted via close human to human contact. It is a common infection that causes disease almost exclusively in AIDS and otherwise immunocompromised patients [16]. Polyomaviruses remain latent in the urinary tract. IgG prevalence rates were 58% for Swiss healthy blood donors and asymptomatic urinary shedding was 19% [17].

Cryptococcosis *Cryptococcus neoformans* meningitis used to be the most common opportunistic infection in AIDS. Sporadical cryptococcal infection of the CNS may occur in otherwise immunocompromised patients.

Adenovirus Adenovirus infections are very common and usually cause a mild upper respiratory tract infection, gastroenteritis, and/or conjunctivitis especially in infants and young children. Severe disease may occur in immunocompromised patients and is mainly associated with serotypes 3 and 7 [18].

Ear, nose, and throat infections

Ear, nose, and throat (ENT) infections with less than 4 weeks of symptoms

Frequently found microorganisms and conditions	Rare microorganisms and conditions	Very rare microorganisms
Acute otitis media Streptococcal throat infection Epstein–Barr virus (EBV) Herpes virus (type I and II)	Peritonsillar abscess[a] Tuberculosis Necrotizing fasciitis[a] Lemierre's syndrome[a]	

[a]Require acute ENT evaluation.

Acute otitis media Acute otitis media is most commonly caused by *Streptococcus pneumoniae*, *Haemophilus influenzae*, and *Moraxella catarrhalis*.

Bacterial infections of the ENT area Group A beta-hemolytic *Streptococcus pyogenes* infections of the throat are common in Western Europe, peaking during the winter. Ample use of antibiotics has reduced the incidence of rheumatic fever. Severe bacterial infection of the cervical regions, necrotizing fasciitis and Lemierre's syndrome, caused by fusobacteria, are rare conditions.

Diphtheria Diphtheria is not endemic in Western Europe anymore.

EBV infections rank third among the causes of tonsillitis in Europe after *Streptococcus* and adenovirus infections. There is no seasonal fluctuation.

Herpes labialis, caused by HSV-1, is common in Western Europe. Seroprevalence of HSV-1 is high, in most countries over 50% among the general population. HSV-2 seroprevalence is low.

Ear, nose, and throat infections with symptoms for more than 4 weeks and in the immunocompromised host

Microorganisms and conditions with symptoms for more than 4 weeks	Microorganisms in the immunocompromised host
Tuberculosis	*Candida* Herpes virus

Cardiopulmonary infections

Pneumonia with less than 4 weeks of symptoms

Frequently found microorganisms	Rare microorganisms and conditions	Very rare microorganisms and conditions
Streptococcus pneumoniae *Mycoplasma pneumoniae* *Chlamydia pneumoniae*	*Legionella* Influenza, parainfluenza and RSV	Diphtheria

Streptococcus pneumoniae   Pneumococcal pneumonia is a rather common disease in Western Europe. Underlying (pulmonary) disease, alcohol abuse, compromised immune system, and recent viral respiratory tract infections are risk factors.

Atypical pneumonia   *Mycoplasma pneumoniae* is the most common cause of primary atypical pneumonia. It is typically a disease of crowding and that explains why the incidence in young children increases parallel to the increase of attending day care centers [19]. *Chlamydia pneumoniae* is a rather common cause of mild respiratory tract infections.

(Para) influenza   The epidemiology of influenza in Western Europe follows that of influenza in the northern hemisphere. The peak season is in winter time, from October to April. Influenza A (H1N1) virus circulates in Western Europe since 2009–2010. Oseltamivir-resistant H1N1 influenza virus has been isolated in Western Europe.

Human H5N1 influenza were not reported from Western Europe, but infected birds have been isolated. An outbreak of H7N7 avian flu in the poultry industry led to a series of human infections in 2003, among which a few with fatal outcome.

Q fever   *Coxiella burnetii* is a gram-negative intracellular coccobacillus. Ruminants are the main zoonotic reservoir. Humans become infected by inhalation of infectious spores. The rapidly expanded goat industry in the Netherlands caused the largest and longest outbreak of Q fever in history starting in 2007. Incidence of human disease peaks in the months following the birth of lambs, especially when weather conditions are dry. Vaccination and culling measures have been put in place to curb the epidemic.

Legionellosis   *Legionella pneumophila* and other *Legionella* species may cause atypical pneumonia. They are ubiquitous gram-negative bacteria that live in water and moist conditions. Aspiration of aerosolized water such as in showers is the most common mode of infection. Regulations for and inspection of prevention of water infection in public spaces have been put in place in Western Europe. The notification rates, however, are still rather stable, ranging from approximately 10 to 20 per million population [2,20].

Tuberculosis   Tuberculosis is rare in Western Europe. Notification rates of tuberculosis in Western Europe are below or at the European average of 8 per 100,000 population. The proportion of HIV-infected patients among TB patients is not exactly known for all countries.

Endocarditis with less than 4 weeks of symptoms

Frequently found microorganisms	Rare microorganisms	Very rare microorganisms
Staphylococcus aureus	*Neisseria gonorrhoeae*	*Bartonella*
Nonhemolytic streptococci	*C. burnetii*	*Brucella*
Coagulase-negative staphylococci (*Staphylococcus epidermidis*)	*Propionibacterium*	
S. pneumoniae	HACEK group	
Enterococcus		

Endocarditis for more than 4 weeks and in the immunocompromised host

Microorganisms and diseases with symptoms for more than 4 weeks	Microorganisms in the immunocompromised host
Coagulase-negative staphylococci Nonhemolytic streptococci	*Aspergillus*

Endocarditis Infective endocarditis with underlying rheumatic heart disease declines whereas the proportion of patients undergoing valve surgery increased over the last decades. Intravenous drug use is a separate risk factor. The causative agents of endocarditis do not show an epidemiological pattern that is particular for Western Europe, except Q fever. Non-HACEK gramnegative endocarditis is rare and associated with intravascular medical devices and IV drug use.

Pulmonary symptoms for more than 4 weeks and in the immunocompromised host

Microorganisms and conditions with symptoms for more than 4 weeks	Microorganisms in the immunocompromised host
Chronic obstructive pulmonary disease (COPD) Tuberculosis *Aspergillus*	*Pneumocystis jirovecii* CMV *Aspergillus, Candida*

COPD-associated infections The most important geographical difference is the variable antibiotic susceptibility reported by country. This is, however, outweighed by individual factors such as previous use of antibiotics, recent hospitalization, and living in nursing homes.

Pneumocystis pneumonia *Pneumocystis jirovecii* is an ubiquitous agent with exposure in early life [21]. There is geographic variation in prevalence but no particular ecologic niche. Colonization is more common among patients with chronic disorders such as COPD. Pneumocystis pneumonia (PCP) occurs in patients with untreated AIDS and other immunodeficiencies.

Pulmonary aspergillosis *Aspergillus* infections of the lungs occur in immunocompromised patients, especially patients with hematological disorders and after bone marrow transplantation.

Gastrointestinal infections

Gastrointestinal infections with less than 4 weeks of symptoms

Frequently found microorganisms	Rare microorganisms and conditions	Very rare conditions
Norovirus and calicivirus *Campylobacter* ETEC/VTEC *Giardia intestinalis* *Salmonella* (nontyphi) *Enterobius vermicularis* (threadworm)	*Cryptosporidium* spp. *S. aureus* toxin *Bacillus cereus* toxin *Ascaris lumbricoides*	Tuberculosis Morbus Whipple

Frequently found microorganisms

Norovirus infections Norovirus infections (family Caliciviridae) of the gastrointestinal tract are highly contagious and secondary infections are frequent [22]. Outbreaks are a bit more prominent in the cold season but there is little seasonality.

Campylobacter *infections* *Campylobacter jejuni* is one of the most common causative agents of food-borne illness in Western Europe, with notification rates approaching 70 per 100,000 population predominantly in the younger age groups [23,24]. Infections often come in outbreaks associated with consumption of infected poultry and meat products. The highest incidence is reported during summer.

ETEC/VTEC Enterohemorrhagic or verocytoxin-producing *Escherichia coli* (ETEC and VTEC) infections are rare with a peak during the summer and young children being most vulnerable. Occasional outbreaks are associated with a common infected source of infected food. VTEC serogroup O 157 infections that predispose for hemolytic uremic syndrome (HUS) are prevalent in Western Europe. Infections are usually acquired through consumption of infected meat or mutton, but handling infected (pet) animals has also been reported.

Giardia intestinalis (duodenalis) Reported *G. intestinalis* infections are uncommon, but prevalence of carriership may be high in child day care centers. There is some seasonality, with most of the cases being reported during late summer and early autumn.

Salmonellosis *Salmonella typhi* and *Salmonella paratyphi* infections are almost exclusively imported from outside Western Europe. Intestinal *Salmonella* infections are common with peaks during the summer season. Infants and children are most affected. The majority of infections is caused by the serovars *Salmonella enteritidis* and *Salmonella typhimurium*, is associated with certain food products such as poultry/eggs and tends to come in outbreaks.

Enterobius vermicularis Infections by *E. vermicularis* (oxyuriasis) are not routinely notified. However, this infection is very common among infants and children in day care centers and primary schools.

Cryptosporidium spp. Cattle is the main reservoir of *Cryptosporidium* spp. Oocysts are particularly resistant, also against several disinfectants, and can be found in fresh surface water in Western Europe. Ingestion of contaminated swimming or drinking water is the route of infection. Cryptosporidiosis is usually a self-limiting disease. Immunosuppression, notably AIDS, may seriously aggravate the disease.

Staphylococcus aureus toxin food poisoning *S. aureus* growth is inhibited in the presence of other bacteria. Proliferation of *S. aureus* occurs in partially heated and not cool stored protein-rich food; this may lead to production of one of the 21 currently known heat-stable enterotoxins [25]. It is a rare event in the professional food industry because of strict regulations and control. Domestic infections do occur.

Bacillus cereus toxin food poisoning Survival of *B. cereus* endospores in improperly cooked food is another source of food poisoning with a short incubation time. *B. cereus* is considered a biohazard group 2 organism by the European Commission. Several *B. cereus* toxins have been identified that cause diarrhea or vomiting. The latter is associated with consumption of improperly cooked and stored rice. Outbreaks of *B. cereus* toxin-mediated food poisoning are rare.

Gastrointestinal infections with symptoms for more than 4 weeks and in the immunocompromised host

Microorganisms and conditions with symptoms for more than 4 weeks	Microorganisms in the immunocompromised host
Tuberculosis Morbus Whipple *Blastocystis* *Dientamoeba fragilis*	*Candida* Herpes virus

Tuberculosis   *Mycobacterium bovis* infections of cattle are rare. The Netherlands and Belgium received the "officially tuberculosis-free bovine herd" status (http://www.oie.int/eng/normes/mcode/en_chapitre_1.11.6.htm) [26]. Cattle infection rates in the other Western European countries are very low and pasteurization of milk effectively prevents transmission to humans. *M. bovis* also occurs in wild animals. *M. bovis* infections in AIDS patients may present as *Mycobacterium tuberculosis* infections and may occasionally spread from human to human [27].

Whipple's disease   This is a rare disease in Western Europe caused by the ubiquitous *Tropheryma whipplei*. There is no known geographic limitation [28].

Blastocystis hominis   *B. hominis* is an ubiquitous intestinal protozoan. Pathogenicity may depend on genotype. Carrier rates are rather high (30%) [24].

Dientamoeba fragilis   *D. fragilis* can be acquired in Europe. Transmission is probably through food but person to person transmission is also possible. Infection may be asymptomatic but also cause diarrhea or a chronic syndrome resembling irritable colon syndrome. Carrier rates are lower than for *B. hominis* (15%).

Candidiasis   Candida infections of the gastrointestinal tract occur mainly in immunocompromised patients (see earlier). Candida oesophagitis used to be a frequent problem of patients with untreated AIDS.

Herpes Simplex Virus (HSV) and CMV enteritis   HSV and CMV enteritis are rare complications of advanced immunosuppression.

Infections of the liver

Infections of the liver with symptoms for less than 4 weeks

Frequently found microorganisms	Rare microorganisms and conditions	Very rare microorganisms
	EBV CMV Hepatitis A Hepatitis E Leptospirosis	Varicella

Infections of the liver with symptoms for more than 4 weeks

Frequently found microorganisms	Rare conditions	Very rare microorganisms and conditions
	Hepatitis B	Hepatitis D
	Hepatitis C	*Fasciola hepatica*

Hepatitis A   Hepatitis A is not endemic anymore in Western Europe since more than a generation. Elderly people are also often seronegative. Small outbreaks occur after the holiday season, associated with introduction from immigrants who visited friends and relatives in endemic countries.

Hepatitis E   Hepatitis E is mainly seen as a rare travel-related disease, but locally acquired infections by rare zoonotic strains are repeatedly reported. Especially pigs serve as a zoonotic reservoir.

EBV   EBV infections are common (see earlier). Mild hepatic involvement is frequent, overt hepatitis is relatively rare but to date one of the most common causes of community-acquired hepatitis in Western Europe.

CMV   CMV infections in immunocompetent patients almost always involve the liver as indicated by slightly elevated blood transaminase concentrations. Overt hepatitis is rare.

Hepatitis B   Hepatitis B is a rare disease in Western Europe and confined to certain risk groups and behavior. IV drug users, MSM, hemodialysis patients and immigrants belong to the most affected groups. Most countries introduced hepatitis B vaccination, except the Netherlands, which caused a further decline of notification rates.

Hepatitis C   The notification of hepatitis C is slightly higher than for hepatitis B. This is mainly due the late diagnosis
   Transfusion hepatitis does not occur anymore due to thorough screening of blood products.

Hepatitis D (delta agent)   an incomplete virus that depends on the presence of hepatitis B virus (HBV), is very rare in Western Europe.

Other viral infections of the liver   Varicella used to be an infection of childhood. Immigrants from low endemic countries may develop chicken pox at later age. This may be complicated by hepatitis. Since the introduction of varicella vaccination, local transmission will soon come to a halt with the exception of regions with religious objections against vaccination such as the "bible belt" in the Netherlands.

Fascioliasis   In Europe *F. hepatica* infections are very rare due to the fact that wild water plants are not used for consumption. Cattle infections are still common in Western Europe (see following: Eosinophilia).

Genitourinary infections

Cystitis, pyelonephritis, and nephritis with less than 4 weeks of symptoms

Frequently found microorganisms	Rare microorganisms and conditions	Very rare microorganisms and conditions
E. coli *Klebsiella pneumoniae*	Perirenal abscess Hantavirus	Tuberculosis Leptospirosis

Cystitis, pyelonephritis, and nephritis with symptoms for more than 4 weeks and in the immunocompromised host

Conditions with symptoms for more than 4 weeks	Microorganisms in the immunocompromised host
Bacterial infections in patients with long-term catheters and renal stones Tuberculosis	*Candida*

Common bacterial infections of the genitourinary tract   The incidence of urinary tract infections in Western Europe does not show any difference from other regions. Common pathogens are *E. coli*, *Proteus* spp., and *Klebsiella* spp. Underlying disease and invasive procedures are risk factors. Hospitalization, living in nursery homes, or preceding antibiotic therapy increase the risk of antimicrobial resistance.

Hantavirus infection   There are three hantaviruses known to cause hemorrhagic fever with renal syndrome (HFRS) in Europe [29]. The predominant virus is Puumala virus (PUUV), causing nephropathia epidemica. The rodent reservoir, the bank vole, is prevalent in all countries of Western Europe except the Mediterranean coast. Rodent infestation rates are variable [9].

Tula virus, Seoul virus, Dobrava virus, and Saaremaa virus have been identified in rodents in various parts of Western Europe but human infections have not been confirmed unequivocally [30].

Leptospirosis   Leptospirosis is a relatively rare disease in Europe [31]. The most virulent serotype is *Leptospira icterohaemorrhagiae*, the causative agent of Weil's syndrome, but other serotypes such as *Leptospira grippotyphosa* and *Leptospira hardjo* have also been recognized. Leptospirosis is acquired through leisure activities, mainly by exposure to contaminated fresh surface water, or through occupational exposure (slaughter house workers, farmers, rat catchers, etc.). Active screening programs for cattle and dairy products are in place.

Sexually transmitted infections with less than 4 weeks of symptoms

Frequently found microorganisms	Rare conditions	Very rare microorganisms
Chlamydia *N. gonorrhoeae*	Lymphogranuloma venereum	

Chlamydia infections *Chlamydia* infections are the most frequently reported sexually transmitted disease (STI) in Europe. For Western Europe the notification rates are much lower than from Scandinavia and the United Kingdom. The age group of 15–44 years is most affected with a slight overrepresentation of females.

Lymphogranuloma venereum Lymphogranuloma venereum (LGV) is caused by *Chlamydia trachomatis* serotypes L1, L2 and L3. LGV is a rarely imported disease in Western Europe. LGV proctitis caused by serotype L2 occurs among men having sex with men, mostly HIV positive [32,33].

Neisseria gonorrhoeae Gonorrhea notification rates are approximately fourfold lower than for *C. trachomatis* but with the highest incidence in the same age groups. Rates are slightly higher for males than for females.

Sexually transmitted infections with symptoms for more than 4 weeks and in the immunocompromised host

Conditions with symptoms for more than 4 weeks	Microorganisms in the immunocompromised host
Syphilis	

Joint, muscle, and soft tissue infections

Joint, muscle, and soft tissue infections with less than 4 weeks of symptoms

Frequently found microorganisms and conditions	Rare microorganisms and conditions	Very rare microorganisms and conditions
S. aureus	Necrotizing fasciitis Group G streptococci	Fournier's gangrene (perineum and urogenital)
S. pneumoniae	Septic arthritis: *N. gonorrhoeae*, *B. burgdorferi*	Septic arthritis: *M. tuberculosis*, *P. aeruginosa*, *Mycoplasma hominis*, *Sporothrix schenckii* (fungal infection)
Viral arthritis: parvovirus B19	Hepatitis B Rubella Mumps	Reactive arthritis: *Campylobacter*, *Yersinia*, salmonellae, shigellae, *C. trachomatis*

Joint, muscle, and soft tissue infections with more than 4 weeks of symptoms and in the immunocompromised host

Microorganisms with symptoms for more than 4 weeks	Microorganisms and conditions in the immunocompromised host
Borreliosis (Lyme disease) Tuberculosis, trichinellosis	

Parvovirus B19   Parvovirus B19 infections may cause long-standing arthropathy, especially in adults. Seroprevalence is high in Western Europe [34]. Most acute infections occur during childhood and peak during late winter and spring.

Necrotizing fasciitis   The incidence of invasive streptococcal infections varies over time, suggesting a variation in virulence. In Europe the overall crude incidence rate is 2.79 per 100,000 population with slightly higher rates in the North than in the South [35].

Group G streptococci   Group G streptococci may cause skin infections and serious systemic infections that are predominantly seen in patients with underlying disease such as cancer, alcoholism, and diabetes mellitus.

Fournier's gangrene   Fournier's gangrene is a rare polymicrobial necrotizing infection or gangrene of the perineum that predominantly occurs in elderly patients with concurrent disease.

Staphylococcus aureus   Pyomyositis is very rare in Western Europe.

Reactive arthritis   Reactive arthritis is a mono or oligoarthritis of large joints or spine, often with other symptoms, in response to a previous infection of other organs. Risk factors are HLA-B27 positivity and HIV seropositivity. Especially white young adult males are at risk. Chlamydia infections are probably the most common trigger in Western Europe, but bacillary enteritis by *Campylobacter*, *Salmonella*, and *Yersinia* spp. have also been reported.

Trichinellosis   *Trichinella* spp. infections have become rare in Western Europe and are mostly of foreign origin. In Europe, especially horses, but also pigs, may still be infected where meat inspection does not detect all cases. In Western Europe however, infections are mainly associated with (imported) meat or eating wild animals (boar) [36].

Skin infections

Skin infections with less than 4 weeks of symptoms

Frequently found microorganisms	Rare microorganisms and conditions	Very rare microorganisms and conditions
Erysipelas, *S. pneumoniae*	Scabies	Rat-bite fever (*Spirillum minus*)
S. aureus	Varicella	Anthrax
Borrelia (erythema migrans)	Trichobilharzia	
Viral exanthematous infections		

Frequent skin infections

Erysipelas   Erysipelas is a rather common infection in Western Europe. In contrast to streptococcal pharyngitis, skin infections peak in the summer.

Staphylococcus aureus   *S. aureus* infections of the skin are common in Western Europe. Less than 5% of *S. aureus* isolates are Panton-Valentine leukocidin (PVL) positive, an exotoxin that is associated with severe disease. However, the majority of isolates from hospitalized patients with abscesses are PVL positive.

Scabies   Scabies, caused by *Sarcoptes scabiei*, is rare in Western Europe. Outbreaks in nursing homes or other institutions are repeatedly reported. Lindane resistance has been reported but the drug has been redrawn by the European Medicines Agency [37]. Permethrin, benzyl benzoate, sulfur, and ivermectin are available in Western Europe.

Trichobilharzia (swimmer's itch)   Avian *Schistosoma* species are endemic in Western Europe, Swimming in open waters, lakes and ponds, during the summer may cause acute cercarial dermatitis.

Rat-bite fever   Rat-bite fever is a zoonosis caused by *Streptobacillus moniliformis* or *S. minus*. Rats and other rodents, but sometimes also non-rodent mammals, are the source of infection. Infections may be acquired either by consumption of contaminated water, milk, or other foods (Haverhill fever) or after direct contact with rats, by scratches or bites. Rat bite is a sporadic ubiquitous infection with no specific geographic distribution [38].

Anthrax   Outbreaks of *Bacillus anthracis* infections are repeatedly reported, mainly in France. Incidental human infections occur, mostly limited to skin infection after handling infected animals.

Skin infections with more than 4 weeks of symptoms and in the immunocompromised host

Microorganisms and conditions with symptoms for more than 4 weeks	Microorganisms and conditions in the immunocompromised host
Syphilis Tuberculosis	*Candida tuberculosis*

Lymphadenopathy

Adenopathy of less than 4 weeks' duration

Frequently found microorganisms	Rare microorganisms and conditions	Very rare microorganisms and conditions
EBV	Tularemia	*Ehrlichia*
CMV	*Bartonella*	*Babesia*
Parvovirus B19	*B. burgdorferi*	Measles (rubeola)
Toxoplasma gondii	*Treponema pallidum* (syphilis)	Varicella zoster
HIV		

Toxoplasmosis   *Toxoplasma gondii* infections are common in Western Europe and a common cause of generalized lymphadenopathy. Seropositivity rates are the highest in France and Belgium ranging up to 90%. It is much lower in Switzerland, Austria, and the Netherlands (up to 54%). Notification of acute disease is incomplete. Toxoplasmosis during pregnancy and immunosuppression are the most important disease presentations. Screening during pregnancy is in place. Risk factors are eating of not well done meat products or contact with cats excreta, especially of young cats.

Tularemia Human tularemia, glanders, caused by *Francisella tularensis*, has become very rare in Western Europe, despite the prevalence of *F. tularensis* (subsp. Holarctica) [39]. Transmission takes place after contact with infected (dead) animals or by consumption of contaminated food or water.

Cat scratch disease *Bartonella henselae*, the causative organism of cat scratch disease, is endemic in Western Europe. Acute locoregional lymphadenitis after a cat scratch is a very classical presentation. Extensive chronic infection may mimic lymphoreticular disease.

Fever without focal symptoms

Fever less than 4 weeks without focal symptoms

Frequently found microorganisms	Rare microorganisms and conditions	Very rare microorganisms and conditions
Endocarditis	Tuberculosis	Tularemia
EBV	*C. burnetii*	*Ehrlichia*
CMV		Babesiosis
Parvovirus B19		
T. gondii		
HIV		

Most of the causes of acute fever offer some specific clue for the experienced clinician. Endocarditis is difficult to diagnose but the recent history of exposure (e.g., dental procedures, IV drug use) may offer a clue.

Cytomegalovirus (CMV) The nonspecific presentation of CMV infections in immunocompetent individuals may reveal its cause to the skilled clinician. The seroprevalence in Western Europe is among the lowest in the world with an overall seroprevalence between 40% and 50% [40]. This increases with age and is slightly higher for females. Blood transaminase concentrations are almost always slightly elevated indicative of minor hepatitis.

Rare organisms that may cause fever Tuberculosis, Q fever, trench fever, and tularemia are rare causes of prolonged fever (see earlier).

Human granulocytic anaplasmosis (ehrlichiosis) Anaplasmosis is a tick-borne zoonosis caused by the pathogen *Anaplasma phagocytophilum* (formerly named *Ehrlichia phagocytophila* and *Ehrlichia equi*). In Western Europe it is transmitted by *I. ricinus*. It has infrequently been reported from Western Europe, but not all human infections may have been detected [41,42].

Babesiosis In Western Europe three species have been identified as the cause of human babesiosis: *Babesia microti*, *Babesia divergens*, and *Babesia* spp. EU1, also called *B. venatorum*. *I. ricinus* is thought to be the main vector.

Dengue and Chikungunya The geographic distribution of *Aedes albopictus* comprises the cote d'Azur and southern parts of France and Switzerland. The first locally acquired cases of dengue and chikungunya have been reported in 2010 [43].

Mosquitoes are being imported together with ornamental flowers from Asia, but this not yet lead to acquisition of dengue in Europe.

Fever for more than 4 weeks without focal symptoms and in the immunocompromised host

Microorganisms with symptoms for more than 4 weeks	Microorganisms in the immunocompromised host
T. gondii Tuberculosis	CMV Adenovirus Q fever *Bartonella quintana* *Leishmania infantum*

Chronic fever due to infections that are not diagnosed within 4 weeks are rare and their approach should be that of fever of unknown origin. The differential diagnosis includes endocarditis, Q fever, abscesses, brucellosis, tuberculosis, and bartonellosis.

Bartonella quintana, the causative agent of trench fever, has become a very rare disease since its vector, the body louse, is almost absent in Western Europe.

Leishmaniasis *Leishmania infantum* is endemic in the Mediterranean region. Historically, it were mainly children who became infected, but immunocompromised adult patients are also at risk. Since the introduction of anti-retroviral treatment therapy, HIV–leishmania co-infection has become rare. Mobile patients with immunosuppressant medication at form an increasing risk group.

Eosinophilia and elevated IgE

Eosinophilia and elevated IgE for less than 4 weeks

Frequently found microorganisms	Rare microorganisms and conditions	Very rare microorganisms and conditions
	Toxocara	Anisakiasis *Ascaris lumbricoides* and *A. suum*

Eosinophilia and elevated IgE for more than 4 weeks and in the immunocompromised host

Microorganisms and conditions with symptoms for more than 4 weeks	Microorganisms and conditions in the immunocompromised host
A. *lumbricoides* and *A. suum* Anisakiasis *Echinococcus granulosus*	Strongyloidiasis

(Continued)

Microorganisms and conditions with symptoms for more than 4 weeks	Microorganisms and conditions in the immunocompromised host
Echinococcus multilocularis *Dirofilaria repens* Fascioliasis Hookworm-related cutaneous larva migrans *Toxocara*	

Eosinophilia is a sign of invasive helminthic infection. Intestinal nematode infections cause eosinophilia only during their initial tissue invasion (Loeffler's syndrome). Helminth infections have become rare in Europe.

Ascariasis   Prohibition to use human waste(water) as fertilizer effectively eliminated *Ascaris lumbricoides* infections in Western Europe. *A. suum* infection of pigs is rather common in Western Europe. Morphologically indistinguishable from *A. lumbricoides*, most presumed human *A. suum* infections were probably *A. lumbricoides* infections.

Toxocariasis   *Toxocara canis* infection of pet animals is very common in Western Europe. Transmission to humans occurs by ingestion of eggs, especially by children who play in contaminated sandboxes.

Anisakiasis   Deep freezing sea fish effectively prevents human infection by *Anisakis* spp. (herring worm). Since professional fishing industry adheres to these EU laws, anisakiasis has become a very rare disease. Rare infections may occur by consumption of self-caught fish or fish imported through uncontrolled channels.

Subcutaneous nodules   *Dirofilaria repens*, is a rare infection in humans, causing subcutaneous nodules. It occurs in the southern parts of France. *D. repens* is transmitted by, *Aedes, Culex* and *Anopheles* mosquitoes.

Fascioliasis   Human *Fasciola hepatica* infections are rare (see previous). Cattle, especially sheep, are not free from *F. hepatica*, despite massive treatment. Infection is acquired by eating contaminated water plants or ingestion of contaminated water. Triclabendazole-resistant *F. hepatica* has been reported in sheep in the Netherlands and in an occasional human infection (unpublished observation).

Strongyloidiasis   *Strongyloides stercoralis* is not endemic in Western Europe. Because under immune suppression *S. stercoralis* may proliferate long after the infection was acquired, all people with past exposure who are to undergo immunosuppresive therapy should be screened for the presence of *S. stercoralis*.

Hookworm-related cutaneous larva migrans   Cutaneous larva migrans is rare. An incidental infection has been reported from as north as the southern shores of Bretagne [44].

Echinococcosis   *Echinococcus multilocularis* has been demonstrated in wild animals (foxes) all over Western Europe with the highest endemicity in the Northern Alpine region and the mountainous areas of the middle region. Infection rates of foxes in the Netherlands and Northern Germany are low, but the geographic distribution is expanding [45]. Human infection, alveolar echinococcosis, is a sporadic infection in Western Europe and is acquired by eating wild berries contaminated by fox dung.

Echinococcus granulosus, the causative agent of hydatid echinococcosis, used to be prevalent in Western Europe, but locally acquired human infections have not been reported since a long time.

Antibiotic resistance

Antimicrobial resistance is variable in the region of Western Europe and changes over time. Most recent aggregated data are available from the European Antimicrobial Resistance Surveillance System (EARSS, http://www.rivm.nl/earss/) [46].

The driving forces of selecting resistant microbes are the unrestricted use of antimicrobials for human and veterinary infections. Use of antifungal agents in agriculture may select resistant fungi that are pathogenic for humans.

There are large differences in prescribing practices in Western Europe. The most extreme example is the Netherlands where restricted use of antibiotics in medical practice parallels the low frequency of resistant microorganisms in human infections but where the use of anti-microbial agents in the extremely intensive bioindustry problems is still a common practice.

The lowest rates of penicillin-resistant pneumococci are found in the Netherlands and Southeast Austria (<1%) [47,48]. Rates in Belgium are a little bit higher (4%) but in other regions can be much higher, up to 38% [49–51]. In most instances, amoxicillin–clavulanic acid is still effective.

The proportion of pneumococci not susceptible to both penicillin and to macrolides varies significantly. The two correspond because penicillin resistance induces macrolide prescription which subsequently selects for macrolide resistance. In France reported rates were 30% whereas in the Netherlands and Austria this was less than 5%.

The prevalence of methicillin-resistant *Staphylococcus aureus* (MRSA) varies over Western Europe. Hospital-acquired MRSA is very common in France, Belgium, Luxembourg, Germany, and Switzerland (rates up to 25% of clinical isolates), less common in Austria (5–10%), and rare in the Netherlands (<1%). Dutch hospitals still maintain a search and destroy policy which means that patients attending Dutch hospitals after recent hospitalization in any other country will be admitted in strict isolation until MRSA carriage has been excluded by repeated culturing skin and orifices. Community-acquired MRSA, which seems to be less virulent, is rather common in cattle industry so that patients with exposure to these animals will also be subjected to MRSA isolation policies.

Invasive *Enterococcus faecalis* infections are far more frequent than *Enterococcus faecium* infections, but both show high rates of resistance to aminoglycosides in Western Europe, between 25% and 50%.

Reported rates of vancomycin-resistant enterococci are low in Western Europe; the highest rates are found in the Alpine countries (<5%).

Antimicrobial resistance of *E. coli* to third-generation cephalosporins is generally below 5% in Western Europe. EARSS 2008 reported rates of fluoroquinolone-resistant *E. coli* ranges between 10% and 25% in Western Europe but are increasing. Multiple resistant *E. coli* is an increasingly frequent finding.

In general, the frequency of resistant gram-negative bacteria is slightly higher than in Scandinavia and lower than in Southern and Central-Eastern Europe. A similar geographic north-south axis is seen for resistance rates of *P. aeruginosa*.

Extended spectrum Beta-lactamase-producing *K. pneumoniae*, and increasingly also *E. coli*, are being reported. Carbapenem-resistant *K. pneumoniae* (associated with the KPC-2-carbapenemase-gene and the New-Delhi-metallo-carbapenemase-gene, NDM-1) has been reported from patients in Western Europe who acquired these outside the region.

Multidrug-resistant TB is very rare and in most cases of foreign origin.

Vaccine-preventable diseases in children [52]

Country	DTP, IPV, MMR	Hib	HBV	HAV	PCconj	PCps	HPV	MenC	Varicella	Influenza	TBE	Rotavirus
Austria	Yes	Yes	Yes		Yes		Girls	Yes		Elderly and risk groups	Risk areas	Yes
Belgium	Yes	Yes	Yes		Yes		Girls	Yes		Elderly and risk groups		Yes[a]
France	Yes	Yes	Yes		Yes		Girls	Yes		Elderly and risk groups		Yes[b]
Germany	Yes	Yes	Yes		Yes	>60	Girls	Yes		Elderly and risk groups	Risk areas	
Luxembourg	Yes	Yes	Yes		Yes	≥60	Girls	Yes	Yes	Elderly and risk groups		Yes
Netherlands	Yes	Yes	Risk groups		Yes		Girls	Yes		Elderly and risk groups		
Switzerland	Yes	Yes	Yes		Yes	>65	Girls	Yes	Adolescents	Elderly and risk groups	Risk areas	
Monaco	Yes	Yes	Yes	Risk groups		2 months	Girls	Yes		Elderly and risk groups		

DTP, diphtheria, tetanus, and acellular pertussis vaccine; IPV, parenteral polio vaccine; MMR, measles, mumps, and rubella; Hib, *H. influenzae* vaccine; HBV, hepatitis B virus vaccine; HAV, hepatitis A vaccine; HPV, Human Papilloma Virus vaccine; Menc, conjugated Meningococcus C vaccine; PCconj, conjugated pneumococcal vaccine; PCps, polysaccharide pneumococcal vaccine; TBE, tick-borne encephalitis vaccine.
[a] Some differences between Flanders/Wallony and German-speaking community.
[b] Recommended but not or partially reimbursed.

Basic economic and demographic data

	GNI per capita (USD)	Life expectancy at birth (total, years)	School enrollment, primary (% net)
Austria	46,260	80	97
Belgium	44,330	80	98
France	42,250	81	99
Germany	42,440	80	98
Liechtenstein	NA	NA	89
Luxembourg	84,890	79	97
Monaco	NA	NA	NA
The Netherlands	50,150	80	98
Switzerland	65,330	82	89

World Bank, 2008.

GNI, gross national income; NA, not available.

Causes of death in children under 5 years—regional average

Neonatal causes	44
Pneumonia	13
Diarrheal diseases	10
HIV/AIDS	0
Measles	0
Injuries	6
Others	25

WHO, 2000–2003 data.

Most common causes of death in all ages in Western Europe [53]

	Austria	Belgium	France	Germany	Luxembourg	Monaco	the Netherlands	Switzerland
					%			
Ischemic and hypertensive heart disease	22	15	9	21	13	10	14	18
Neoplasms	27	28	30	28	27	28	30	26
Cerebrovascular disease	11	9	7	10	11	8	9	7
Lower respiratory infections	2	5	4	3	3	4	6	4
Alzheimer and other dementias	0	4	3	1	3	0	4	5
COPD	3	5	3	3	3	3	5	3
Falls	1	1	2	1	1	2	1	1
Diabetes mellitus	0	1	2	0	1	2	1	1

References

1. Wilson A, Mellor P. Bluetongue in Europe: vectors, epidemiology and climate change. Parasitol Res 2008;103:69–77.
2. European Centre for Disease Prevention and Control. Annual Epidemiological Report on Communicable Diseases in Europe—2009. Stockholm, Sweden: European Centre for Disease Prevention and Control, 2010.
3. Irani DN. Aseptic meningitis and viral myelitis. Neurol Clin 2008;26(3):635–55.
4. Chambon M, Archimbaud C, Bailly JL, et al. Circulation of enteroviruses and persistence of meningitis cases in the winter of 1999–2000. J Med Virol 2001;65(2):340–7.
5. Mailles A, Stahl JP. Infectious encephalitis in France in 2007: a national prospective study. Clin Infect Dis 2009;49(12):1838–47.
6. Blanc F. [Epidemiology of Lyme borreliosis and neuroborreliosis in France]. Rev Neurol (Paris) 2009;165(8–9):694–701.
7. Jouda F, Perret JL, Gern L. *Ixodes ricinus* density, and distribution and prevalence of *Borrelia burgdorferi* sensu lato infection along an altitudinal gradient. J Med Entomol 2004;41(2):162–9.
8. Jouda F, Perret JL, Gern L. Density of questing *Ixodes ricinus* nymphs and adults infected by *Borrelia burgdorferi* sensu lato in Switzerland: spatio-temporal pattern at a regional scale. Vector Borne Zoonotic Dis 2004;4(1):23–32.
9. Linard C, Lamarque P, Heyman P, et al. Determinants of the geographic distribution of Puumala virus and Lyme borreliosis infections in Belgium. Int J Health Geogr 2007;6(1):15.
10. Allerberger F, Wagner M. Listeriosis: a resurgent foodborne infection. Clin Microbiol Infect 2010;16(1):16–23.
11. Goulet V, Hedberg C, Le Monnier A, de Valk H. Increasing incidence of listeriosis in France and other European countries. Emerg Infect Dis 2008;14(5):734–40.
12. Kent ME, Romanelli F. Reexamining syphilis: an update on epidemiology, clinical manifestations, and management. Ann Pharmacother 2008;42(2):226–36.
13. Lindquist L, Vapalahti O. Tick-borne encephalitis. Lancet 2008;371(9627):1861–71.
14. Visvesvara GS, Moura H, Schuster FL. Pathogenic and opportunistic free-living amoebae: *Acanthamoeba* spp., *Balamuthia mandrillaris*, *Naegleria fowleri*, and *Sappinia diploidea*. FEMS Immunol Med Microbiol 2007;50(1):1–26.
15. de Boer MG, Lambregts PC, van Dam AP, van't Wout JW. Meningitis caused by *Capnocytophaga canimorsus*: when to expect the unexpected. Clin Neurol Neurosurg 2007;109(5):393–8.
16. Boothpur R, Brennan DC. Human polyoma viruses and disease with emphasis on clinical BK and JC. J Clin Virol 2010;47(4):306–12.
17. Egli A, Infanti L, Dumoulin A, et al. Prevalence of polyomavirus BK and JC infection and replication in 400 healthy blood donors. J Infect Dis 2009;199(6):837–46.
18. Hakim F, Tleyjeh I. Severe adenovirus pneumonia in immunocompetent adults: a case report and review of the literature. Eur J Clin Microbiol Infect Dis 2008;27(2):153–8.
19. Atkinson TP, Balish MF, Waites KB. Epidemiology, clinical manifestations, pathogenesis and laboratory detection of *Mycoplasma pneumoniae* infections. FEMS Microbiol Rev 2008;32(6):956–73.
20. Joseph CA, Ricketts KD. Legionnaires' disease in Europe 2007–2008. Euro Surveill 2010;15:pii=19493.
21. Catherinot E, Lanternier F, Bougnoux ME, Lecuit M, Couderc LJ, Lortholary O. *Pneumocystis jirovecii* pneumonia. Infect Dis Clin North Am 2010;24(1):107–38.
22. Glass RI, Parashar UD, Estes MK. Norovirus gastroenteritis. N Engl J Med 2009;361(18):1776–85.
23. Horrocks SM, Anderson RC, Nisbet DJ, Ricke SC. Incidence and ecology of *Campylobacter jejuni* and *coli* in animals. Anaerobe 2002;15(1–2):18–25.
24. de Wit MA, Koopmans MP, Kortbeek LM, van Leeuwen NJ, Vinje J, van Duynhoven YT. Etiology of gastroenteritis in sentinel general practices in The Netherlands. Clin Infect Dis 2001;33(3):280–8.
25. Ostyn A, De Buyser ML, Guillier F, et al. First evidence of a food poisoning outbreak due to staphylococcal enterotoxin type E, France, 2009. Euro Surveill 2010;15(13):19528.
26. Reviriego Gordejo FJ, Vermeersch JP. Towards eradication of bovine tuberculosis in the European Union. Vet Microbiol 2006;112(2–4):101–9.
27. Bouvet E, Casalino E, Mendoza-Sassi G, et al. A nosocomial outbreak of multidrug-resistant *Mycobacterium bovis* among HIV-infected patients. A case–control study. AIDS 1993;7(11):1453–60.

28. Desnues B, Al Moussawi K, Fenollar F. New insights into Whipple's disease and *Tropheryma whipplei* infections. Microbes Infect 2010 (in press).

29. Olsson GE, Dalerum F, Hornfeldt B, et al. Human hantavirus infections, Sweden. Emerg Infect Dis 2003;9(11):1395–401.

30. Schlegel M, Klempa B, Auste B, et al. Dobrava-belgrade virus spillover infections, Germany. Emerg Infect Dis 2009;15(12):2017–20.

31. Baranton G, Postic D. Trends in leptospirosis epidemiology in France. Sixty-six years of passive serological surveillance from 1920 to 2003. Int J Infect Dis 2006;10(2):162–70.

32. Stary G, Meyer T, Bangert C, et al. New *Chlamydia trachomatis* L2 strains identified in a recent outbreak of lymphogranuloma venereum in Vienna, Austria. Sex Transm Dis 2008;35(4):377–82.

33. Stary G, Stary A. Lymphogranuloma venereum outbreak in Europe. J Dtsch Dermatol Ges 2008;6(11):935–40.

34. Mossong J, Hens N, Friederichs V, et al. Parvovirus B19 infection in five European countries: seroepidemiology, force of infection and maternal risk of infection. Epidemiol Infect 2008;136(8):1059–68.

35. Lamagni TL, Darenberg J, Luca-Harari B, et al. Epidemiology of severe *Streptococcus pyogenes* disease in europe. J Clin Microbiol 2008;46 (7):2359–67.

36. Dupouy-Camet J. Trichinellosis: still a concern for Europe. Euro Surveill 2006;11(1):5.

37. van den Hoek JA, van de Weerd JA, Baayen TD, et al. A persistent problem with scabies in and outside a nursing home in Amsterdam: indications for resistance to lindane and ivermectin. Euro Surveill 2008;13(48):19052.

38. Gaastra W, Boot R, Ho HT, Lipman LJ. Rat bite fever. Vet Microbiol 2009;133(3):211–28.

39. Foley JE, Nieto NC. Tularemia. Vet Microbiol 2010;140(3–4):332–8.

40. Cannon MJ, Schmid DS, Hyde TB. Review of cytomegalovirus seroprevalence and demographic characteristics associated with infection. Rev Med Virol 2010;20(4):202–13.

41. Blanco JR, Oteo JA. Human granulocytic ehrlichiosis in Europe. Clin Microbiol Infect 2002;8(12):763–72.

42. Strle F. Human granulocytic ehrlichiosis in Europe. Int J Med Microbiol 2004;293(Suppl. 37):27–35.

43. La Ruche G, Souares Y, Armengaud A, Peloux-Petiot F, Delaunay P, Despres P, et al. First two autochthonous dengue virus infections in metropolitan France, September 2010. Euro Surveill 2010;15:19676.

44. Tamminga N, Bierman WF, de Vries PJ. Cutaneous larva migrans acquired in Brittany, France. Emerg Infect Dis 2009; 15: 1856–1858.

45. Romig T, Dinkel A, Mackenstedt U. The present situation of echinococcosis in Europe. Parasitol Int 2006;55(Suppl. 1):S187–91.

46. European Antimicrobial Resistance Surveillance System. Annual Report 2008. European Antimicrobial Resistance Surveillance System; 2008.

47. Nethmap 2010. Consumption of antimicrobial agents and antimicrobial resistance among medically important bacteria in the Netherlands. Annual report of the Dutch Foundation of the Working Party for Infectious Disease Control, SWAB.

48. Hoenigl M, Fussi P, Feierl G, et al. Antimicrobial resistance of *Streptococcus pneumoniae* in Southeast Austria, 1997–2008. Int J Antimicrob Agents 2010;36(1):24–7.

49. Kempf M, Baraduc R, Bonnabau H, et al. Epidemiology and antimicrobial resistance of *Streptococcus pneumoniae* in France in 2007: data from the Pneumococcus Surveillance Network. Microb Drug Resist 2011;17:31–36.

50. Vanhoof R, Camps K, Carpentier M, et al. 10th Survey of antimicrobial resistance in non-invasive clinical isolates of *Streptococcus pneumoniae* collected in Belgium during winter 2007–2008. Pathol Biol 2010;58(2):147–51.

51. Jaecklin T, Rohner P, Jacomo V, Schmidheiny K, Gervaix A. Trends in antibiotic resistance of respiratory tract pathogens in children in Geneva, Switzerland. Eur J Pediatr 2006;165 (1):3–8.

52. http://apps.who.int/immunization_monitoring/en/globalsummary/ScheduleResult.cfm.

53. World Health Statistics 2010. Geneva, World Health Organization;2010.

Chapter 20
Caribbean

Jana I. Preis[1,2] and Larry I. Lutwick[1,2]
[1]Infectious Diseases, VA New York Harbor Health Care System, Brooklyn, NY, USA
[2]State University of New York (SUNY) Downstate Medical School, Brooklyn, NY, USA

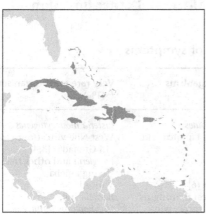

Antigua and Barbuda	Jamaica
Aruba	Netherlands Antilles
Bahamas	Puerto Rico
Barbados	St. Kitts and Nevis
Bermuda	St. Lucia
Cayman Islands	St. Vincent and
Dominica	the Grenadines
Dominican Republic	Trinidad and Tobago
Grenada	Virgin Islands
Haiti	

The purpose of this chapter is to provide a concise review of common infections in the Caribbean region. The Caribbean consists of an archipelago of islands with large variations in life expectancy and economy. The most important acute infection with an incubation time of less than 4 weeks is dengue fever. In Haiti, an outbreak of cholera was seen after the 2010 earthquake, and falciparum malaria is endemic but still fully sensitive to chloroquine. Over the last decade, malaria has spread from Haiti to the Dominican Republic and is now established on the eastern part of the island (Punta Cana) and an outbreak, which has been difficult to control, is ongoing in Kingston, Jamaica. Even though malaria outside Haiti is rare, these outbreaks illustrate that malaria should be considered in persons with residence or a travel history from the Caribbean. Typhoid and other *Salmonella* infections are common in less affluent parts of the region and may cause diarrhea or just fever without focal symptoms and leptospirosis can be seen in any part of the region. The Caribbean has been more heavily affected by HIV than any other region outside sub-Saharan Africa and has the second highest level of HIV prevalence. In 2008, an estimated 240,000 people were living with HIV in the Caribbean region, while an estimated 20,000 people were newly infected and some 12,000 died of AIDS-related illnesses (Adams EB, Macleod

Infectious Diseases: A Geographic Guide, First Edition.
Edited by Eskild Petersen, Lin H. Chen & Patricia Schlagenhauf.
© 2011 John Wiley & Sons, Ltd. Published 2011 by John Wiley & Sons, Ltd.

IN, Medicine (Baltimore) 1987;56:315–23). Tuberculosis with or without coinfection with HIV should always be considered in patients with slowly evolving symptoms over weeks and months. Schistosomiasis is now rare and filariasis due to *Wuchereria bancrofti* is rare except in Haiti. *Ascaris* and *Strongyloides* are found throughout the region. At the end of the chapter, comments about antibiotic resistance patterns and list of vaccine-preventable diseases are provided.

CNS infections: meningitis, encephalitis, and other infections with neurological symptoms

Acute infections with less than 4 weeks of symptoms

Frequently found microorganisms (>5%)	Rare microorganisms (1–5%)	Very rare microorganisms (<1%)
Viral meningitis (enteroviruses)	*Angiostrongyloides* (endemic in Jamaica and Cuba) [1,2]	*Listeria monocytogenes*
Pneumococcal meningitis	Neurosyphilis	West Nile virus (four cases in Grenada) [3,4]
Ciguatera fish poisoning	Rabies	*Naegleria* and other free-living ameba
HTLV (endemic in Jamaica) [5]	Dengue fever [6]	Varicella
Human immunodeficiency virus (HIV)	Meningococcal meningitis	*Borrelia* spp.
Herpes virus group I and II	Leptospirosis (especially in Jamaica)	*Haemophilus influenzae* type b meningitis
		Tick-borne encephalitis (five cases described in Cayman Islands) [6]

Rabies is generally transmitted by bat, mongoose, and dog. Islands where rabies is found in wildlife include Puerto Rico, Trinidad, Cuba, Antigua, and Grenada. West Nile virus has been found in birds and horses in Cuba and Puerto Rico, but has not yet been reported from humans.

CNS infections: meningitis and encephalitis with symptoms for more than 4 weeks and in the immunocompromised host

Microorganisms with symptoms for more than 4 weeks	Microorganisms in the immunocompromised host
HIV	*Nocardia*
Tuberculosis	Polyomavirus
	Cryptococcus spp.
Polio myelitis [1,7]	Varicella zoster virus (VZV), cytomegalovirus (CMV)
	Adenovirus
Neurosyphilis	Toxoplasmosis [2,5]
	Polio myelitis

An outbreak of polio myelitis was reported from Haiti and the Dominican Republic in 2000–2001, but no further cases have been found. In the midst of the 2010–2011 cholera epidemic on Haiti, several paralytic poliomyelitis-like cases were reported but not shown to be due to the polio virus.

Ear, nose, and throat infections

Ear, nose, and throat infections with less than 4 weeks of symptoms

Frequently found microorganisms	Rare microorganisms and conditions	Very rare microorganisms
Group A streptococcus Epstein–Barr virus (EBV) Herpes virus (type I and II)	Peritonsillar abscess Tuberculosis Necrotizing fasciitis Diphtheria [3] Mumps (in Jamaica) [4] Rubella	

Ear, nose, and throat infections with symptoms for more than 4 weeks and in the immunocompromised host

Tuberculosis should be considered in immunocompetent patients with symptoms for more than 4 weeks, and *Candida* and herpes virus are seen in immunocompromised patients.

Cardiopulmonary infections

Pneumonia with less than 4 weeks of symptoms

Frequently found microorganisms	Rare microorganisms and conditions	Very rare microorganisms
Streptococcus pneumoniae	*Histoplasmosis Corynebacterium diphtheriae* *Bordetella pertussis* Influenza [8]	*Legionella* spp. [9] Measles *Mycoplasma pneumoniae*

Histoplasmosis is found on many islands in the Caribbean basin. These include Cuba, Trinidad, Puerto Rico, Martinique, and Barbados.

Endocarditis with less than 4 weeks of symptoms

Frequently found microorganisms	Rare microorganisms and conditions	Very rare microorganisms
Staphylococcus aureus Alpha or nonhemolytic streptococci Coagulase-negative staphylococcus *Enterococcus* spp.	*Neisseria gonorrhoeae* HACEK group *S. pneumoniae*	*Bartonella* spp. *Brucella* spp. *Coxiella burnetii* *Propionibacterium* spp.

H *Haemophilus*
A *Aggregatibacter* (formerly *Actinobacillus*)
C *Cardiobacterium*
E *Eikenella*
K *Kingella*

Pulmonary symptoms for more than 4 weeks and in the immunocompromised host

Tuberculosis, histoplasmosis, and *Aspergillus* should be considered in both immunocompetent and immunodeficient host with symptoms for more than 4 weeks.

Endocarditis for more than 4 weeks and in the immunocompromised host

Microorganisms and diseases with symptoms for more than 4 weeks	Microorganisms in the immunocompromised host
Coagulase-negative staphylococci Alpha or nonhemolytic streptococci	*Aspergillus* Gram-negative bacilli [4]

Gastrointestinal infections

Gastrointestinal infections with less than 4 weeks of symptoms

Frequently found microorganisms	Rare microorganisms and conditions	Very rare microorganisms

Norovirus
Hepatitis A, B, C, D, E
Ciguatera fish poisoning [5]
S. aureus enterotoxin
Shigella
 	
Strongyloides stercoralis
Campylobacter
Enterotoxigenic *E. coli*
Giardia spp.
Salmonella enterica serotype
  Typhi and non-Typhi
Ascaris lumbricoides
	Cryptosporidium spp.
	
	Bacillus cereus toxin
	Vibrio cholerae (2010 Haiti outbreak) [2,5]
	Escherichia coli O157:H7 (and other
	  verotoxin-producing *E. coli*)
		Tuberculosis
		Whipple's disease [1]

Starting in October 2010 and continuing until manuscript preparation, an epidemic of cholera beginning in the Artibonite valley of Haiti occurred which spread throughout Haiti and to some extent to the Dominican Republic. As of February 25, 2011, almost 250,000 cases were reported in Haiti with over 4,600 deaths. In the Dominican Republic, about 250 cases were reported, most acquired locally, with several deaths.

There has been little transmission of *Schistosoma mansoni* in Puerto Rico since the first half of the 1990s, and the infection is now probably eradicated from the island as no new cases have been reported since 2001. Schistosomiasis is rare but can still be seen in Saint Lucia, Antigua, Montserrat, Martinique, Guadeloupe, and the Dominican Republic.

Gastrointestinal infections with symptoms for more than 4 weeks and in the immunocompromised host

Microorganisms and diseases with symptoms for more than 4 weeks	Microorganisms in the immunocompromised host
Tuberculosis	*Candida*
Whipple's disease	Herpes virus
Blastocystis hominis (unclear if pathogenic)	CMV
Dientamoeba fragilis (unclear if pathogenic)	

Infections of liver, spleen, and peritoneum

Acute infections of liver, spleen, and peritoneum with less than 4 weeks of symptoms

Frequently found microorganisms	Rare microorganisms
Hepatitis A virus, hepatitis B virus (alone or delta virus coinfection/superinfection), hepatitis C virus, dengue virus	Herpes viruses (CMV, EBV, HSV, VZV), adenovirus, HIV, hepatitis E virus
Leptospirosis (especially in Jamaica), *Salmonella Typhi, Mycobacterium tuberculosis*	Rickettsia, nontuberculous mycobacteria, *Brucella, Salmonella, Burkholderia pseudomallei*
	Toxocara (larva migrans), *Fasciola hepatica, A. lumbricoides, Plasmodium falciparum*[a]

[a]In Haiti, eastern part of the Dominican Republic and recent outbreaks in Kingston, Jamaica and in Great Exuma, Bahamas.

Chronic infections of liver, spleen, and peritoneum with more than 4 weeks of symptoms

Frequently found microorganisms	Rare microorganisms	Microorganisms in the immunocompromised host
Hepatitis B virus (with or without delta virus coinfection/superinfection), hepatitis C virus		Herpes viruses: CMV, EBV, HSV, VZV, HIV
Salmonella Typhi, M. tuberculosis	Nontuberculous mycobacteria, *Salmonella, Brucella, Borrelia*, syphilis Amebic liver abscess, *F. hepatica, Toxocara* (visceral larva migrans)	*Salmonella, M. tuberculous,* Nontuberculous mycobacteria, syphilis *Histoplasma, Cryptococcus, Candida, Cryptosporidium, Microsporidium*

Yellow fever in humans has not been currently reported in the area. However, yellow fever has been found in 2009 in dead monkeys in Trinidad. The autopsy was conducted by CAREC (Caribbean Epidemiology Centre)/PAHO (Pan American Health Organization). It should be noted that in 1988, 1989, and 1995 the yellow fever virus was also found in monkeys. Special note: although yellow fever is not endemic in the Caribbean, proof of vaccination is required of travelers returning from yellow fever-endemic areas.

Genitourinary infections

Cystitis, pyelonephritis, and nephritis with less than 4 weeks of symptoms

Frequently found microorganisms	Rare microorganisms and conditions	Very rare microorganisms
E. coli *Klebsiella pneumoniae* and other enteric gram-negative bacilli	Perineal abscess Tuberculosis	

Sexually transmitted infections with less than 4 weeks of symptoms

Frequently found microorganisms	Rare microorganisms and conditions	Very rare microorganisms
Chlamydia spp., *Ureaplasma* *N. gonorrhoeae*	Lymphogranuloma venereum [3] *Entamoeba histolytica* [10–12]	Chancroid

Cystitis, pyelonephritis, and nephritis with symptoms for more than 4 weeks and in the immunocompromised host

Bacterial infections are common in patients with long-term catheters and renal stones, and tuberculosis should be considered in patients with persistent finding of white blood cells in the urine with negative culture. *Candida* is particularly a problem in the immunocompromised host.

Sexually transmitted infections with symptoms for more than 4 weeks and in the immunocompromised host

Syphilis can give symptoms months after infection (secondary and tertiary syphilis and neuro-syphilis). The incubation period for human papilloma virus from infection until cancer is years.

Joint, muscle, and soft tissue infections

Joint, muscle, and soft tissue infections with less than 4 weeks of symptoms

Frequently found microorganisms	Rare microorganisms and conditions	Very rare microorganisms

S. aureus
 	
Group A streptococcus
	Necrotizing fasciitis,
	  group G streptococci
	S. pneumoniae
		Fournier's gangrene
		  (perineum and urogenital)
		Trichinella spp. [7]
		Filarial infections [15] (especially in Haiti)
		Tetanus

Joint, muscle, and soft tissue infections with more than 4 weeks of symptoms and in the immunocompromised host

Tuberculosis should be considered in patients with long-term symptoms and *Candida* in the immunocompromised.

Skin infections

Skin infections with less than 4 weeks of symptoms

Frequently found microorganisms	Rare microorganisms and conditions	Very rare microorganisms
Erysipelas, group A streptococcus	Measles	Cutaneous anthrax (Haiti) [13]
S. aureus	Rat-bite fever (*Streptobacillus* spp.)	
Group C streptococcus	Cutaneous larva migrans	
VZV	Scabies [1]	

Skin infections with more than 4 weeks of symptoms and in the immunocompromised host

Microorganisms with symptoms for more than 4 weeks	Microorganisms in the immunocompromised host
Syphilis [4]	*Candida*
Tuberculosis	Histoplasmosis
Histoplasmosis [3]	Coccidioidomycosis (island of Martinique) [2]

Adenopathy

Adenopathy of less than 4 weeks' duration

Frequently found microorganisms	Rare microorganisms and conditions	Very rare microorganisms
EBV	Tularemia [14]	Lymphogranuloma inguinale
CMV	*Bartonella* [9]	
Parvovirus B19		
Toxoplasma gondii		
HIV		
Rubella		
Mumps		

Adenopathy of more than 4 weeks' duration and in the immunocompromised host

Microorganisms with symptoms for more than 4 weeks	Microorganisms in the immunocompromised host
T. gondii	Adenovirus
Tuberculosis	CMV

Toxoplasma gondii is highly endemic in the Caribbean and genotype I and III and the so-called exotic genotypes are common. Thus, patients with fever and adenopathy whether for 4 weeks less or longer should be tested for antibodies to *T. gondii*. The so-called exotic genotypes usually present with a more severe clinical symptoms and may cause eye disease (retinochoroiditis) more often than genotype I, II, and III.

Fever without focal symptoms

Fever for less than 4 weeks without focal symptoms

Frequently found microorganisms	Rare microorganisms and conditions	Very rare microorganisms
Endocarditis	Tuberculosis	Tularemia
EBV	C. burnetii	Brucellosis
CMV		
Parvovirus B19		
T. gondii		
Dengue [3]		
Leptospirosis [5]		
Malaria[a]		
Enteric fever from salmonellosis		
HIV		

[a]Haiti, Dominican Republic, Jamaica, Bahamas.

Health officials across the Caribbean are concerned about the near epidemic level of mosquito-borne dengue fever, saying it could get more severe as rainy season progresses. Last 2 years have also been active in terms of dengue epidemics in the Caribbean. The highest toll of this infection is documented in Jamaica with more than 1,000 cases last September 2010, and the island of St. Martin with more than 2,000 cases [3,4].

As we know, currently there is no vaccine to prevent HIV/AIDS infections. However, the epidemic of HIV infection is significant in this geographic region. In 2008, an estimated 240,000 people were living with HIV in the Caribbean region, while an estimated 20,000 people were newly infected and some 12,000 died of AIDS-related illnesses [11]. The Caribbean has been more heavily affected by HIV than any region outside sub-Saharan Africa and has the second highest level of HIV prevalence. The Dominican Republic has experienced a decline in HIV prevalence due to changes in sexual behavior, including increased condom use and partner reduction.

Fever for more than 4 weeks without focal symptoms and in the immunocompromised host

Microorganisms with symptoms for more than 4 weeks	Microorganisms and in the immunocompromised host
T. gondii Tuberculosis Amebic liver abscess Brucellosis Q fever	CMV Adenoviruses

Eosinophilia with elevated IgE

Eosinophilia and elevated IgE for less than 4 weeks

Frequently found microorganisms	Rare microorganisms and conditions	Very rare microorganisms
A. lumbricoides *S. stercoralis* *S. mansoni*	*Toxocara* spp.	*A. cantonensis*

Eosinophilic meningitis has been described in a group of American tourists visiting Jamaica and serological evidence of infection was found with *A. cantonensis*. The infection was probably transmitted by salad.

Eosinophilia and elevated IgE for more than 4 weeks and in the immunocompromised host

Microorganisms with symptoms for more than 4 weeks	Microorganisms in the immunocompromised host
A. lumbricoides and *Ascaris suum* Zoonotic hookworms *F. hepatica* [5] Lymphatic filariasis[a]	*Toxocara* spp. *Gnathostoma* spp. Cysticercosis (*Taenia solium*) *Hymenolepis* spp. [1]

[a]Lymphatic filariasis caused by *Wuchereria bancrofti* is common and widespread in Haiti and is seen sporadically in the Dominican Republic. *W. bancrofti* has previously been found also in Trinidad and has not been reported in humans over the past few years [13].

Antibiotic resistance patterns

Similar to the rest of the world, when choosing appropriate treatment options, physicians should be aware of local antimicrobial resistance patterns. In the Caribbean region there is a high degree (around 10%) of penicillin resistance in pneumococci and increasing fluoroquinolone resistance in *S. enterica* and *E. coli*. However, unlike USA and Western Europe, MRSA is still rarely represented in the region (less than 1%) and further epidemiological studies are suggested to explore further such pattern.

Regarding *M. tuberculosis* drug resistance patterns, less than 0.6% of cases were described as MDR-TB.

Vaccine-preventable infections

In 2006, WHO estimated that close to 2 million of death among children less than 5 years of age and more than 20 million of death among adults were due to diseases that could have been prevented by routine vaccination. Due to overall poverty in the Caribbean, this area of preventive medicine remains a significant problem requiring continuous global attention. Among list of vaccine-preventable diseases applicable to this geographic region are: diphtheria, HiB, hepatitis B, measles, streptococcal infections, mumps, tetanus, poliomyelitis, rubella, pertussis.

Although yellow fever is not particularly endemic in the region, and although no human cases of yellow fever have been reported from Trinidad since 1979, recent yellow fever case in monkeys indicate that the virus is circulating in forested areas of the island [11].

An outbreak of paralytic poliomyelitis occurred in the Dominican Republic (13 confirmed cases) and Haiti (eight confirmed cases, including two fatal cases) during 2000–2001 [1]. All but one of the patients were either unvaccinated or incompletely vaccinated. The outbreak was associated with the circulation of a derivative of the type 1 OPV strain, probably originating from a single OPV dose given in 1998–1999 [7,15].

Significant epidemics of rubella have been documented in the Caribbean countries since the 1960s with cases of congenital rubella syndrome being diagnosed following such outbreaks. For the last 5 years there were no documented cases of rubella. Grenada reported 648 cases in 1982, and Trinidad and Tobago reported 1,159 cases in 1983. Twenty cases of CRPS, including sudden deaths, were documented in Grenada between April 1982 and July 1983 [3,7]. Beginning in 1995, renewed rubella activity was observed in Jamaica. Between 1996 and 1997, 31 cases of CRS were reported from Jamaica, Barbados, Trinidad and Tobago, and Bahamas.

Diphtheria is endemic in the Caribbean as well. During the last 10 years, a large epidemic has occurred again in Haiti due to the earthquake conditions with more than 100 cases documented [15]. The outbreak of diphtheria, which precise numbers are not known as this writing, has prompted the WHO to support Haitian health authorities in a targeted vaccination campaign for about 5,000 people thought to be exposed to diphtheria. Pediatric vaccination against *Haemophilus influenzae* type b became more common in 2003 and beyond. Cases have decreased since.

Basic economic and demographic data

Basic demographics*	GNI per capita (USD)	Life expectancy at birth (total, years)	School enrollment, primary (% net)
Antigua and Barbuda	13,620	75	74
Aruba	NA	75	99
Bahamas	17,160	73	91
Barbados	9,330	77	97
Bermuda	NA	79	92

Basic demographics*	GNI per capita (USD)	Life expectancy at birth (total, years)	School enrollment, primary (% net)
Cayman Islands	NA	NA	81
Cuba	NA	78	99
Dominica	4,770	77	77
Dominican Republic	4,390	72	78
Grenada	5,710	69	76
Haiti	660	61	NA
Jamaica	4,870	73	86
Netherland Antilles	NA	75	97
Puerto Rico	10,960	78	NA
St. Kitts and Nevis	10,960	71	87
St. Lucia	5,530	74	98
St. Vincent and the Grenadines	5,140	72	91
Trinidad and Tobago	16,540	70	94
Vigin Islands (United States)	NA	79	NA

*GNI, gross national income; NA, not available.
[*] World Bank.

Causes of death in children under 5 years—regional average

	%
Neonatal causes	44
Pneumonia	13
Diarrheal diseases	12
Malaria	1
HIV/AIDS	4
Measles	0
Injuries	3
Others	21

WHO, 2006 data.

Most common causes of death in all ages in three countries selected for a low (Haiti), middle (Dominican Republic), and high (Trinidad and Tobago) GNI (gross national income) per capita

	Haiti	Dominican Republic	Trinidad and Tobago
HIV/AIDS	22	15	16
Lower respiratory infections	7	NS	3
Cerebrovascular disease	6	4	11
Meningitis	5	NS	NS

(Continued)

	Haiti	Dominican Republic	Trinidad and Tobago
Perinatal conditions	4	3	2
Tuberculosis	4	2	NS
Anemia	3	NS	NS
Diabetes mellitus	3	4	11
Liver cirrhosis	NS	2	NS
Ischemic and hypertensive heart disease	3	17	22
Road traffic accidents	NS	4	1
Cancers	NS	NS	2
Injuries	NS	NS	2

WHO, 2006.
NS, not stated.

References

1. Jong EC, Sanford C (eds). The Travel and Tropical Medicine Manual, 4th edn. Philadelphia, PA: Saunders/Elsevier, 2008.
2. http://wwwnc.cdc.gov/travel/destinations/list.
3. Cook GC, Zumla AI, Weir J (eds) Manson's Tropical Diseases. Philadelphia, PA: Saunders/Elsevier, 2008.
4. Eddleston M, Davidson R, Brent A. Oxford Handbook of Tropical Medicine. Wiley Blackwell, 2008.
5. www.who.int/countries.
6. García-Rivera EJ, Vorndam V, Rigau-Párez JG. Use of an enhanced surveillance system for encephalitis and aseptic meningitisfor the detection of neurologic manifestations of dengue in Puerto Rico, 2003. P R Health Sci J 2009;28:114–20.
7. Edlow JA, McGillicuddy DC. Tick paralysis. Infect Dis Clin North Am 2008;22:397–413.
8. Gill G, Nick B. Tropical Medicine. Oxford: Wiley-Blackwell, 2009.
9. Dennis DT, Inglesby TV, Henderson DA, et al.; Working Group on Civilian Biodefense. Tularemia as a biological weapon: medical and public health management. JAMA 2001;285(21): 2763–73.
10. Adal KA, Kress K, Petri WA Jr. Determination of the pathogenicity of *Entamoeba histolytica*. Clin Infect Dis 1993;16:340.
11. Adams EB, Macleod IN. Invasive amebiasis. I. Amebiasis liver abscess and its complications. Medicine 1987;56:315–23.
12. Ahmed M, McAdam KP, Sturm AW, Hussain R. Systemic manifestations of invasive amebiasis. Clin Infect Dis 1992;15:974–82.
13. Orihel TC, Eberhard ML. Zoonotic filariasis. Clin Microbiol Rev 1998;11(2):366–81.
14. Peck RN, Fitzgerald DW. Cutaneous anthrax in the Artibonite valley of Haiti, 1992–2002. Am J Trop Med Hyg 2007;77:806–11.
15. Ellis J, Oyston PC, Green M, Titball RW. Tularemia. Clin Microbiol Rev 2002;15(4):631–46.

Chapter 21
Central America

Julius B. Salamera[1,2] and Larry I. Lutwick[1,2]
[1]Infectious Diseases, VA New York Harbor Health Care System, Brooklyn, NY, USA
[2]State University of New York (SUNY) Downstate Medical School, Brooklyn, NY, USA

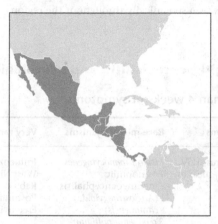

Belize
Costa Rica
El Salvador
Guatemala
Honduras
Nicaragua
Panama

There are quite a few neglected tropical pathogens in Central America, which needed serious attention in the hope of achieving a near total eradication in the future. This chapter will focus on the profiles of certain infectious agents which are potentially problematic in exposed individuals residing or traveling to Belize, Costa Rica, El Salvador, Guatemala, Honduras, Nicaragua, and Panama.

Bacterial infections: Typhoid fever, leptospirosis, listeriosis, and rickettsial infections are all common. Tuberculosis is common and whenever tuberculosis is diagnosed coinfection with HIV should be considered.

Viral infections: Dengue fever is common in Central America where it gives rise to repeated outbreaks. Hantavirus infections give rise to Hantavirus pulmonary syndrome and hemorrhagic fever with renal syndrome. West Nile virus is seen in Mexico, but has the potential to spread further south. Human exposure to rabies infected dogs is reported throughout the region. HIV is a risk in all countries in the region.

Parasitic infections: Malaria in most areas is predominantly due to *Plasmodium vivax* in more than 90% but varies within regions, including altitudes below 1,000–1,500 m (in Honduras and Guatemala) (World Health Organization, International Travel Health 2010, http://www.who.int/ith/ITH2010countrylist.pdf). Although *Plasmodium falciparum*

Infectious Diseases: A Geographic Guide, First Edition.
Edited by Eskild Petersen, Lin H. Chen & Patricia Schlagenhauf.
© 2011 John Wiley & Sons, Ltd. Published 2011 by John Wiley & Sons, Ltd.

is seen only in less than 10% of cases, chloroquine-resistant strains have been reported in Darien and San Blas provinces of Panama (United States Center for Disease Control (CDC), Malaria, http://www.cdc.gov/malaria/). Hookworms are endemic as are the two tapeworms *Taenia saginata* and *Taenia solium* which also cause cysticercosis. American trypanosomiasis (Chagas disease) and leishmaniasis (cutaneous, mucosal, and visceral forms) are seen throughout the region, and onchocerciasis (river blindness) is found mainly in Guatemala. Recently, *Trichinella* has been reported from pigs in Mexico.

Fungal infections: Pulmonary coccidioidomycosis is seen in dry and dessert-like environments, and histoplasmosis is seen sporadically throughout the region.

CNS infections: meningitis, encephalitis, and neurological syndromes

CNS infections with less than 4 weeks of symptoms

Frequently found microorganisms	Rare microorganisms	Very rare microorganisms
Viruses (enterovirus, dengue virus, HSV, VZV, CMV, EBV, HIV, mumps, measles, rubeola) *Streptococcus pneumoniae* *Neisseria meningitidis* *Haemophilus influenzae* type b *Mycobacterium tuberculosis* *Plasmodium falciparum*	*Listeria monocytogenes* Eosinophilic meningoencephalitis (*Angiostrongyloides cantonensis*) *Treponema pallidum* *Leptospira* *Brucella* *Salmonella enterica*	Influenza West Nile virus Rabies Postimmunization/vaccine Free-living amebae

CNS infections with symptoms for more than 4 weeks and in the immunocompromised host

Microorganisms with symptoms for more than 4 weeks	Microorganisms in the immunocompromised host
M. tuberculosis *Taenia solium* (neurocysticercosis) HIV/AIDS *C. neoformans* *T. pallidum*	*C. neoformans* *M. tuberculosis* *T. gondii* CMV, JC virus, VZV, EBV *Nocardia, Actinomyces* *Aspergillus* *T. pallidum* Free-living amebae

Cysticercosis: Humans, the usual definitive host of the parasite, may also become an intermediate host by direct ingestion of *T. solium* eggs in food contaminated by human feces. This is particularly dangerous since the larval forms of the parasite cause cysticercosis, presenting with varying CNS symptoms including seizures which is seen in <0.1% throughout Central America [1].

Rabies continue to be reported throughout Central America, and a Mexican women died in the United States in 2010 from rabies and another fatal case was reported from Guatemala in 2007. In May and August 2008, cases in 1 dog and 2 horses, respectively, were confirmed in Belize [2]. The occurrence of rabies in dogs, cows and in wildlife, such as vampire bats and foxes, represents an ongoing public health threat.

Ear, nose, and throat infections

Ear, nose, and throat infections with less than 4 weeks of exposure

Frequently found microorganisms	Rare microorganisms and conditions	Very rare microorganisms
Group A streptococci Influenza, parainfluenza, rhinovirus Herpes simplex EBV, CMV, HIV *Neisseria gonorrhoeae*	Peritonsillar abscess Necrotizing fasciitis *M. tuberculosis*	Diphtheria

Ear, nose, and throat infections with more than 4 weeks and in the immunocompromised host

Microorganisms with symptoms for more than 4 weeks	Microorganisms in the immunocompromised host
M. tuberculosis *Mycobacterium leprae* Mucocutaneous leishmaniasis	*Candida albicans* HSV, EBV Human herpes virus 8 *Pseudomonas aeruginosa* *Aspergillus, Mucor, Rhizopus*

Mucosal leishmaniasis can affect the nasal, oral, and pharyngeal mucosa which lead to a disabling and mutilating disease.

Cardiopulmonary infections

Cardiopulmonary infections with less than 4 weeks of symptoms

Frequently found microorganisms	Rare microorganisms and conditions	Very rare microorganisms

Pulmonary symptoms
  S. pneumoniae
  H. influenzae b
	Influenza
	Staphylococcus aureus	

(Continued)

Frequently found microorganisms	Rare microorganisms and conditions	Very rare microorganisms

Legionella pneumophila
Mycoplasma pneumoniae
Chlamydophila pneumoniae
Respiratory viruses
Histoplasma capsulatum
Coccioides immitis
Endocarditis, pericarditis, and
  myocarditis
  Viridans streptococci
  S. aureus
  Enterococcus
  Coagulase-negative
  staphylococci
  Coxsackievirus
	Aerobic Gram-negative bacilli
	  (e.g., *Klebsiella pneumoniae*)
	Ascaris lumbricoides (Loeffler's
	  syndrome)
	Wuchereria bancrofti
	Hantavirus pulmonary syndrome
	S. pneumoniae
	N. gonorrhoeae
	HACEK group
	Nutritionally variant streptococci
	Brucella
		Bartonella
		Coxiella burnetii

The pandemic strain of influenza A H1N1 was spread to the rest of Central America after appearing in Mexico [2]. The H5N1 avian-origin influenza has not spread to the Western Hemisphere but low pathogenic strains have been found.

Pulmonary symptoms and endocarditis for more than 4 weeks and in the immunocompromised host

Microorganisms and diseases with symptoms for more than 4 weeks	Microorganisms in the immunocompromised host

Pulmonary symptoms
  M. tuberculosis
  C. neoformans
  Aspergillus
  Nocardia
  Nontuberculous mycobacteria
	M. tuberculosis
	Pneumocystis jirovecii
	Aspergillus, Candida
	Mycobacterium avium complex
	CMV
	H. capsulatum
	P. aeruginosa
	C. immitis

Endocarditis, pericarditis, and myocarditis
  Coagulase-negative staphylococci
  Viridans streptococci
  Bartonella
  Candida
  Trypanosoma cruzi
	Aspergillus
	T. gondii

Infection from *C. immitis* is transmitted by inhalation of fungal conidia from dust, can be asymptomatic or present in a range of patterns from influenza-like illness, to overwhelming pulmonary and disseminated disease. Activities that increase the risk are those that result in exposure to dust, as in construction, excavation, or dirt biking.

Infection associated with *H. capsulatum* is transmitted via inhalation of spores from soil contaminated with bat guano or bird droppings and is found throughout Central America. It is particularly seen in persons who are exposed to bird droppings and bat guano, including high-risk activities in the form of spelunking, mining, and construction and excavation works.

This infection caused by *T. cruzi* is transmitted by blood-sucking triatomine bugs ("kissing bugs"). The vector is found mainly in rural areas of Central America where it lives in the walls of poorly constructed housing. There are reported cases of oral transmission by ingestion of unprocessed freshly squeezed sugarcane or fruit juice in areas where the vector is present. It causes a chronic illness with progressive myocardial damage leading to cardiac arrhythmias and cardiac dilatation, and gastrointestinal involvement leading to mega esophagus and mega colon. Across Central America, a prevalence rate of 1.6% has been reported [3].

Gastrointestinal infections

Gastrointestinal infections with less than 4 weeks of symptoms

Frequently found microorganisms	Rare microorganisms and conditions	Very rare microorganisms
Escherichia coli (enterotoxic, enterohemorrhagic, enteroinvasive)		*Tropheryma whipplei*
		Yersinia enterocolitica
Nontyphoidal *Salmonella* enterica serotypes		
Campylobacter spp.	*Isospora*	
Shigella spp.	*Cryptosporidium*	
Salmonella Typhi	*Cyclospora*	
Giardia intestinalis		
Entamoeba histolytica		
S. aureus enterotoxin disease		
A. lumbricoides		
Enterobius vermicularis		
Norovirus, rotavirus		

Giardia intestinalis infection usually occurs through ingestion of cysts in water or food contaminated by the feces of infected humans or animals. *Cyclospora cayetanensis* has been the source of outbreaks from consuming fruits and berries contaminated with cysts.

Gastrointestinal infections with symptoms for more than 4 weeks and in the immunocompromised host

Microorganisms with symptoms for more than 4 weeks	Microorganisms in the immunocompromised host
Giardia	*Candida* spp.
Cryptosporidium	*Cryptosporidium*
Cyclospora	*Isospora*
A. lumbricoides	Microsporidia spp.
Hookworms	*Salmonella*
T. solium and *Taenia saginata*	CMV
M. tuberculosis	*M. tuberculosis*
HIV Strongyloides stercoralis	*S. stercoralis*
	HSV
	HHV 8

The tapeworm *T. saginata* is acquired by consumption of raw or undercooked beef from cattle that harbor the larval form of the parasite. *T. solium* is similarly acquired from raw or undercooked pork. Cattle and pigs become infected with the larval stages of tapeworm as a result of access to human feces, from which they ingest tapeworm eggs, spread by human tapeworm carriers.

Infection may also be acquired by handling soil-contaminated foods, in street markets, or by contaminated water. Guatemala has the highest prevalence of ascariasis and trichuriasis which may partly explain why the nation has the highest prevalence of underweight children [3].

Infections of liver, spleen, and peritoneum

Acute infections of liver, spleen, and peritoneum with less than 4 weeks of symptoms

Frequently found microorganisms	Rare microorganisms
Hepatitis A virus, hepatitis B virus (isolated or delta virus coinfection/superinfection), hepatitis C virus, dengue virus	Herpes viruses (CMV, EBV, HSV, VZV), adenovirus, HIV, hepatitis E virus
Leptospira	*Rickettsia*, nontuberculous mycobacteria, *Brucella*, *Salmonella*
M. tuberculosis	*Toxocara* (larva migrans), *Fasciola hepatica*, *A. lumbricoides*
S. Typhi	*P. falciparum*

Chronic infections of liver, spleen, and peritoneum with more than 4 weeks of symptoms

Frequently found microorganisms	Rare microorganisms	Microorganisms in the immunocompromised host
Hepatitis B virus (with or without delta virus coinfection/superinfection), hepatitis C virus	Torque teno (TT) virus, hepatitis G virus	Herpes viruses (CMV, EBV, HSV, VZV), HIV
S. typhi	Nontuberculous mycobacteria, *S. typhi*, *Brucella*, *Borrelia*, *T. pallidum*	*S. typhi*, *M. tuberculosis*, nontuberculous mycobacteria, *T. pallidum*
M. tuberculosis	*E. histolytica*, *F. hepatica*, *Toxocara* (larva migrans)	*Histoplasma*, *Cryptococcus*, *Candida*, *Cryptosporidium*, *Microsporidium*

Genitourinary infections

Genitourinary symptoms with less than 4 weeks' duration

Frequently found microorganisms	Rare microorganisms and conditions	Very rare microorganisms
Cystitis, pyelonephritis, and nephritis *E. coli*	*Enterococcus* spp.	

Frequently found microorganisms	Rare microorganisms and conditions	Very rare microorganisms
Staphylococcus saprophyticus	*S. aureus*	
K. pneumoniae	Perirenal abscess	
Proteus spp.		
Chlamydia trachomatis		
P. aeruginosa		
Leptospira spp.		
Sexually transmitted infections		
Chlamydia spp.	LGV	
N. gonorrhoeae	*E. histolytica* Haemophilus ducreyi	
T. pallidum	Granuloma inguinale	
HSV II		
HPV		
Trichomonas vaginalis		
Parasites (scabies, lice)		

Genitourinary symptoms for more than 4 weeks and in the immunocompromised host

Microorganisms with symptoms for more than 4 weeks	Microorganisms in the mmunocompromised host
Cystitis, pyelonephritis, and nephritis	
Bacterial infections (catheters, renal stones)	*Candida* spp.
M. tuberculosis	*M. tuberculosis*
HIV-associated nephropathy	HHV 8
Sexually transmitted infections	
T. pallidum	Same in immunocompetent host
HPV	
HSV	
HIV	
H. ducreyi	
C. trachomatis	
N. gonorrhoeae	
T. vaginalis	

Sexually transmitted infections

There is inadequate data on sexually transmitted infections (STIs) in most areas in Central America. The inability to determine trends are thought to be related to emphasis on HIV disease, and thus neglecting the other infections acquired through unsafe sexual contacts. Data from 2007 revealed that *Trichomonas* infections in women, and nonspecific genital infections in both sexes, were the most commonly reported STIs [4].

Joint, muscle, and soft tissue infections

Joint, muscle, and soft tissue infections with less than 4 weeks of symptoms

Frequently found microorganisms	Rare microorganisms and conditions	Very rare microorganisms and conditions
S. aureus N. gonorrhoeae	Necrotizing fasciitis Vibrio vulnificus Clostridium perfringens Echinococcus spp. S. pneumoniae Trichinella spiralis Virus (parvovirus, rubella, HBV, enterovirus) Salmonella spp.	Fournier's gangrene

Joint, muscle, and soft tissue infections with more than 4 weeks of symptoms and in the immunocompromised host

Microorganisms with symptoms for more than 4 weeks	Microorganisms in the immunocompromised host
M. tuberculosis Brucella spp. Virus (influenza, dengue fever, HBV, enterovirus, HIV) Postviral myopathy, chronic fatigue syndrome C. immitis	Candida spp. M. tuberculosis M. avium complex Cryptococcus spp.

Skin infections

Skin infections with less than 4 weeks of symptoms

Frequently found microorganisms	Rare microorganisms and conditions	Very rare microorganisms and conditions
S. aureus	Leishmania spp.	Erysipelothrix rhusiopathiae
Beta-hemolytic streptococci Dermatophytoses Cutaneous larva migrans	C. neoformans S. stercoralis	Yaws Rat-bite fever (Spirillum minus, Streptobacillus moniliformis)
T. pallidum N. gonorrhoeae Spotted fever group rickettsioses Sarcoptes scabiei Helminths Tinea versicolor (Malassezia furfur) HIV Candida spp. Leptospira spp.	T. spiralis Onchocerca volvulus	

Skin infections with more than 4 weeks of symptoms and in the immunocompromised host

Microorganisms with symptoms for more than 4 weeks	Microorganisms in the immunocompromised host
T. pallidum	*Candida* spp.
M. tuberculosis	HHV 8
M. leprae	*H. capsulatum*
Nontuberculous mycobacteria	*M. tuberculosis*
Pityriasis versicolor	*C. neoformans*
Candida spp.	*Bartonella* spp.
Mycetoma (actinomycosis)	*M. avium* complex
Nocardia	*S. scabiei*
HIV	

Leishmaniasis is transmitted by the bite of female phlebotomine sand flies. Dogs, rodents, and other mammals, including humans, are reservoir hosts for leishmaniasis. Sand flies acquire the parasites by biting infected reservoirs. Transmission from person to person by infected blood or contaminated syringes and needles is also possible.

Cutaneous leishmaniasis is the most common presentation and causes skin sores and chronic ulcers. It is one of the highest disease burdens among the neglected tropical diseases in Central America, with 62,000 infected populations presenting mainly as cutaneous disease, and 5,000 cases as mucocutaneous disease [3].

Lymphadenopathy

Adenopathy of less than 4 weeks' duration

Frequently found microorganisms	Rare microorganisms and conditions	Very rare microorganisms and conditions
Regional adenopathy		
T. pallidum	*Leishmania* spp.	
Staphylococci, streptococci	*Bartonella* spp.	*Babesia microti*
Fungal infections	*W. bancrofti*	Rat-bite fever (*S. minus*, *S. moniliformis*)
Nontuberculous mycobacteria	*Brucella* spp.	
Systemic adenopathy		
HIV		
EBV, CMV, enterovirus		
Parvovirus B19		
Rickettsioses		
M. tuberculosis		

Adenopathy of more than 4 weeks' duration and in the immunocompromised host

Microorganisms with symptoms for more than 4 weeks	Microorganisms in the immunocompromised host
HIV	HIV
M. tuberculosis	*M. tuberculosis*
T. pallidum	*M. avium* complex
	T. gondii
	EBV, CMV
	HHV 8
	Fungal infections (*H. capsulatum*)

Tuberculosis remains a major health threat in persons living with HIV/AIDS with prevalence of coinfection of about 12.4% in 2008 [5]. It has started to decline over the past several years due to improved strategy in screening, treatment by directly observed therapy, and effective anti-retroviral therapy. Political commitment is also strongly reinforced in the hope of curbing the infection rates and emergence of drug-resistant tuberculosis.

Global surveillance of HIV and AIDS through the joint effort of WHO and UNAIDS has developed a core framework of national-level indicators to monitor the availability, coverage, outcomes, and impact of health sector interventions for prevention, treatment, and care of people living with this disease. In general, there is a steady increase of new cases per year with HIV. Adult prevalence is highest in Belize among all countries in Central America and the third highest in the Carribean [2]. The main mode of transmission is through heterosexual contact.

Fever without focal symptoms

Fever for less than 4 weeks without focal symptoms

Frequently found microorganisms	Rare microorganisms and conditions	Very rare microorganisms and conditions
Viral infections (HIV, EBV, CMV, enterovirus, parvovirus B19)	*Brucella*	*Rickettsia prowazekii*
M. tuberculosis	Nontuberculous mycobacteria	
P. falciparum, Plasmodium vivax	*Bartonella*	
Dengue fever	*C. burnetii*	
Leptospira spp.		
Rickettsioses		
T. gondii		
Salmonella spp.		

Rickettsia rickettsii infections have been identified in northern Mexico, Costa Rica, and Panama and is known in Mexico as fiebre manchada. *Rickettsia prowazekii* cause louse-borne typhus, and are transmitted by the human body louse. Louse-borne typhus fever is the only rickettsial disease that can cause explosive epidemic. Although rare, it can be seen in colder regions of Central and South America, and in conditions of overcrowding and poor hygiene, such as prisons and refugee camps.

Dengue fever (DF) transmission often occurs in both rural and urban areas; dengue infections are most often reported from urban settings with lower risk at altitudes above 1,000 m. Usually

DF causes a mild illness, but it can be severe and lead to dengue hemorrhagic fever (DHF) which can be fatal if not treated. People, especially children, who have had a different serotype of DF before are more at risk of getting DHF.

In 2002, WHO has reported an increase in endemic dengue disease in El Salvador. About 1,200 cases of DF and 101 cases of DHF from serotype 1 have been laboratory confirmed, with children between the ages of 5 and 9 years were most affected. During the same year, Honduras experienced an outbreak with reports of 3,993 cases of DF including 8 deaths and 545 cases of DHF. About 3 years later, a smaller outbreak in Belize with 652 cases, including the first confirmed case of the hemorrhagic type, was reported [2].

West Nile virus is found in Mexico and may spread in other parts of Central America, presenting as febrile syndrome and/or encephalitis.

Malaria occurs at least 7–9 days after being bitten up by an infected anopheline mosquito. Malaria in most parts of Central America is predominantly due to *P. vivax* in more than 90% but varies within regions, including altitudes below 1,000–1,500 m (in Honduras and Guatemala) [2]. Although *P. falciparum* is seen only in less than 10% of cases, chloroquine-resistant strains have been reported in the eastern Darien and San Blas provinces of Panama [6].

Leptospirosis is acquired through contact between the skin or mucous membranes and water, wet soil, or vegetation contaminated by the urine of infected animals, notably rats. Occasionally, it may also result from direct contact with urine or tissues of infected animals or from consumption of food contaminated by the urine of infected rats.

Leptospirosis is present throughout Central America, and outbreaks have occurred in whitewater rafters in Costa Rica and US troops training in Panama [2].

Hantavirus infection is found in tropical and subtropical regions of Central America. Hantaviruses are carried by various species of rodents, and infection occurs through direct contact with the feces, saliva, or urine of infected rodents or by inhalation of the virus in rodent excreta. It causes damage to the vascular endothelium leading to increased vascular permeability, hypotension, bleeding, and shock. Two distinct syndromes are well-known associations, hemorrhagic fever with renal syndrome and Hantavirus pulmonary syndrome.

World Health Organization reported 12 suspected cases including three deaths from Hantavirus pulmonary syndrome in March of 2000 around some locales of Panama particularly from Las Tablas and Guarare districts, and Los Santos Province. The diagnosis has been confirmed by serological tests (positive IgM and IgG) on samples from three surviving patients [2].

Fever for more than 4 weeks without focal symptoms and in the immunocompromised host

Microorganisms with symptoms for more than 4 weeks	Microorganisms in the immunocompromised host
M. tuberculosis	*M. tuberculosis*
HIV	*M. avium* complex
T. gondii	*C. neoformans*
Salmonella	EBV
Leishmania	CMV
Brucellosis	*H. capsulatum*

Brucellosis have been reported from Mexico after consumption of unpasteurized cheese. *Mycobacterium bovis* has also been reported in humans after consuming cheese from Mexico produced from unpasteurized milk.

Eosinophilia and elevated IgE

Eosinophilia and elevated IgE for less than 4 weeks

Frequently found microorganisms	Rare microorganisms and conditions	Very rare microorganisms and conditions
S. stercoralis	T. spiralis	Anisakis spp.
Hookworms (Ancylostoma, Necator)	HIV	
W. bancrofti	Echinococcus granulosus	
Schistosoma spp.	Drug hypersensitivity reaction	
Neurocysticercosis (T. solium)		
Trichuris trichiura		
Toxocara spp.		

Eosinophilia and elevated IgE for more than 4 weeks and in the immunocompromised host

All helminthic infections can present with chronic eosinophilia in immunocompetent and immunocompromised host. Advanced HIV infection with CD4 count of less than 200/µl can also cause some degree of eosinophilia.

Filariasis is transmitted through the bite of infected mosquitoes, which introduce larval forms of the nematodes during a blood meal [3]. The prevalence of filariasis in Central America is approximately 0.1%. Typical manifestations in symptomatic cases include filarial fever, lymphadenitis, and retrograde lymphangitis. Chronic cases can present as lymphedema, hydrocele, chyluria, tropical pulmonary eosinophilic syndrome, and in rare instances, renal damage.

Hookworms, particularly *Necator* and *Ancylostoma* species, may be a risk for humans especially in places where beaches are polluted by human or canine feces. Humans become infected by larval forms of the parasite which penetrate the skin. The non-human species produce a characteristic skin rash, cutaneous larva migrans.

Onchocerca volvulus, onchocerciasis, is transmitted through the bite of infected blackflies. The adult worms are found in fibrous nodules under the skin where they discharge microfilaria which migrates through the skin causing dermatitis, and can reach the eye causing damage that results in blindness. Although this disease is mainly seen in Western and Central Africa, sporadic cases can be found in Central and South America in less than 5% of cases characterized by low worm burden with little eye disease presenting as classical kerato-irido-cyclitis [1]. Guatemala has the greatest number of cases, with 0.2 million at risk [3].

Trichinella is found throughout the region in wild animals and appear occasionally in domesticated pigs.

Antimicrobial resistance in Central America

Resistance of certain pathogens to current pharmacologic armamentarium presents therapeutic dilemmas to clinicians worldwide, and particularly troublesome in developing countries. Resistance is an ecological phenomenon stemming from the response of a microorganism to the widespread use of antimicrobials and their presence in the environment. The underlying problems are economic and societal, and no ready solutions are available. The Environmental Protection Agency (EPA) reported that hundred and thousand pounds of antibiotics were being sprayed onto fruit trees all across the globe, including Central America [7,8]. The end result is excellent conditions for the selection of drug resistance. Compounding with this problem is the widespread and inappropriate use of antimicrobials in the setting where its use is likely to be futile.

Malaria

Chloroquine-resistant strains have been reported in Darien and San Blas provinces of Panama [9].

Tuberculosis

The Americas have been reported as one with the lowest proportion of new cases of multidrug-resistant tuberculosis (MDR-TB) with the notable exception of Guatemala with 3.0% [5]. In general, absolute numbers of extensively drug-resistant tuberculosis (XDR-TB) are low in Central America.

Staphylococcus aureus

Methicillin-resistant *Staphylococcus aureus* (MRSA) is a growing problem in the Americas. Information gathered by the Pan American Health Organization (PAHO)-sponsored program on nosocomial infections demonstrated the prevalence of MRSA as follows: Costa Rica, 58%; Guatemala, 64%; Honduras, 12%; Panama, 28%; and Nicaragua, 20% [10,11].

Gram-negative enteric bacteria

During the last 25 years, outbreaks of disease due to multidrug-resistant strains of enteric bacterial pathogens have occurred with alarming frequency in less affluent areas of the world. The outbreaks have involved most of the important etiologic agents of bacterial diarrhea. Drug-resistant *Shigella* and *Salmonella* species are widespread in Central America [12]. The problem was brought dramatically to the world's attention in 1969, when a pandemic of bacillary dysentery began in Guatemala and eventually spread to involve six Central American countries and southern Mexico before subsiding the following year [13,14]. The epidemic strain was resistant to sulfonamides, streptomycin, tetracycline, and chloramphenicol.

The rate of multidrug-resistant enterobacteriaceae is sporadically seen mostly in countries around Latin America with efficient surveillance system. The mechanism is mainly related to extended-spectrum beta-lactamases (ESBL) among isolates from both the community and hospital setting.

Vaccine-preventable infections in children

Immunization is one of the most successful and cost-effective interventions which has shown significant reduction of mortality rates. Children should be considered for vaccination at all times against the same diseases as adults, although take into consideration the specific product, dose, and administration details may vary.

As programs around the nation are reinforcing basic vaccination schedules, global health agencies as well as local health sectors have joined effort in the hope of controlling disease outbreaks in the future.

The risk of major vaccine-preventable diseases has been reduced through a steady increase in vaccination coverage against measles, mumps, rubella, diphtheria, tetanus, pertussis, poliomyelitis, hepatitis B, *H. influenzae* type b, pneumococcal disease, and varicella. Each has a coverage level above 90%. Depending on the risk involved, rabies and influenza vaccines may be given. Rotavirus vaccine has been included in the immunization schedule, but will be in effect starting October 2010 [15,16].

There have been no reported cases of measles, diphtheria, and poliomyelitis in the last decade. Overall, all Central America have significant number of reported cases of mumps in 2009 except Belize and Guatemala. Likewise, pertussis is still prevalent in Costa Rica, Guatemala, Nicaragua, and Panama [2].

Basic economic and demographic data

	GNI per capita (PPP, USD)	Life expectancy at birth (years)	Health life expectancy at birth (years)	Adult mortality rate (per 1,000 adults, 15–59 years)	Under-five mortality rate (per 1,000 live births)	Prevalence of HIV (per 1,000 adults, 15–49 years)	Prevalence of tuberculosis (per 100,000 population)
Belize	5,940	72	60	178	19	21	43
Costa Rica	10,960	78	69	97	11	4	3
El Salvador	6,630	72	61	214	18	8	18
Guatemala	4,690	69	60	228	34	8	110
Honduras	3,830	70	62	179	31	7	79
Nicaragua	2,620	74	64	165	27	2	26
Panama	12,630	76	67	112	23	10	14

GNI, gross national income.
World Health Organization [17].

Causes of death in children under 5 years, 2008 (%)

	Causes	Percentage
Belize	Prematurity	18
	Congenital abnormalities	15
	Pneumonia	11
	Injuries	11
	Birth asphyxia	9
	Diarrhea	7
	Neonatal sepsis	4
	Malaria	0
	Measles	0
	Others	
Costa Rica	Congenital abnormalities	30
	Prematurity	23
	Birth asphyxia	9
	Neonatal sepsis	6
	Pneumonia	5
	Injuries	3
	Diarrhea	1
	Malaria	0

	Causes	Percentage
	Measles	0
	Others	
El Salvador	Prematurity	21
	Congenital abnormalities	19
	Pneumonia	14
	Birth asphyxia	9
	Injuries	7
	Diarrhea	4
	Neonatal sepsis	1
	Malaria	0
	Measles	0
	Others	
Guatemala	Pneumonia	20
	Diarrhea	19
	Prematurity	19
	Congenital abnormalities	5
	Injuries	5
	Birth asphyxia	5
	Neonatal sepsis	1
	Malaria	0
	Measles	0
	Others	
Honduras	Prematurity	22
	Pneumonia	18
	Birth asphyxia	12
	Diarrhea	10
	Congenital abnormalities	9
	Neonatal sepsis	5
	Injuries	4
	Malaria	0
	Measles	0
	Others	
Nicaragua	Prematurity	22
	Pneumonia	20
	Congenital abnormalities	13
	Diarrhea	9
	Birth asphyxia	8
	Injuries	4
	Neonatal sepsis	2
	Malaria	0
	Measles	0
	Others	
Panama	Congenital abnormalities	24
	Prematurity	16
	Pneumonia	13
	Birth asphyxia	6
	Injuries	6
	Diarrhea	6
	Neonatal sepsis	5
	Malaria	0
	Measles	0
	Others	

World Health Organization, 2008.

All top 10 causes of death in all ages

	Causes
Belize	Diabetes
	Hypertension
	Diseases of the pulmonary circulation and other forms of heart disease
	HIV/AIDS
	Cerebrovascular diseases
	Transport accidents
	Ischemic heart disease
	Acute respiratory disease
	Injury, undetermined
	Injury, purposely inflicted
Costa Rica	Ischemic heart disease
	Cerebrovascular diseases
	HIV/AIDS
	COPD
	Road traffic accidents
	Stomach cancer
	DM
	Hypertensive heart disease
	Lower respiratory tract infections
	Perinatal conditions
El Salvador	Ischemic heart disease
	Lower respiratory tract infections
	Violence
	HIV/AIDS
	Perinatal conditions
	Road traffic incidents
	Nephritis and nephrosis
	Cerebrovascular diseases
	DM
	Alcohol use disorders
Guatemala	COPD
	HIV/AIDS
	Lower respiratory tract infections
	Violence
	Perinatal conditions
	Diarrheal diseases
	Ischemic heart diseases
	Cerebrovascular diseases
	DM
	Cirrhosis of liver
Honduras	Ischemic heart disease
	HIV/AIDS
	Perinatal conditions
	Cerebrovascular diseases
	DM
	Diarrheal diseases
	Lower respiratory tract infections
	Nephritis and nephrosis
	Hypertensive heart disease
	Protein energy malnutrition
Nicaragua	Ischemic heart disease
	Cerebrovascular disease
	Lower respiratory tract infections

	Causes
Panama	Perinatal conditions Diarrheal diseases DM Nephritis and nephrosis Road traffic accidents Hypertensive heart disease Self-inflicted injuries Ischemic heart disease Cerebrovascular disease DM Perinatal conditions Lower respiratory tract infections COPD Road traffic accidents Prostate cancer Violence Stomach cancer

References

1. Mandell G, Bennett G, Dolin R. Principles and Practice of Infectious Diseases, 7th edn. Philadelphia, PA: Elsevier, 2010:3593.
2. World Health Organization. International Travel Health 2010. Accessed March 2010 at http://www.who.int/ith/ITH2010countrylist.pdf.
3. Hotez PJ, Bottazzi ME, Franco-Paredes C, Ault S, Periago MR. The neglected tropical diseases of Latin America and the Carribean: a review of disease burden and distribution and a roadmap for control and elimination. PLoS Negl Trop Dis 2008;2(9):e300.
4. US CDC Online Health Information for International Travel (The Yellow Book). Accessed March 2010 at http://cdc.gov/travel/yb/index.htm.
5. World Health Organization. Anti-tuberculosis drug resistance in the world. The WHO/IUATLD Global Project on Anti-tuberculosis Drug Resistance Surveillance 2008. Accessed August 2010 at http://www.who.int/tb/publications/drs_report4.htm.
6. United States Center for Disease Control (CDC). Malaria. Accessed March 2010 at http://www.cdc.gov/malaria/.
7. Kunin C. Resistance to antimicrobial drugs—a worldwide calamity. Ann Intern Med 1993; 118:557–61.
8. Levy S. Antibiotic resistance: consequences of inaction. Clin Infect Dis 2001;33(Suppl.3): S124–9.
9. Bloland P. Drug resistance in malaria. World Health Organization Department of Communicable Diseases Surveillance and Response. Accessed July 2010 at http:www.who.int/emc.
10. Wertheim H, Verbrugh H. Global prevalence of methicillin-resistant *Staphylococcus aureus*. Lancet 2006;368:1866.
11. Guzman-Blanco M, Mejia C, Isturiz R, et al. Epidemiology of methicillin-resistant *Staphylococcus aureus* (MRSA) in Latin America. Int J Antimicrob Agents 2009;34:304–8.
12. Pan American Health Organization. Annual Report of the Monitoring/Surveillance Network for Resistance to Antibiotics, 2004. Accessed August 2010 at http://www.paho.org/English/AD/DPC/CD/amr-2004.htm.
13. Farrar WE. Antibiotic resistance in developing countries. J Infect Dis 1985;152(6):1103–6.
14. Guzman-Blanco M, Casellas JM, Sader HS. Bacterial resistance to antimicrobial agents in Latin America. Infect Dis Clin North Am 2000; 14(1):67–81.
15. World Health Organization. Vaccine-preventable diseases: monitoring system. Global Summary 2010. Accessed July 2010 at http://apps.who.int/immunization_monitoring/en/globalsummary/countryprofileselect.cfm.
16. US CDC Traveler's Health Home. Accessed March 2010 at http://www.cdc.gov/travel/index.htm.
17. World Health Organization. Global Health Indicators 2010. Accessed July 2010 at http://www.who.int/whosis/indicators/en/.

Chapter 22
South America

Rodrigo Nogueira Angerami[1] and Luiz Jacintho da Silva[2]
[1]Infectious Diseases, Unicamp, State University of Campinas, Brazil
[2]Dengue Vaccine Initiative, International Vaccine Institute, Seoul, Republic of Korea

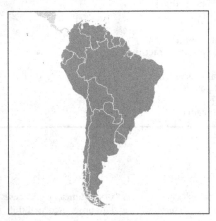

Argentina
Bolivia
Brazil
Chile
Colombia
Ecuador
French Guyana
Guyana
Paraguay
Peru
Suriname
Uruguay
Venezuela

South America is a large and heterogeneous subcontinent that extends from 12°27′ north to 53°54′ south, islands excluded from consideration, and from 34°77′ west to 81°19′ west, islands also excluded.

Its landmass is of 17,840,000 km^2 (6,890,000 mi^2), or almost 3.5% of the Earth's surface, with a population of roughly 370 million.

The intense urbanization occurred during the twentieth century and still ongoing, as well as increasing migration has contributed to the present distribution of infectious disease in the subcontinent.

Although there has been significant improvement in the health conditions, several infectious diseases are still endemic and epidemic in South America. Their distribution is far from homogeneous and considerable differences in disease surveillance account for much of this distribution.

Infectious Diseases: A Geographic Guide, First Edition.
Edited by Eskild Petersen, Lin H. Chen & Patricia Schlagenhauf.
© 2011 John Wiley & Sons, Ltd. Published 2011 by John Wiley & Sons, Ltd.

South America travel and travelers

Data from the World Tourism Organization show a significant increase in the number of arrivals to South American countries over the years. In 2008, of 922 million of international arrivals around the world, 20.8 million had a South American country as destiny. More expressive, however, is the increase from 2007 to 2008, 3.9% against 1.7% for the Americas overall. The greatest increases were in Uruguay (10%), Chile (8%), Peru (7%), and Ecuador (7%) [1].

Fever is the most frequent clinical sign of illness acquired among returned travelers [2,3]. In ill travelers returning from the Caribbean and Central and South America, fever was reported in 3–18% of cases [2,3]. Other retrospective study identified fever as the most important clinical sign in 8.5% of patients [3]. Fever is usually associated with a nonspecific clinical picture, a challenge during etiological investigation of febrile acute disease in this increasing group of patients.

Among acute febrile patients, malaria is one of the most common specific diagnoses when an endemic area is visited [2–4]. However, in South America, the reemergence of dengue fever in all countries except Uruguay [5] figures as the most important vector-borne disease and one of the most relevant differential diagnosis of acute nonspecific, exanthematic, or hemorrhagic febrile syndromes. According to WHO data from 2008, there were 826,535 notified cases of dengue fever, 16,737 of those dengue hemorrhagic with 225 deaths. This explains why since 1980s dengue fever is more frequent than malaria in travelers returning from any region except Africa and Central America [4,6].

Other vector-borne diseases (arbovirosis, rickettsial diseases, trypanosomiasis) are endemic in many regions of South America, although mostly rural or sylvatic, and with a lower incidence [2–4,7].

Although tropical diseases are important differential diagnosis, diseases with universal distribution (e.g., herpes viruses, HIV, toxoplasmosis, influenza, leptospirosis, salmonellosis, pneumococcosis) account for the majority of travel-related illnesses, and for this reason should be always considered and, if the clinical and epidemiological picture are consistent, investigated [3,6,7].

A large retrospective study using GeoSentinel database observed the most frequent clinical syndromes among ill travelers returning from countries of South America as following: dermatologic disorders (264/1,000 patients), acute diarrhea (219/1,000 patients), systemic febrile illness (143/1,000 patients), and respiratory disorders (50/1,000 patients).

When considering the interval of time from returning to the first medical evaluation, many retrospective studies show that most patients sought medical assistance within a month after travel, the majority within 2 weeks (77–84.4%) [2,4,7], but a significant proportion (10%), because an indolent disease or a longer incubation period, were first evaluated after 6 months or more [3,4].

Reported disease activity in the last 10 years (isolated cases, clusters, and epidemics)

Country	Disease
Argentina	Anthrax (cutaneous)
	Arenavirus (Junin)
	Chagas' disease (vector-borne)
	Dengue fever
	Hantavirus
	Malaria
	Measles
	Mucocutaneous leishmaniasis
	Coccidioidomycosis
	Saint Louis encephalitis
	Trichinellosis
	Visceral leishmaniasis
	West Nile virus
	Yellow fever (jungle)
Bolivia	Arenavirus (Chapare, Machupo)
	Chagas' disease (vector-borne)
	Dengue
	Hantavirus
	Malaria
	Mucocutaneous leishmaniasis
	Visceral leishmaniasis
	Plague
	Yellow fever
Brazil	Bat-transmitted rabies
	Brazilian spotted fever (*Rickettsia rickettsii*)
	Chagas' disease (oral infection)
	Dengue fever
	Diphyllobothriasis
	Filariasis (*Wuchereria bancrofti*)
	Hantavirus
	Hepatitis Delta
	Leptospirosis
	Malaria (*Plasmodium falciparum, Plasmodium vivax, Plasmodium malariae*)
	Mayaro
	Oropouche
	Measles
	Melioidosis (Ceará State)
	Meningococcal disease
	Mucocutaneous leishmaniasis
	Onchocerciasis
	Oropouche
	Plague
	Saint Louis encephalitis
	Schistosomiasis (*Schistosoma mansoni*)
	Visceral leishmaniasis
	Yellow fever
Chile	Coccidioidomycosis
	Dengue (Easter Island)
	Hantavirus
	Listeriosis
	Trichinellosis
	Vibrio parahaemolyticus

Country	Disease
Colombia	Anthrax (cutaneous)
	Bartonellosis (Carrion's disease; Oroya fever)
	Bat-transmitted rabies
	Chagas' disease (oral infection)
	Mucocutaneous leishmaniasis
	Onchocerciasis
	Spotted fever (*R. rickettsii*)
	Visceral leishmaniasis
Ecuador	*Angiostrongylus* meningitis
	Histoplasmosis
	Bartonellosis (Carrion's disease; Oroya fever)
	Bat-transmitted rabies
	Dengue fever
	Malaria
	Onchocerciasis
	Oropouche
French Guyana	Measles
	Yellow fever
Guyana	Dengue fever
	Leptospirosis
	Malaria
	Mucocutaneous leishmaniasis
Paraguay	Diphteria
	Hantavirus pulmonary syndrome
	Malaria
	Visceral leishmaniasis
	Yellow fever
Peru	Bartonellosis (Carrion's disease; Oroya fever)
	Bat-transmitted rabies
	Epidemic typhus (*Rickettsia prowazekii*)
	Leptospirosis
	Oropouche
	Plague
	Spotted fever (*R. rickettsii*)
	Yellow fever
Suriname	Dengue
	Schistosomiasis
	Yellow fever
Uruguay	Anthrax (cutaneous)
	Coccidioidomycosis
	Hantavirus
	Histoplasmosis
	Meningococcal disease
	Rickettsia parkeri
Venezuela	Arenavirus
	Chagas' disease (oral infection)
	Dengue
	Eastern equine encephalitis
	Malaria
	Mayaro
	Onchocerciasis
	Venezuelan equine encephalitis
	Yellow fever

Source: Promed (www.promedmail.org), September 9, 2010; WHO (www.who.org), July 30, 2010; CDC (www.cdc.gov), July 30, 2010; Pan American Health Organization (PAHO) Epidemiological alerts (http://new.paho.org/hq/index.php?option=com_content&task=view&id=1239&Itemid=1091& lang=en).

Universal distribution: Amebiasis, cryptosporidiosis, histoplasmosis, leptospirosis, salmonellosis, viral hepatitis (A, B, C), mononucleosis syndromes, influenza, tuberculosis.

Emerging issues in South America are as follows:

Acute Chagas' disease acquired through oral transmission [8–10]

Dengue and dengue hemorrhagic fever [11–13]

Expansion and urbanization of visceral (Calazar) leishmaniasis

Increasing yellow fever activity (nonhuman primate epizooty, clusters of human cases in expanding transmission area) [14]

For information about South American malaria-risk areas, see http://cdc-malaria.ncsa.uiuc.edu/, for information about dengue epidemiological activity in South America, Dengue map http://healthmap.org/dengue, and for yellow fever risk and vaccine recommendation, http://wwwnc.cdc.gov/travel/yellowbook/2010/chapter-2/yellow-fever-vaccine-requirements-and-recommendations.aspx.

CNS infections: meningitis and encephalitis

Acute infections with less than 4 weeks of symptoms

Frequently found microorganisms	Rare microorganisms	Very rare microorganisms
Virus: arboviruses (dengue, yellow fever[a]), enteroviruses (echoviruses, coxsackieviruses, parvovirus), mumps, herpes simplex viruses (HSV1, HSV2, varicella, cytomegalovirus), HIV	Virus: arboviruses (Saint Louis, Rocio), rabies, measles, influenza virus	Virus: West Nile, alphaviruses (eastern equine encephalitis, western equine encephalitis, Venezuelan equine encephalitis)
Bacteria: pneumococcus, meningococcus, *Haemophilus influenzae*, leptospirosis	Bacteria: neurosyphilis, *Staphylococcus aureus*, *Streptococcus pyogenes*, *Salmonella, Rickettsia, Brucella*	Bacteria: *Listeria monocytogenes*
Other agents: *Toxoplasma, P. falciparum*	Other agents: *Cryptococcus*, American trypanosomiasis (acute)	Other agents: *Naegleria* and other free-living ameba, *Angiostrongylus cantonensis*

[a]Only jungle cycle. Bolivia and Paraguay had possible urban transmission in the last 10 years.

CNS infections: meningitis, and encephalitis with symptoms for more than 4 weeks and in the immunocompromised host

Microorganisms with symptoms for more than 4 weeks	Microorganisms in the immunocompromised host
Virus: HIV, rabies, HTLV-1 (tropical spastic paraparesis)	Virus: polyomavirus, JC virus, cytomegalovirus, poliovirus
Bacteria: *Mycobacterium tuberculosis, Borrelia*, neurosyphilis	Bacteria: *Nocardia, M. tuberculosis, Borrelia*, neurosyphilis, *Listeria*

Microorganisms with symptoms for more than 4 weeks	Microorganisms in the immunocompromised host
Other agents: *S. mansoni, Toxoplasma, Taenia solium* (cysticercosis), *Lagochilascaris minor*	Other agents: *Cryptococcus* spp., American trypanosomiasis, *Toxoplasma, Strongyloides stercoralis*

Consider noninfectious causes like vasculitis and lymphoma.

Ear, nose, and throat infections

Ear, nose, and throat infections with less than 4 weeks of symptoms

Frequently found microorganisms	Rare microorganisms and conditions	Very rare microorganisms
Common cold: rhinovirus, adenovirus, parainfluenza virus, respiratory syncytial virus, influenza virus	Pharyngitis: HSV 1 and 2, coxsackievirus A, Cytomegalovirus, HIV-1, *Corynebacterium diphtheriae, Neisseria gonorrhoeae, Chlamydophila pneumoniae, Mycoplasma pneumoniae*	Common cold: coronavirus, human metapneumovirus
Pharyngitis: rhinovirus, adenovirus, parainfluenza virus, influenza virus, Epstein–Barr virus, group A β-hemolytic streptococcus	Laryngitis: *C. pneumoniae, M. pneumoniae*	Pharyngitis: coronavirus, *Yersinia enterocolitica, Francisella tularensis*
Peritonsillar abscess[a]: *C. pneumoniae, M. pneumoniae*	Epiglotitis: *H. influenzae*	Laryngitis: coronavirus, human metapneumovirus
Laryngitis: rhinovirus, influenza virus, parainfleunza virus, adenovirus	Otitis externa: *Pseudomonas aeruginosa*	Vincent's angina[a]: Mixed infection
Acute otitis media: *Streptococcus pneumoniae, Moraxella catarrhalis*, group A streptococcus, *S. aureus*		Ludwig's angina[a]
Otitis externa: *S. aureus, Staphylococcus epidermidis, Corynebacterium*, anaerobics		
Acute sinusitis: rhinovirus, influenza virus, adenovirus, parainfluenza virus, *S. pneumoniae, M. catarrhalis, S. pyogenes, S. aureus, H. influenzae* (unencapsulated), gram-negative bacteria, anaerobic bacteria		Lemierre disease[a]: *Fusobacterium necrophorum*

[a]Requires acute ENT evaluation.

Ear, nose, and throat infections with symptoms for more than 4 weeks and in the immunocompromised host

Microorganisms with symptoms for more than 4 weeks	Microorganisms in the immunocompromised host
Sinusitis: *Aspergillus, Zygomycetes (Mucor* spp., *Rhizopus* spp.), *S. pneumoniae, H. influenzae,* gram-negative bacteria Laryngitis: *Paracoccidioides brasiliensis,* tegumentary leishmaniasis, *M. tuberculosis,* human papillomaviruses (HPVs), *C. diphtheriae* Nose/oral ulcers: *P. brasiliensis,* tegumentary leishmaniasis, *M. tuberculosis,* syphilis, HSV, *Candida* spp., *C. diphtheriae, Actinomyces, Streptococcus,* anaerobic bacteria, *Mycobacterium leprae*	Bacteria: *S. pneumoniae, H. influenzae,* gram-negative bacteria, *M. tuberculosis,* nontuberculous mycobacterium, syphilis Viral: HSV, HPV, cytomegalovirus Other pathogens: *Aspergillus, Zygomycetes (Mucor* spp., *Rhizopus* spp.), *Candida, Fusarium*

Consider noninfectious causes like vasculitis and lymphoma.

Cardiopulmonary infections

Pneumonia with less than 4 weeks of symptoms

Frequently found microorganisms	Rare microorganisms and conditions	Very rare microorganisms
Viral: influenza virus, respiratory syncytial virus (in children) Bacteria: *S. pneumoniae, S. pyogenes, S. aureus, H. influenzae, P. aeruginosa, M. pneumonia, Chlamydia pneumonia, M. tuberculosis*	Viral: adenovirus, parainfluenza virus, hantavirus, varicella zoster virus Bacteria: *M. catarrhalis, Legionella, Leptospira* spp., *Chlamydia psittaci,* nontuberculous mycocabterium, *Bordetella pertussis* Other agents: *Aspergillus* spp., *P. brasiliensis, Histoplasma capsulatum, Toxoplasma gondii, Ascaris lumbricoides, S. stercoralis, Toxocara canis*	Virus: coronavirus, metapneumovirus, measles, adenovirus Bacteria: *Bacillus* spp., *Corynecabterium, Coxiella, Burkholderia pseudomallei*[a], *Yersinia pestis*

[a]Only reported in Ceara State, Brazil.

Endocarditis with less than 4 weeks of symptoms

Frequently found microorganisms	Rare microorganisms and conditions	Very rare microorganisms
S. aureus, Coagulase-negative staphylococci (*S. epidermidis*), Viridans streptococci, *S. pneumoniae, Enterococcus* spp., other streptococci	*N. gonorrhoeae, Coxiella burneti,* HACEK group (*Haemophilus parainfluenzae, H. aphrophilus, Actinobacillus, Cardiobacterium, Eikenella, Kingella*), *Propionibacterium, Candida* spp.	*Bartonella* spp., *Brucella* spp.

Selected *cardiac infections (myocarditis) other than infectious endocarditis*

• Viral: hantavirus, coxsackieviruses, dengue virus, yellow fever virus, arenavirus, and influenza virus.
• Bacteria: *Leptospira, Rickettsia, Borrelia, Mycoplasma, Chlamydia, Salmonella, Coxiella, C. diphtheriae, S. pyogenes, S. aureus.*
• Other agents: American trypanosomiasis (acute presentation), *Toxoplasma, Trichinella.*

Pulmonary symptoms for more than 4 weeks and in the immunocompromised host

Microorganisms and diseases with symptoms for more than 4 weeks	Microorganisms in the immunocompromised host
Bacteria: *M. tuberculosis, B. pertussis, Chlamydia* Other agents: COPD, *Aspergillus* spp., *H. capsulatum, P. brasiliensis, T. gondii, A. lumbricoides, S. stercoralis, T. canis*	Virus: cytomegalovirus Bacteria: *M. tuberculosis*, nontuberculous mycobacterium, *Rhodococcus equi, Nocardia* Other agents: *Pneumocystis jirovecii, Aspergillus, Cryptococcus, Toxoplasma, Strongyloides*
Consider noninfectious causes like lung cancer, autoimmune lung fibrosis, Wegener's granulomatosis, allergic pneumonitis, sarcoidosis.	

Endocarditis for more than 4 weeks and in the immunocompromised host

Microorganisms and diseases with symptoms for more than 4 weeks	Microorganisms in the immunocompromised host
Coagulase-negative staphylococci (*S. epidermidis*), nonhemolytic streptococci	*Aspergillus, Candida* spp.
Consider noninfectious causes like sarcoidosis, systemic lupus.	

Gastrointestinal infections

Gastrointestinal infections with less than 4 weeks of symptoms

Frequently found microorganisms	Rare microorganisms and conditions	Very rare microorganisms
Viral: calicivirus (norovirus), rotavirus	Bacteria: *Bacillus cereus* toxin, *Vibrio cholera, Clostridium perfringens, S. typhi,* Invasive *Escherichia coli, E. coli* O157, *V. parahaemolyticus, Listeria*	Bacteria: *Y. enterocolitica, M. tuberculosis*
Bacteria: *Campylobacter*, VeroToxin producing E Coli (VTEC), Enterotoxigenic *E. coli, Salmonella* (nontyphi), *S. aureus* toxin, *Shigella*, group A streptococcus Other agents: *Giardia intestinalis, Enterobius vermicularis* (threadworm)	Other agents: *Cryptosporidium* spp., *Cyclospora, Trichinella, A. lumbricoides, S. mansoni*, chemical agents (toxins, heavy metals)	

Gastrointestinal infections with symptoms for more than 4 weeks and in the immunocompromised host

Microorganisms with symptoms for more than 4 weeks	Microorganisms in the immunocompromised host
Bacteria: *M. tuberculosis, S. typhi* Other agents: *Blastocystis* (b), *Dientamoeba fragilis* (b), *Cryptosporidium, Entamoeba histolytica, Giardia, Trichinella*	Bacteria: *Clostridium difficile, Campylobacter jejunii*, nontuberculous mycobacterium, *M. tuberculosis, Listeria* Other agents: *Candida*, herpes viruses, *S. stercoralis, Cryptosporidium, Cyclospora,* Microsporidia, *Isospora, Histoplasma*

Infections of liver, spleen, and peritoneum

Acute infections of liver, spleen, and peritoneum with less than 4 weeks of symptoms

Frequently found microorganisms	Rare microorganisms
Virus: hepatitis A virus, dengue virus, yellow fever virus, hepatitis B virus (isolated or delta virus coinfection/superinfection), hepatitis C virus Bacteria: leptospirosis, hepatic abscess, cholecystitis, cholangitis, *S. typhi, M. tuberculosis* Other agents: *Toxoplasma, P. falciparum*	Virus: herpes viruses (cytomegalovirus, Epstein–Barr virus, HSV, varicella zoster virus), adenovirus, HIV, hepatitis E virus, arenavirus, hantavirus, influenza virus Bacteria: *Rickettsia*, nontuberculous mycobacterium, *Brucella, Salmonella, Rickettsia, Chlamydia, L. monocytogenes, B. pseudomallei* Other agents: *Leishmania* spp. (visceral Leishmaniasis), amebic abscess, *S. mansoni*, American trypanosomiasis (acute), *Toxocara* (larva migrans), *Fasciola hepatica, A. lumbricoides*

Chronic infections of liver, spleen, and peritoneum for more than 4 weeks of symptoms

Frequently found microorganisms	Rare microorganisms	Microorganisms in the immunocompromised host
Virus: hepatitis B virus (isolated or delta virus coinfection/ superinfection), hepatitis C virus Bacteria: hepatic abscess, *S. typhi, M. tuberculosis* Other agents: *P. falciparum, S. mansoni*	Virus: TT virus, hepatitis G virus Bacteria: Nontuberculous mycobacterium, *Salmonella, Brucella, Borrelia*, syphilis Other agents: *T. gondii, Leishmania* spp. (visceral Leishmaniasis), Amebic abscess, *P. brasiliensis, F. hepatica, Echinococcus* (hydaticcyst), *Toxocara* (larva migrans)	Virus: herpes viruses (cytomegalovirus, Epstein–Barr virus, HSV, Varicella zoster virus), HIV Bacteria: *Salmonella, M. tuberculosis*, nontuberculous mycobacterium, syphilis Other agents: *Leishmania* spp. (visceral Leishmaniasis), *Histoplasma, Cryptococcus, Candida, Cryptosporidium, Microsporidium*

Genitourinary infections

Cystitis, pyelonephritis, and nephritis with less than 4 weeks of symptoms

Frequently found microorganisms	Rare microorganisms and conditions	Very rare microorganisms
E. coli (most frequent), *Klebsiella, Proteus, Pseudomonas, Enterobacter*	*Staphylococci, M. tuberculosis,* Perirenal abcess	Adenovirus, *Ureaplasma, Mycoplasma*

Sexually transmitted infections with less than 4 weeks of symptoms

Frequently found microorganisms	Rare microorganisms and conditions
Urethritis, vulvovaginitis: *N. gonorrhoeae, Chamydia trachomatis, Ureaplasma urealyticum, Trichomonas vaginalis, Mycoplasma genitalium,* HSV, *Candida (vulvovaginitis), Gardnerella vaginalis* (bacterial vaginosis) Epididymitis/orchitis: mumps, *N. gonorrhoeae, C. trachomatis, E. coli, Klebsiella pneumoniae, P. aeruginosa,* staphylococci, streptococci Ulcers: syphilis, HSV 1 and 2, *Haemophilus ducreyi* (cancroid) Wart: HPV	*C. trachomatis (Lymphogranuloma venereum), Calymmobacterium granulomatis (Granuloma inguinale)* Orchitis: coxsackie virus, lymphocytic choriomeningitis virus, *Brucella*

Cystitis, pyelonephritis, and nephritis with symptoms for more than 4 weeks and in the immunocompromised host

Microorganisms with symptoms for more than 4 weeks	Microorganisms in the immunocompromised host
Bacterial infections in patients with long-term catheters and renal stones, *M. tuberculosis*	*Candida, M. tuberculosis,* JC virus, BK virus

Sexually transmitted infections with symptoms for more than 4 weeks and in the immunocompromised host

Microorganisms with symptoms for more than 4 weeks	Microorganisms in the immunocompromised host
Ulcers: syphilis Wart: HPV	Cytomegalovirus, mycobacteria, *Candida, Cryptococcus, Salmonella*

(Continued)

Microorganisms with symptoms for more than 4 weeks	Microorganisms in the immunocompromised host
Epididymitis/Orchitis: *M. tuberculosis, P. brasiliensis* Prostatitis: *Enterococcus faecalis, Staphylococcus saprophyticus, E. coli, N. gonorrhoeae, C. trachomatis, U. urealyticum, T. vaginalis, M. genitalium, M. tuberculosis, P. brasiliensis*	

Joint, muscle, skin, and soft tissue infections

Joint, muscle, and soft tissue infections with less than 4 weeks symptoms

Frequently found microorganisms	Rare microorganisms and conditions	Very rare microorganisms and conditions
Skin and soft tissues[a]: *S. aureus*, group A streptococci, scabies	Skin and soft tissues[a]: *P. aeruginosa, Pasteurella multocida* (postanimal bites), *Leishmania* species, *P. brasiliensis, Borrelia*	Skin and soft tissues[a]: *C. diphtheriae, Bartonella, Bacillus anthracis, Sporothrix,* nontuberculous mycobacterium, *B. pseudomallei, Spirillum minus*
Arthritis: *S. aureus, N. gonorrhoeae, Neisseria meningitidis, S. pneumoniae*	Arthritis: *Brucella, Parvovirus* B19, HIV (acute infection), dengue virus, *Borrelia*[b]	Arthritis: Mayaro virus, *Bartonella*
Myositis: dengue virus, *Leptospira, S. aureus,* group A streptococci	Necrotizing fasciitis: Group A/G streptococci	Fournier's gangrene
	Myositis: Group B/C/G streptococci, echovirus, influenza virus, coxsackie virus, *Rickettsia, Toxoplasma*	Myositis: *Trichinella, T. solium,* influenza virus, *Mycobacterium*
	Tropical pyomyositis: *S. aureus* Scarlet fever syndromes: *S. aureus,* group A streptococci Gas gangrene: *C. perfringens*	

[a]Impetigo, folliculitis, furuncles, paronychia, ecthyma, erysipelas, cellulitis, and ulcers.
[b]Transmission, epidemiology, and clinical picture not completely known in South America.

Joint, muscle, and soft tissue infections for more than 4 weeks of symptoms and in the immunocompromised host

Microorganisms with symptoms for more than 4 weeks	Microorganisms in the immunocompromised host
Skin and soft tissues: syphilis, yaws[a] (*Treponema pertenue*), Pinta[b] (*Treponema carateum*), Onchocerciasis[c], Paracoccidiodomycosis, Verruga Peruana (*Bartonella bacilliformis*), *M. tuberculosis, M. leprae, Sporothrix, Leishmania*	Skin and soft tissues: *Candida, Histoplasma, Cryptococcus, Fusarium, Bartonella hensellae, M. tuberculosis,* nontuberculous mycobacterium, varicella virus, herpes virus

Microorganisms with symptoms for more than 4 weeks	Microorganisms in the immunocompromised host
Arthritis: *Borrelia*[a], *M. tuberculosis*, syphilis, *Nocardia*, *Brucella*, nontuberculous mycobacterium (including *M. leprae*), *Sporothrix*, *P. brasiliensis*, reactive arthritis (Reiter's syndrome—post-*Chlamydia trachomatis* and enterobacteriaceae infection)	

Consider other inflammatory noninfectious arthritis: Still's disease, rheumatic fever, rheumatoid arthritis, and Kawasaki syndrome.
[a]Rare: Ecuador, Colombia, Suriname, and Guyana.
[b]Rare: Amazon region, cases reported almost exclusively in Indians.
[c]Limited area: Brazil (Roraima State), Venezuela (most cases in Yanomami Indians).

Adenopathy

Adenopathy of less than 4 weeks' duration

Frequently found microorganisms	Rare microorganisms and conditions	Very rare microorganisms and conditions
Virus: Epstein–Barr virus, cytomegalovirus, parvovirus, HIV, rubella, adenovirus	Virus: dengue virus	Filariaisis, Onchocerciasis, *F. tularensis*, *Y. pestis*, Ehrlichia
Bacteria: *M. tuberculosis*, *Treponema pallidum* Other agents: *T. gondii*, *P. Brasiliensis*	Bacteria: *Bartonella*, *H. ducreyi*, *R. parkeri* Other agents: *Trypanossoma cruzi* (acute infection), *S. mansoni* (acute infection), Leishmaniasis calazar	

Adenopathy of more than 4 weeks' duration and in the immunocompromised host

Microorganisms with symptoms for more than 4 weeks	Microorganisms in the immunocompromised host
T. gondii, *P. brasiliensis*, *M. tuberculosis*, *Leishmania chagasi*, Kikuchi's disease	Cytomegalovirus, parvovirus, HIV, adenovirus, *M. tuberculosis*, nontuberculous mycobacterium, histoplasmosis, *Bartonella*, *Leishmania chagasi*

Fever without focal symptoms

Fever for less than 4 weeks without focal symptoms

Frequently found microorganisms	Rare microorganisms and conditions	Very rare microorganisms and conditions
Viral: Epstein–Barr virus, cytomegalovirus, dengue virus, HIV	Viral: oropouche virus, parvovirus B19, herpes virus 6, mayaro virus, Guaroa virus[a], Venezuelan equine encephalitis virus, Saint Louis virus	*F. tularensis, Y. pestis*[b], *Ehrlichia, Babesia, R. prowazekii*[c]
Bacterial: *M. tuberculosis*, *Salmonella* (typhoid and paratyphoid fevers), infective endocarditis	Bacterial: *C. burnetti*, organ abscess	
Other agents: *P. vivax, P. falciparum, Leishmania chagasi, T. gondii*	Other agents: *Trichinella spiralis*[d]	

[a]Amazon region.
[b]Peru, Bolivia, and Colombia reported recent human cases.
[c]Remote high-altitude Andean region. No recent activity.
[d]Argentina and Chile, mostly. Exposed to locally produced pork or wild boar meat.

Fever for more than 4 weeks without focal symptoms and in the immunocompromised host

Microorganisms with symptoms for more than 4 weeks	Microorganisms in the immunocompromised host
T. gondii Tuberculosis	Cytomegalovirus Adenovirus

Eosinophilia and elevated IgE

Eosinophilia and elevated IgE for less than 4 weeks

Frequently found microorganisms	Rare microorganisms and conditions	Very rare microorganisms and conditions
A. lumbricoides and *Ascaris suum*[a], *S. stercoralis*[a], *Necator americanus*[a]	*Toxocara* spp., *S. mansoni*[b], *P. brasiliensis*[c], *T. spiralis*	*W. bancrofti* (lymphatic filariasis)

[a]Larval phase.
[b]Acute phase.
[c]Disseminated (juvenile) form.

Eosinophilia and elevated IgE for more than 4 weeks and in the immunocompromised host

Microorganisms with symptoms for more than 4 weeks	Microorganisms in the immunocompromised host
A. lumbricoides and A. suum, Angiostrongylus costaricensis	Toxocara spp., S. stercoralis

Hemorrhagic and leptospirosis fever

Hemorrhagic fever	leptospirosis fever
Viral: dengue virus, arenavirus, hantavirus[a] Bacteria: meningococci, staphylococci, R. rickettsii Other agents: P. falciparum	Virus: yellow fever virus, arenavirus, hepatitis A virus, hepatitis B/D Bacteria: R. rickettsii, Leptospira, Salmonella Other agents: P. falciparum, P. vivax (uncommon)

[a]In South America, cardiopulmonary syndrome.

Selected endemic tropical infections in South America

Disease	Transmission	Clinical picture	Clinical alert signs and complications	Laboratorial diagnosis
Dengue fever (DENV1, DENV2, DENV3, DENV4)	Vectorial (Aedes aegypti); urban transmission—Endemic/epidemic	*Incubation period:* Median 5–6 days (3–15 days) *General signs and symptoms:* Fever, headache, prostration, ocular pain, exanthema, joint and muscle pain, diarrhea, vomiting, pruritus	*Alert signs:* Abdominal pain, vomiting, hypothermy, altered mental status, hemorrhagic signs, hemoconcentration, hepatomegaly, thrombocytopenia *Complications* Dengue hemorrhagic fever: hypoalbuminemia, hypovolemic hypotension, cavitary effusion, hemorrhage, thrombocytopenia Dengue shock syndrome	–Viral isolation –PCR –Antigen NS1 detection –IgM detection –Immunohistochemistry (tissue)

(Continued)

Disease	Transmission	Clinical picture	Clinical alert signs and complications	Laboratorial diagnosis
Malaria (*P. falciparum*, *P. vivax*, and *P. malariae*)	Vectorial (*Anopheles* spp.) Jungle, rural, and, rarely, urban transmission Endemic	*Incubation period*[a]: –*P. falciparum*: 8–12 days –*P. vivax*: 13–17 days –*P. malariae*: 18–30 days *General signs and symptoms*: Fever, headache, joint and muscle pain, prostration, chills, diarrhea, vomiting	Unusual: encephalitis, myocarditis, idiopathic thrombocytopenic purpura, hepatitis (including fulminant forms) Alert signs: hypoglycemia, anemia, thrombocytopenia, jaundice, hemorrhagic signs, altered mental status, oliguria *General Complication* Respiratory distress, disseminated intravascular coagulation, hemorrhages, severe anemia, cerebral edema, seizures, hypotension, shock, acute renal failure	–Blood films (including tick films) (parasite observation) –Rapid test antigen detection –PCR
Yellow fever	Vectorial (*Haemagogus*, *Sabethes*, *Aedes*) Sylvatic (jungle) transmission Recent outbreaks and epidemics in many countries	*Incubation period*: 3–6 days *General signs and symptoms*: fever, headache, joint and muscle pain, low-back pain, prostration, vomiting, diarrhea	*Alert signs* Intense nausea and vomiting, hematemesis, oliguria, albuminuria, thrombocytopenia, jaundice, hemorrhagic signs, altered mental status *Complication* Respiratory distress, disseminated intravascular coagulation, hemorrhages, enchephalopathy, coma, hypotension, shock, acute renal failure, liver failure	–Viral isolation –PCR –IgM detection –Immunohistochemistry (tissues)
Acute Chagas' disease (*Trypanosoma cruzi*)	Vectorial, food-borne, vertical, parenteral (e.g., transfusion) Sporadic clusters and outbreaks	*Incubation period*: –Vectorial: 4–15 days –Enteral/oral: 3–22 days *General signs and symptoms*: prostration, diarrhea, vomiting, lymphadenopathy, hepatomegaly, splenomegaly, diarrhea, muscle pain, exhantema	*Complication* Acute: facial edema, anasarca, myocarditis, pericarditis, cardiomegaly, arrhythmia, cough, dyspnea, congestive heart insufficiency, digestive hemorrhage, meningoencephalitis Chronic: –Myocardiopathy (dilatation, aneurysms, arrhythmia, cardiac congestive insufficiency) –Digestive tract dysfunction (megacolon, megaesophagus) –Reactivation in immunocompromised patients (mostly cardiac and neurologic damage)	–Blood films (parasite observation) –IgM detection –IgG increasing antibodies titers (paired samples) –PCR

[a]The use of antimalarial chemoprophylaxy may extend the incubation period.

Special considerations

Malaria

As observed in many endemic areas, the observation of emergence of *Plasmodium* species has increased in South America. *P. falciparum* should always be considered chloroquine-resistant [15].

Antibiotic resistance

As observed worldwide, the emergence of an increasing number of pathogens resistant to a wide spectrum of antimicrobials is a critical issue in many countries of South America. Despite the heterogeneous information among countries, some systems of surveillance and information have been contributing for the best knowledge of frequency, distribution, clinical, and therapeutics implications.

Pneumococcus: The SIREVA (*Sistema Regional de Vacunas—Regional System of Vaccines*), a multicenter, international laboratory-based surveillance project on invasive *S. pneumoniae*, monitors circulating serotypes and susceptibility pattern to antibiotics. From 2000 to 2005, SIREVA determined 38.8% as the continental index of *S. pneumoniae* strains with diminished susceptibility to penicillin (21.5% intermediate; 17.3% high) for pneumonia, sepsis, and bacteremia; for meningitis, 30.5% (19.3% intermediate; 17.3% high) [16–18].

Other gram-positive bacteria: In a SENTRY study, including Brazilian hospital, from 2005 to 2008, 31% oxacillin (MRSA) resistance among *S. aureus* strains was also resistant to clindamycin, ciprofloxacin, levofloxacin, and trimethoprim/sulfamethoxazole (68.1%); all strains were susceptible to vancomycin, daptomycin, and linezolid [19]. Among coagulase-negative staphylococci, 80% were resistant to oxacillin. A significant increase in vancomycin resistance has been observed in enterococci. Despite the strong evidence of spread of MRSA in Latin America with a wide range of clones, especially in Brazil, Argentina, Chile, Colombia, and Paraguay, more consistent data including prevalence studies is lacking [20].

Meningococcus: SIREVA II (2000–2005) found 65.8% and 99.2% susceptibility to penicillins and rifampicin, respectively; 34.1% intermediate resistance to penicillin and only 0.2% resistant [16–18].

Salmonella: Nalidixic acid-resistant *Salmonella* strains are common. According to SENTRY Antimicrobial Surveillance Program, from 1997 to 2004, the overall *Salmonella* resistance to Nalidixic acid with reduced susceptibility to ciprofloxacin in Latin America was 15% [21]. In the same study it was observed that all strains were susceptible to cefepime, carbapenems, gentamicin, and fluoroquinolones.

Vaccine-preventable diseases in children

The childhood vaccination programs in South America are above the average of developing countries in other continents, both in number of vaccines available and coverage.

Only 2 of the 12 countries and one overseas department (French Guyana) qualify as Global Alliance for Vaccines and Immunizations (GAVI)-dependent countries.

The work of the PAHO has been fundamental in achieving high quality standards. Polio and measles have been eliminated. Occasional imported cases of measles with secondary cases may occur; however, no wild polio cases have been detected since the early 1990s.

Most countries have a vaccination schedule that includes ID-BCG, DPT, Hib, OPV, HepB, Rotavirus, measles, and rubella. Pneumococcal conjugate vaccine has been introduced in several countries and many have annual influenza vaccination for the elderly.

Updated vaccination schedules, as well as vaccine coverage in children and incidence of selected vaccine-preventable disease, by country can be found in PAHO's web site (http://new. paho.org/hq/index.php?option=com_content&task=view&id=2043&Itemid=259).

Yellow fever vaccines is part of the childhood schedule in children above 1 year of age in risk areas (areas where yellow fever has been detected in humans or monkeys) in Argentina, Brazil, Bolivia, Peru, Paraguay, Ecuador, and Colombia. Venezuela vaccinates only travelers to risk areas.

HPV has not yet been introduced in public programs in South American countries.

In 2008, the region reported 16 cases of neonatal tetanus, a good indicator of the effectiveness of vaccination program, from five countries (Brazil, Colombia, Ecuador, Paraguay, and Peru), down from 130 cases in seven countries reported 10 years earlier, in 1999.

Basic economic and demographic data

Basic demographics[a]	GNI[b] per capita (USD)	Life expectancy at birth (total, years)	School enrollment, primary (% net)
Argentina	7,200	75	98
Bolivia	1,460	66	94
Brazil	7,350	73	93
Chile	9,400	78	94
Columbia	4,660	73	87
Ecuador	3,640	75	97
French Guyana	NA	NA	NA
Guyana	1,420	67	NA
Paraguay	2,180	72	94
Peru	3,990	73	96
Suriname	4,990	69	94
Uruguay	8,260	76	97
Venezuela	9,230	74	90

NA, not available.
[a]World Bank.
[b]Gross National Income.

Causes of death in children under 5 years—regional average

	%
Neonatal causes	44
Pneumonia	12
Diarrheal diseases	10
Malaria	0
HIV/AIDS	1
Measles	0
Injuries	5
Others	28

WHO, 2006.

The top most causes of deaths in all ages in three countries elected for a low (Guyana), middle (Bolivia), and high (Brazil) gross national income (GNI) per capita

	%		
	Guyana	Bolivia[a]	Brazil
HIV/AIDS	19	1	12
Lower respiratory infections	3	9	4
Diarrheal diseases	4	6	NS
Violence	NS	NS	5
Perinatal conditions	4	8	6
Malaria	NS	NS	b
Tuberculosis	3	4	7[c]
Cerebrovascular diseases	12	4	11
Ischemic heart disease	11	5	11
Inflammatory heart disease	NS	NS	2
Road traffic accidents	NS	NS	3
Measles	NS	NS	NS
Hypertensive heart disease	4	NS	3
Diabetes mellitus	4	2	4
Cirrhosis of the liver	NS	3	NS
Genitourinary system diseases	NS	3	NS
All cancers	NS	2	NS
Anemia	2	NS	NS
Chronic obstructive lung disease	NS	NS	4

NS, not stated.
WHO, 2006.
[a]WHO, 2002.
[b]30 deaths reported in 2006.
[c]Of which 29% were HIV-positive persons.

References

1. World Tourism Organization. Tourism Highlights 2009 Edition. Available from http://www.unwto.org/facts/eng/pdf/highlights/UNWTO_Highlights09_en_HR.pdf. Accessed September 15, 2010.
2. Antinori S, Galimberti L, Gianelli E, et al. Prospective observational study of fever in hospitalized returning travelers and migrants from tropical areas, 1997–2001. J Travel Med 2004;11:135–42.
3. Wilson ME, Weld LH, Boggild A, et al. Fever in returned travelers: results from GeoSentinel Surveillance Network. Clin Infect Dis 2007;44:1560–8.
4. Freedman DO, Weld LH, Kozarsky PE, et al. Spectrum of disease and relation to place of exposure among ill returned travelers. N Engl J Med 2006;354:119–30.
5. Pan American Health Organization. Epidemiological Alert: Update on Dengue Outbreaks in the Americas (September 8, 2010). Available from http://new.paho.org/hq/index.php?option=com_content&task=view&id=3409&Itemid=2206. Accessed September 8, 2010.
6. Askling HH, Lesko B, Vene S, et al. Serologic analysis of returned travelers with fever, Sweden. Emerg Infect Dis 2009;15:1805–8.
7. Ansart S, Perez L, Vergely O, Danis M, Bricaire F, Caumes E. Illnesses in travelers returning from the tropics: a prospective study of 622 patients. J Travel Med 2005;12:312–18.
8. Bastos CJ, Aras R, Mota G, et al. Clinical outcomes of thirteen patients with acute Chagas disease acquired through oral transmission from two urban outbreaks in Northeastern Brazil. PLoS Negl Trop Dis 2010;15:e711.

9. Pereira KS, Schimidt FL, Barbosa RL, et al. Transmission of Chagas disease (American Trypanosomiasis) by food. Adv Food Nutr Res 2010;59C:63–85.

10. Miles MA. Orally acquired Chagas disease: lessons from an urban outbreak. J Infect Dis 2010;201:1282–4.

11. Guzmán MG, Kouri G. Dengue: an update. Lancet Infect Dis 2001;2:33–42.

12. Halstead SB. Dengue. Lancet 2007;370:1644–52.

13. Suaya JA, Shepard DS, Siqueira JB, et al. Cost of dengue cases in eight countries in the Americas and Asia: a prospective study. Am J Trop Med Hyg 2009;80:846–55.

14. Barnett ED. Yellow fever: epidemiology and prevention. Clin Infect Dis 2007;44:850–6.

15. World Health Organization. Guidelines for the Treatment of Malaria—2nd edn. Geneva: WHO, 2010.

16. Gabastou JM, Agudelo CI, Brandileone MCC, et al. Caracterización de aislaminetos invasivos de S. pneumoniae, H influenzae y N. meningitidis en America Latina y el Caribe: SIREVA II, 2000–2005. Pan Am J Public Health 2008;24:1–15.

17. Agudelo CI, Castañeda E, Corso A, et al. Resistencia a antibióticos no betalactamicos de aislamientos invasores de *Streptococcus pneumoniae* em niños latinoamericanos. SIREVA II, 2000–2005. Pan Am J Public Health 2009; 25:305–13.

18. Castañeda E, Agudelo CI, Regueira M, et al. Laboratory-based surveillance of *Streptococcus pneumoniae* invasive disease in children in 10 Latin American countries. A SIREVA II project, 2000–2005. Pediatr Infect Dis J 2009;28: e265–70.

19. Gales AC, Sader HS, Ribeiro J, et al. Antimicrobial susceptibility of Gram positive bacteria isolated in Brazilian hospitals participating in the SENTRY Program (2005–2008). Braz J Infect Dis 2009;13:90–8.

20. Rodriguez-Noriega E, Seas C, Guzmán-Blanco M, et al. Evolution of methicillin-resistant *Staphylococcus aureus* clones in Latin America. Int J Infect Dis 2010;14:e560–66.

21. Biedenbach DJ, Toleman M, Walsh TR, Jones RN. Analysis of *Salmonella* spp. With resistance to extended-spectrum cephalosporins and fluoroquinolones isolated in North America and Latin America: report from SENTRY Antimicrobial Surveillance Program (1997–2004). Diagn Microbiol Infect Dis 2006;54:13–21.

Chapter 23
Northern America

Barbra M. Blair,[1,2] Philip R. Fischer,[3] Michael Libman[4] and Lin H. Chen[1,2]

[1]Division of Infectious Diseases, Mount Auburn Hospital, Cambridge, MA, USA
[2]Harvard Medical School, Boston, MA, USA
[3]Department of Pediatric and Adolescent Medicine, Mayo Clinic College of Medicine, Rochester, MN, USA
[4]Division of Infectious Diseases, McGill University and Department of Microbiology, McGill University Health Centre, Montreal, Quebec, Canada

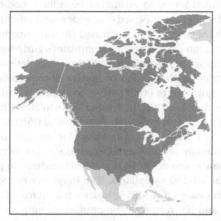

Canada
United States

Northern America consists of two major industrialized nations, Canada and the United States, with populations of 34 million and over 300 million, respectively. Infectious agents in Northern America are typical of those identified in most developed countries, but some regionally specific pathogens exist. Agents and illnesses specific to Northern America (or less commonly recognized in other world regions) include *Babesia*, *Ehrlichia*, *Anaplasma*, Lyme, Rocky Mountain spotted fever, and *Coccidioides*. West Nile virus has become established in the region since its initial identification in 1999. Food-borne outbreaks cause an estimated 76 million illnesses in the United States annually, with the majority attributed to infectious agents including *Salmonella* spp., norovirus, Shiga toxin-producing *Escherichia coli*, *Shigella* spp., and *Clostridium perfringens*. *Giardia* and *Cryptosporidium* cause approximately 30,000 infections annually, many associated with recreational water activities. Community-acquired *Clostridium difficile* diarrhea has emerged,

Infectious Diseases: A Geographic Guide, First Edition.
Edited by Eskild Petersen, Lin H. Chen & Patricia Schlagenhauf.
© 2011 John Wiley & Sons, Ltd. Published 2011 by John Wiley & Sons, Ltd.

whereas previously this had been a consequence of antibiotic therapy. Antimicrobial resistance is a common concern when treating infections in Northern America, especially vancomycin-resistant *Enterococci* and methicillin-resistant *Staphylococcus aureus*.

Acute infections within 4 weeks of exposure

Infectious agents in Northern America are typical of those identified in most developed countries, but some pathogens exist that are less commonly recognized in other world regions, including *Babesia, Ehrlichia, Anaplasma*, Lyme, Rocky Mountain spotted fever, *Coccidioides*, St Louis encephalitis, eastern equine encephalitis, and western equine encephalitis. With the globalization of food procurement within the United States, an estimated 76 million food-borne illness occur annually [1]. Clonal outbreaks have become dispersed over wide geographic areas and sometimes have involved enormous numbers of people. Thus, increased clinical suspicion should be maintained for persons presenting with acute gastrointestinal complaints. Furthermore, diagnosis and reporting of gastrointestinal pathogens has gained importance in detecting outbreaks and implementing control measures. While the burden of human immunodeficiency virus (HIV) infection has not reached the heights seen in other parts of the world, an estimated 1.1 million children and adults were living with HIV within the United States in 2006 [2]. Increased surveillance and recognition especially in major metropolitan areas has identified more acute cases, and given its nonspecific symptoms, HIV should be contemplated in anyone with fever and other nonspecific complaints [3]. Additionally, several bacterial infections have increased prevalence in the community setting within North America and should be considered in patients presenting from this region with compatible clinical complaints. The frequency of community-acquired methicillin-resistant *Staphylococcus aureus* (CA-MRSA) isolates has increased >7× in the United States between 1999 and 2006, and has restricted the options for empiric antibiotic therapy, particularly for skin and soft tissue infection [4]. The incidence of *Clostridium difficile* infections is rising both in hospitalized patients and in the community, and must be considered in the differential diagnosis of diarrhea in Northern America [5,6]. Finally, pertussis has re-emerged, with 11,000–25,000 cases annually in the United States since 2003 [7].

Diversity within the region

Within the subcontinent, some organisms have limited distribution, particularly tick-borne diseases such as babesiosis, ehrlichiosis, anaplasmosis, Lyme disease, and Rocky Mountain spotted fever. Many ecological factors influence vector survival and feeding and pathogen transmission. *Babesia microti* is the most frequently identified *Babesia* species in the United States, primarily parts of New England, New York State, New Jersey, Wisconsin, and Minnesota. In the Northeast, babesiosis occurs in both inland and coastal areas including the islands [7]. The most common type of ehrlichiosis is caused by *Ehrlichia chaffeensis*, transmitted by the tick *Amblyomma americanum*, and mainly occurring in the lower Midwest, Southeast, and East Coast [7]. Anaplasmosis, caused by *Anaplasma phagocytophilum* and transmitted by the tick *Ixodes scapularis*, occurs generally in the upper Midwest and coastal New England [7]. The distribution of these pathogens reflects the range of their tick vectors and the range of preferred animal hosts. Likewise, most cases of Lyme disease (90%) are reported from the Northeast and upper Midwest (Figure 23.1a–d) [7]. Other tick-borne diseases include *Rickettsia parkeri* (Gulf Coast tick vector), southern tick-associated rash illness (STARI, southeastern and eastern United States), 364D rickettsiosis (California), and tick-borne relapsing fever.

(a)

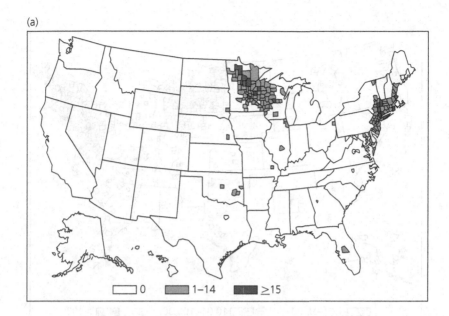

(b)

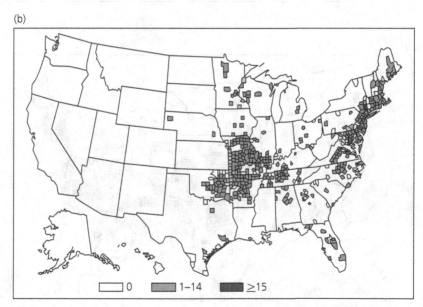

Fig. 23.1 Distribution of some tick-borne diseases in the United States. (a) Ehrlichiosis, *A. phagocytophilum*. Number of reported cases, by county—United States, 2008. (b) Ehrlichiosis, *E. chaffeensis*. Number of reported cases, by county—United States, 2008. (c) Lyme disease. Incidence (per 100,000 population) of reported cases, by county—United States, 2008. (d) Rocky Mountain spotted fever. Number of reported cases, by county—United States, 2008. (Reproduced from CDC [7], with permission from US Department of Health and Human Services.)

(c)

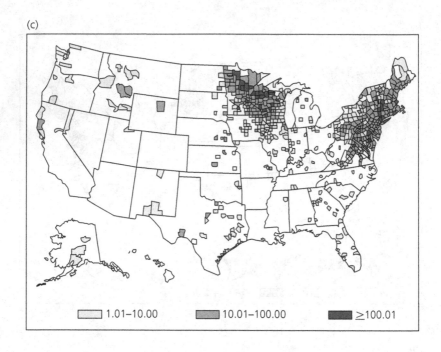

(d)

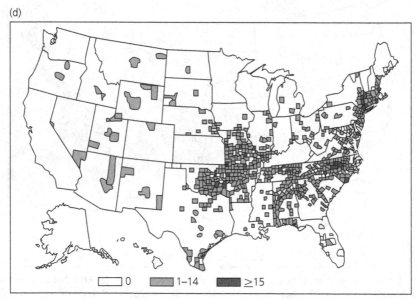

Fig. 23.1 Continued.

Dimorphic fungi, such as *Coccidioides immitis*, *Histoplasma capsulatum*, and *Blastomyces dermatitidis* are acquired via inhalation of the spores. They cause a spectrum of illness from subclinical to disseminated infection, the latter particularly in immunosuppressed hosts. These fungi have demonstrated predominance in certain areas. For example, coccidioidomycosis is endemic to the southwestern states, particularly California and Arizona, although cases have been reported in other states in travelers returning from endemic areas [7]. The alkaline soil

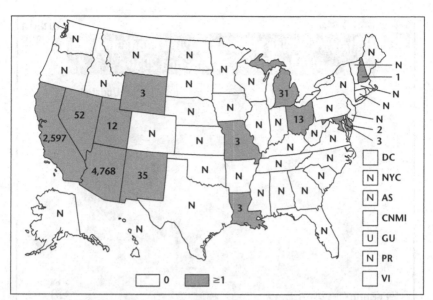

Fig. 23.2 Coccidioidomycosis. Number of reported cases—United States and US territories, 2008. (Reproduced from CDC [7], with permission from US Department of Health and Human Services.)

and climate in southwestern United States support the growth of coccidioidomycosis, and when the soil is disrupted, fungal conidia become airborne (Figure 23.2) [7]. In Northern America, *H. capsulatum* is endemic in the Mississippi and Ohio River valleys. The endemic areas of blastomycosis appear to be the Mississippi and Ohio River valleys of the south central and Midwestern United States, and both American and Canadian sides of the St Lawrence valley.

West Nile virus (WNV) was introduced into New York in 1999, but spread throughout the United States and southern Canada over just a few years (Figure 23.3) [8].

Dengue virus is typically an imported disease in Northern America, acquired when travelers to warmer regions are bitten by the *Aedes* mosquito. One vector, *Aedes albopictus*, is present in many southern states, allowing locally acquired dengue virus infections within Northern America. Such transmissions have occurred in Florida, Texas, and Hawaii, including outbreaks in 2009–2010 in Key West, Florida [9]. Dengue virus should be considered in the differential diagnosis among febrile individuals who have visited these areas within the incubation period of 2 weeks.

Food-borne outbreaks cause an estimated 76 million illnesses in the United States annually, and of those with identifiable causes, 93% are attributed to infectious agents [1]. Recent multistate outbreaks have implicated many commercially processed foods and have identified *Salmonella* (ground beef, peanut butter, eggs), *Escherichia coli* O157:H7 (ground beef, frozen pepperoni pizza), norovirus (raw oysters), and *Clostridium botulinum* toxin (canned hotdog chili sauce) [1].

Infections in the Canadian Arctic and Alaska

The Arctic regions of North America are endemic for several infections which are otherwise rare in the rest of the continent. In addition, several more common types of infections are far more prevalent in northern regions. This is due to the intersection of poverty, which is often extreme among the indigenous peoples of the Arctic, the unique lifecycles of several Arctic fauna and their associated parasites, and the particular hunting and food preferences in the area. The definition of "Arctic" for this discussion is generally the region north of the 10°C July isotherm, which corresponds roughly to the "tree line."

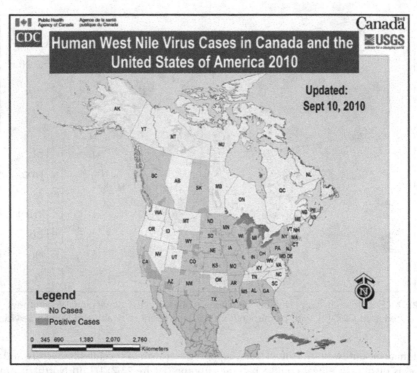

Fig. 23.3 WNV activity in North America, 2010. (Reproduced from http://www.eidgis.com/wnvmonitor [8], with permission from Public Health Agency of Canada.)

Rates of diagnosis of acute otitis media are twofold higher, and hospital admission rates for lower respiratory infection in the Canadian Arctic are 10-fold higher than other Canadian populations. Invasive infections with *Haemophilus influenzae* type A has emerged in Alaska and northern Canada after the success of vaccination against type B. Hepatitis B and C are relatively prevalent in the north, and a seroprevalence rate of 3% for Hepatitis E was reported among the Inuit; *Helicobacter pylori* infection appears to be linked to particularly high rates of iron deficiency anemia [10].

Several helminthic infections are far more common in the north than in the rest of Canada. Trichinellosis outbreaks are common, and are linked to consumption of polar bear and walrus. The organism is generally *Trichinella nativa*, rather than *Trichinella spiralis*. Repeated infection produces a syndrome of chronic diarrhea, rather than the more classic symptoms of this disease. Diphyllobothriasis (fish tapeworm) is still endemic, and occasionally worms are mistaken for tumors on barium enema. Both cystic and alveolar forms of *Echinococcus* still occur. The northern biotype of *Echinococcus granulosus* appears to produce less-virulent disease than elsewhere in the world. *Echinococcus multilocularis* is rare, but a focus may exist in western Alaska. An unusual gastrointestinal infection due to consumption of raw freshwater fish infected with *Metorchis conjunctus* has been described well south of the tree line.

Seroprevalence of toxoplasmosis has been reported to be up to 60%, far higher than the rest of the continent. The Arctic lifecycle of this parasite remains mysterious given the near total absence of felines in the region. Screening programs in pregnancy appear to have rendered congenital infection very rare.

Infections in Southern Canada

The epidemiology of most infectious diseases in southern Canada resembles that described in the United States. Infections which have specific distributions include Lyme disease, which is uncommon in Canada, but appears to be increasing as climate change improves conditions for dissemination. It has moved from a single focus north of Lake Erie to scattered southern parts of Ontario, Nova Scotia, Manitoba, and southeastern New Brunswick. Blastomycosis is endemic in central Canada, with almost all cases originating from Quebec, Ontario, or Manitoba. Histoplasmosis occurs mainly in the central provinces, uncommonly in the Maritimes and the north, and rarely in western Canada.

CNS infections: meningitis, encephalitis, and other infections with neurological symptoms

Infections of the central nervous system (CNS) can be life threatening and associated with a high incidence of morbidity and mortality. Therefore, prompt recognition, diagnosis, and institution of appropriate therapy are mandated to avoid negative consequences. The presentation of infection of the CNS may be acute, subacute, or chronic, and correct identification of the signs and symptoms of a CNS infection involves assessment of the patient's complaints in conjunction with a compatible physical examination. In most cases sampling of the cerebral spinal fluid (CSF) is key in the diagnostic evaluation, in conjunction with imaging.

Acute infections with less than 4 weeks of symptoms

Frequently found microorganisms	Rare microorganisms	Very rare microorganisms
Viral meningitis (enterovirus group)	*Listeria monocytogenes*	*Naegleria* and other free-living ameba
Streptococcus pneumoniae	*Treponema pallidum*	Influenza
Neisseria meningitidis	*Borrelia burgdorferi*	*Baylisascaris procyonis*
Herpes simplex virus (HSV)	Western equine encephalitis	*C. botulinum*
H. influenzae	St Louis encephalitis	Rabies
WNV	Eastern equine encephalitis	Powassan virus

CNS infections: meningitis and encephalitis with symptoms for more than 4 weeks and in the immunocompromised host

Microorganisms with symptoms for more than 4 weeks	Microorganisms in the immunocompromised host
HIV	*Nocardia*
Mycobacterium tuberculosis	JC virus
B. burgdorferi	*Cryptococcus neoformans*
T. pallidum	*Toxoplasma gondii*

Consider noninfectious causes like vasculitis and lymphoma.

Ear, nose, and throat infections

Because of the proximity of the structures in the head and their interconnectedness, the symptoms of the many pathogens that affect this area may be interrelated. The most common illness for which adults visit their physicians is acute pharyngitis. Many organisms both bacterial and viral can cause acute pharyngitis either in isolation of as part of a more widespread disease process [11]. The most often implicated organisms are: group A streptococcus (GAS), Epstein–Barr Virus (EBV), HSV, *N. gonorrheae*, Cytomegalovirus (CMV), HIV, *Mycoplasma pneumoniae*, and very rarely *Corynebacterium diphtheria*. In the immunocompromised host, candidal infections also play a larger role. In addition to pharyngitis, rhinosinusitis and otitis are prominent conditions for which adults seek medical treatment. Rhinosinusitis affects 31 million adults in the United States annually [12]. Most often, viral causes such as rhinovirus predominate and bacteria including *S. pneumoniae, H. influenzae, and Moraxella catarrhalis* only account for 2% of these infections [13].

Cardiopulmonary infections

A leading cause of hospitalization and death in the United States is pneumonia and those aged ≥ 65 years are most susceptible to pneumonia-related morbidity and mortality [14]. Population-based data on community-acquired pneumonia are limited, and data derived from most published studies reflect a variety of selection biases [15–17]. In cases where symptoms have been present for more than 4 weeks and alternative diagnoses such as malignancy, autoimmune disease, and vasculitis are ruled out, organisms such as *M. tuberculosis, H. capsulatum, Aspergillus* spp., and atypical mycobacteria should be considered. In the immunocompromised, consideration should also be give to *Pneumocystis jirovecii*, CMV, *Candida albicans*, and *Aspergillus* spp.

Pneumonia with less than 4 weeks of symptoms

Frequently found microorganisms	Rare microorganisms and conditions	Very rare microorganisms
S. pneumoniae	*Influenza*	*C. diphtheriae*
M. pneumoniae	*S. aureus*	*Francisella tularensis*
H. influenzae	*Chlamydophila pneumoniae*	*Coxiella burneti*
Legionella pneumophila	*Chlamydophila psittaci*	*Hantavirus (southwest)*
C. immitis[a]		

[a]Regional distribution as noted earlier.

Infective endocarditis can be a highly morbid and potentially deadly infection accounting for 1 in 1,000 hospitalizations each year in the United States totaling about 15,000 new cases yearly [18]. Like pneumonia, data on endocarditis trends may be extrapolated from population-based studies [19,20]. While typically most of the organisms listed here will present within 4 weeks, some may cause more protean manifestations and take longer to present to care: Coagulase-negative *Staphylococcus*, nonhemolytic streptococci, *Bartonella* spp. and *Brucella* spp. In addition, in susceptible hosts, fungi such as *Candida* spp., *Aspergillus* spp. may rarely cause endocarditis.

Endocarditis with less than 4 weeks of symptoms

Frequently found microorganisms	Rare microorganisms and conditions	Very rare microorganisms
S. aureus	HACEK group (*Hemophilus* spp., *Actinobacillus* actinomycetemcomitans, *Cardiobacterium hominis*, *Eikenella corrodens*, and *Kingella* spp.)	*Bartonella* spp.
Viridans group streptococci	*C. burneti*	*Brucella* spp.
Coagulase-negative staphylococci[a] (*S. epidermidis*)	*Propionibacterium*	
S. pneumoniae	Beta-hemolytic streptococci	
Enterococcus spp.		

[a]Predominantly on prosthetic valves.

Gastrointestinal infections

Gastroenteritis manifesting as diarrhea is fairly common and can be due to many causes other than just infection. Many times, changes in bowel function caused by gastrointestinal infection are short lived and often resolved without specific treatment. That said, food-borne disease outbreaks especially multistate outbreaks have been attributable to organisms such as *E. coli* O157:H7, *C. botulinum*, *Salmonella*, and norovirus [1]. When investigating for infectious etiologies for gastrointestinal symptoms, repeatedly negative bacterial cultures and microscopy for parasites should lead to the consideration that the symptoms may not be caused by an infection. Inflammatory bowel disease, malabsorption, irritable bowel syndrome, and celiac disease must also be considered.

Gastrointestinal infections with less than 4 weeks of symptoms

Frequently found microorganisms	Rare microorganisms and conditions	Very rare microorganisms
Norovirus and calicivirus	*Cryptosporidium* spp.	*Vibrio*, noncholera (predominantly *Vibrio* parahaemolyticus)[a]
Rotavirus (in children)		
Campylobacter spp.	*Bacillus cereus* toxin	Cyclospora
Enterohemorrhagic *E. coli*	*Ascaris lumbricoides*[b]	Aeromonas
Giardia intestinalis	Shigella	Plesiomonas
Salmonella (nontyphi)	Yersinia	Entamoeba histolytica
C. difficile		
S. aureus toxin		

[a]Infection is associated with saltwater.
[b]Ascaris may cause nonspecific gastrointestinal discomfort but not diarrhea.

Gastrointestinal infections with symptoms for more than 4 weeks and in the immunocompromised host

Microorganisms with symptoms for more than 4 weeks	Microorganisms in the immunocompromised host
M. tuberculosis	Candida
Tropheryma whipplei	HSV
Blastocystis[a]	CMV
Dientamoeba fragilis[a]	Cryptosporidium
Giardia lamblia	Isospora
Salmonella spp.	Microspora
Cryptosporidium	

[a]Of uncertain pathogenicity in humans.

Infections of liver, spleen, and peritoneum

A frequent cause of infection of the liver is viral hepatitis and most frequently caused by hepatitis A, B, or C in North America. The incidences of acute infections are decreasing due to vaccination as within the United States in 2007 the newly identified cases of hepatitis A, hepatitis B, and hepatitis C were only 27,000, 43,000, and 17,000, respectively [21]. Although hepatitis A used to be more prevalent in the western United States, increased vaccination has resulted in similar rates throughout the country [21]. In Canada, the incidence of HAV is low and also declining as is the incidence of HBV, although it is about 20 times more prevalent in northern natives compared to whites in southern Canada [22]. Hepatitis E is considered prevalent but rarely pathogenic in the United States as data from the Third National Health and Nutrition Examination survey (NHANES), 1988–1994, showed that 21% of US residents are seropositive for HEV while the Centers for Disease Control and Prevention (CDC) only reports five cases of acute HEV in the United States from 1997 to 2006 [23]. In contrast, the prevalence of HEV in Canadian Inuits is about 3% [24]. Acute EBV infection may cause hepatitis and splenomegaly and is most common in the United States in teenagers aged 15–19 accounting for about 68% of the cases of acute mononucleosis [25]. Of those awaiting liver transplant in the United States, HBV and HCV account for 4.2% and 35.9%, respectively [26]. In addition to viral infections, the spleen and liver may become infected with bacterial or fungal organisms through hematogenous or embolic spread leading to abscess. Most cases of acute peritonitis are either spontaneous and monobacterial in presence of ascites, or polymicrobial when secondary to a perforated viscus.

Genitourinary infections

Urinary tract infection (UTI), that is infection of the urinary system: urethra, bladder, ureters, or kidneys, is one of the most common bacterial infections, accounting for 7 million office visits in 1997 [27]. However, because UTIs are not reportable, the true incidence is difficult to accurately project. *E. coli* cause 80% of all community-acquired UTI, yet a wide range of bacteria such as *Pseudomonas, Staphylococcus, Proteus mirabilis*, and *Enterobacter* grow well in urine and may successfully invade the urinary system and potentially lead to complications such as perinephric abscess [28]. Rarely, *Candida* spp. can cause infections in immunocompromised hosts. Additionally, *M. tuberculosis* and hantavirus very infrequently can cause symptomatic UTI.

Regardless of one's country of origin, sexually transmitted diseases (STDs) have serious health effects. In the United States, half of STD cases excluding HIV occur among young people under age 25. Cases of *Chlamydia*, gonorrhea, and syphilis are reportable to public health authorities in Canada and the United States [29]. *Chlamydia* is the most frequently reported among all age groups. Gonorrhea is the second most commonly reported followed by syphilis [29]. Between 2000 and 2005, the rate of gonorrhea has increased 42% in western United States, whereas rates had decreased for the remainder of the United States [30]. Overall, the rate of primary and secondary syphilis seems to be decreasing in the United States; however, there are serious racial/ethnic disparities and increased rates documented among blacks [31]. In 2006, the estimated incidence rate of HIV was 22.8 per 100,000 with 45% of infections among blacks and 53% among men who have sex with men [32]. Other causes that should be considered in evaluating a patient with a suspected STD include HSV, *Trichomonas vaginalis*, *Lymphogranuloma venereum*, *Haemophilus ducreyi* (chancroid), human papillomavirus (HPV), and *E. histolytica*. Bacterial vaginosis and *Candida* cause genital symptoms that are generally not sexually transmitted.

Joint, muscle, and soft tissue infections

Several pathogens including bacteria and viruses can precipitate inflammation of the musculoskeletal system. Septic arthritis is rare but most often due to hematogenous spread of bacteria such as *S. aureus*, *Streptococcus pyogenes*, and occasionally *S. pneumoniae*. Rarely these organisms may cause infection of the muscle and fascia and lead to necrotizing fasciitis or in the case of *Clostridium perfringens*, myonecrosis. In patients with joint prostheses, the same pathogens are found, but coagulase-negative *Staphylococcus* and other streptococcal species may also be isolated [33]. Diabetics may present with synergistic gangrene of the perineum that is usually polymicrobial. Lyme (*B. burgdorferi*) disease is a common cause of arthralgia during the summer months especially on the East Coast and upper Midwest [34]. If not recognized and treated early, it can lead to a more chronic arthritis. In sexually active individuals, *Neisseria gonorrheae* may cause an acute monoarticular arthritis. Certain viruses, such as parvovirus B19, rubella, EBV, and CMV, may cause acute arthralgias without frank arthritis. Rarely, *Candida* spp. and *M. tuberculosis* can lead to arthritis that is usually indolent. Finally, several bacterial pathogens including *Campylobacter*, *Salmonella*, and *Shigella* may lead to reactive arthritis and detailed history of recent gastrointestinal symptoms should be sought in those presenting with polyarticular complaints [35].

Skin infections

The most frequently encountered primary skin infection is cellulitis and is a common cause of antibiotic therapy and hospitalization. The table shown below lists the most frequently implicated organisms including organisms that can cause skin findings resembling cellulitis. Less frequent but still important etiologies of skin infections include: *T. pallidum* (syphilis), *Mycobacteria* spp., and *Candida* spp. We have not listed a rash due to viral infections such as varicella zoster, measles, or rubella, as they are not considered infections limited to the skin. Finally, one of the challenges facing each clinician is a noninfectious skin condition mimicking cellulitis. In these cases, consultation with a dermatologist may be necessary.

Skin infections with less than 4 weeks of symptoms

Frequently found microorganisms	Rare microorganisms and conditions	Very rare microorganisms and conditions
	Sarcoptes scabiei (scabies)	*Spirilum minus* and *Streptobacillus* (rat-bite fever)
Beta-hemolytic streptococcus (particularly group A, B[a] and G)	*Vibrio vulnificus*	*Corynebacterium minutissimum* (Erythrasma)
S. aureus	STARI	*Erysipelothrix rhusiopathiae* (Erysipeloid)
Borrelia spp.		*Rickettsia* spp. (*R. parkeri*, 364D)
Gram-negatives in diabetics, particularly Enterobacteriaceae and *Pseudomonas*		

[a]More common in older individuals with underlying comorbidities.

Adenopathy

The potential infectious etiologies causing lymphadenopathy are broad but may be narrowed by anatomic location. Several infectious processes may cause generalized lymphadenopathy. Reactive adenopathy can occur from infections draining to regional nodes. If an infectious diagnosis is not made quickly, then biopsies of a lymph node may be necessary to exclude malignancy which may mimic infection.

Adenopathy of less than 4 weeks' duration

Frequently found microorganisms	Rare microorganisms and conditions	Very rare microorganisms and conditions
EBV	*F. tularensis*	*Ehrlichia* spp.
CMV	*Bartonella*	*Babesia* spp.
Parvovirus B19	Rubella	
T. gondii	Rubeola	
HIV	*T. pallidum*, secondary	

Adenopathy of more than 4 weeks' duration and in the immunocompromised host

Microorganisms with symptoms for more than 4 weeks	Microorganisms in the immunocompromised host
T. gondii	Adenovirus
M. tuberculosis	CMV

Fever without focal symptoms

Fever is a common reason for adults and children to present to medical care. Fever of unknown origin, however is a more rare entity and is usually subdivided into four major categories of which infection is the most common. It is important to be mindful of the potential of less common manifestation of certain diseases such as extrapulmonary tuberculosis or occult abscesses. For newborns, serious bacterial infections (presenting simply with fever or with additional localizing findings) are usually due to group B streptococci, *E. coli*, or, rarely, *Listeria*. For young children, bacteremia is caused by meningococcus, pneumococcus, and *H. influenzae* type b; the latter two organisms have become less common with immunizations widely available.

Fever without focal symptoms

Frequently found microorganisms and conditions	Rare microorganisms and conditions	Very rare microorganisms and conditions
Endocarditis	*M. tuberculosis*	*F. tularensis*
EBV	*C. burneti*	Other *Rickettsia* (*R. parkeri*, 364D)
CMV	*Brucella* spp.	*Borrelia recurrentis* (tick-borne relapsing fever)
Parvovirus B19	WNV	Adenovirus (immunocompromised)
T. gondii	Rocky Mountain spotted fever	Dengue virus (Florida, Texas)
HIV	*Ehrlichia* spp. *Anaplasma* spp. *Babesia* spp.	*Leptospira interrogans*

Eosinophilia and elevated IgE

Eosinophilia may be caused by a number of conditions including fungal infections, parasites, mycobacteria, and malignancy. The fungi within Northern America including coccidioidomycosis, cryptococcosis, and histoplasmosis have been identified as potential etiologies to eosinophilia. While the majority of parasitic diseases within the United States are identified in travelers and immigrants, there are several parasites that are endemic and should be considered in the correct clinical context. While *Trichinella* spp. have declined overall in the subcontinent, there are reservoirs in wild life and noncommercial pork and thus continued case outbreaks [36,37]. *Toxocara* is the most common parasitic worm infection in the United States affecting mostly those living in poverty [38]. *B. procyonis* has caused eosinophilic encephalitis in Illinois and California [39]. *E. granulosus* is endemic to south central Canada and the northern Midwestern United States with reservoirs in wolves and thus also domesticated sheep and dogs. Several reports of human disease in these areas are documented. Isolated foci of strongyloidiasis have been reported in the southeastern United States.

Antibiotic resistance

Resistance patterns vary between continents and within various parts of Northern America. Group A streptococci remain completely susceptible to penicillin. Approximately 7% of clinically isolated strains in Northern America are resistant to macrolides, but macrolide resistance varies geographically and temporally [40]. Clindamycin resistance is much less common (less than 1%).

Transcontinental surveillance suggests that *S. pneumoniae* is uniformly susceptible to vancomycin, 99.6% susceptible to a "respiratory" quinolone, 93% susceptible to cefotaxime, 87% susceptible to tetracycline, and 76% susceptible to penicillin [41]. Over time, pneumococcal strains covered by the 7-valent vaccine have become less common, but multidrug resistance remains stable at about 20% of strains [42]. A decade ago, Canadian pneumococcal isolates were less likely than US isolates to be penicillin-resistant [43].

For 100,000 people living in Northern America, there are approximately 4.9 community-acquired cases of MRSA infection and 0.5 deaths. For the same population, there are 16.8 health care–associated cases of MRSA infection (and 1.6 deaths) [44]. For American children with head and neck infections, the proportion of *S. aureus* that are methicillin-resistant rose from 11.8% in 2001 to 28.1% in 2006 [45]. Although comparative data are scarce, rates of CA-MRSA are lower in Canada than in the United States. About 28% of US respiratory tract isolates of *H. influenzae* produce beta-lactamase [46].

Gram-negative bacteria causing UTIs vary widely in response to antibiotics. Overall, 50% are susceptible to ampicillin, 78% are susceptible to trimethoprim–sulfamethoxazole, and over 90% are susceptible to a quinolone [47]. Cefdinir is effective against more than 95% of urinary tract–based *E. coli*, *Klebsiella*, and coagulase-negative staphylococci.

For approximately one decade, about 1.2% of new cases of tuberculosis in the United States have been multidrug resistant. The majority (80%) of these resistant cases were in individuals born outside of Northern America [48].

Vaccine-preventable diseases in children

Some, but not all, vaccine-preventable illnesses are relatively uncommon in Canada and the United States. In 2007, for instance, the United States' CDC identified no cases of diphtheria, 28 cases of tetanus, 10,454 cases of pertussis, no cases of polio, 4,519 cases of hepatitis B, 22 preschool-aged cases of *H. influenzae* type b, 2,595 preschool-aged cases of invasive *S. pneumoniae*, 43 cases of measles, 800 cases of mumps, 12 cases of rubella, 6 varicella-related deaths, 2,979 cases of hepatitis A, and 77 influenza-related pediatric deaths [49].

Measles is no longer endemic in the United States, but outbreaks have involved groups of adolescents following importation of an index patient from another country [50]. Similarly, the mumps outbreaks that affected thousands of US university students seem to have been introduced from the United Kingdom [51]. A significant number of cases have occurred despite good compliance with recommended vaccination. There is little endemic rubella in the United States, and the majority of children with congenital rubella were delivered by foreign-born Hispanic women. Despite improvements with expanded immunization programs, indigenous populations (such as American Indians and Alaska Natives) who make up only 1–3% of the entire population remain at relatively greater risk of vaccine-preventable illnesses.

Adolescents and adults serve as a reservoir for the spread of pertussis to prevaccinated infants. Adult immunization programs can prevent illness in children.

Pediatric vaccination schedules are similar in Canada [52] and the United States [53], although policies vary by province in Canada. In each country, childhood coverage is provided for diphtheria, tetanus, pertussis, polio, hepatitis B, pneumococcus, *H. influenza* type b, measles, mumps, rubella, and varicella. In the United States, a 13-valent (rather than the 7-valent) pneumococcal vaccine is now recommended [54]. In the United States, but not Canada, rotavirus vaccine is also given to infants. In Canada, meningococcus C vaccine is given to infants whereas US children receive a quadrivalent meningococcal vaccine after the second birthday. Hepatitis A vaccine is given beginning at 1 year of age in the United States and also in some provinces in Canada. The United States and some provinces in Canada have incorporated HPV into childhood vaccinations. Influenza vaccine is recommended for children aged 6 months to 2 years in Canada but to all children and adolescents in the United States. A total of 76% of young US children have received complete vaccine series. In Canada, approximately 85–90% of children at age 2 years have complete vaccine series.

Basic economic and demographic data

Basic demographics[a]	GNI[b] per capita (USD)	Life expectancy at birth (total, years)	School enrollment, primary (% net)
Canada	43,640	81	99.5
United States	47,930	78	98.0

[a]World Bank.
[b]Gross national income.

Causes of death in children under 5 years

	%
Neonatal causes	44
Pneumonia	12
Diarrheal diseases	10
Malaria	0
HIV/AIDS	1
Measles	0
Injuries	5
Others	28

WHO, regional average, 2006 data.

The most common causes of deaths in all ages

	%	
	Canada	United States
Chronic obstructive lung disease	5	5
Lower respiratory infections	3	3
Tracheal, bronchial, and lung cancers	8	7
Breast cancer	3	2
Cerebrovascular diseases	7	7
Ischemic and hypertensive heart disease	19	21
Alzheimer and other dementias	5	4
Diabetes mellitus	3	3
Road traffic accidents	NS	2
Colon and rectal cancers	4	3
Myeloma and lymphomas	2	

NS, not stated
http://www.who.int/countries/en/.

References

1. CDC. Surveillance for foodborne disease outbreaks—United States, 2007. MMWR 2010;59 (31):973–9.
2. CDC. HIV prevalence estimates—United States, 2006. MMWR 2008;57(39):1073–6.
3. CDC. Acute HIV infection—New York City, 2008. MMWR 2009;58(46):1296–9.
4. Klein E, Smith DL, Laxminarayan L. Community-associated methicillin-resistant *Staphylococcus aureus* in outpatients, United States, 1999–2006. Emerg Infect Dis 2009;15(12):1925–30.
5. Mulvey MR, Boyd DA, Gravel D, et al. Hypervirulent *Clostridium difficile* strains in hospitalized patients, Canada. Emerg Infect Dis 2010;16(4):678–81.
6. Kutty PK, Woods CW, Sena AC, et al. Risk factors for and estimated incidence of community-associated *Clostridium difficile* infection, North Carolina, USA. Emerg Infect Dis 2010;16(2):197–204.
7. CDC. Summary of notifiable diseases—United States, 2008. MMWR 2010;57(54):1–94.
8. Public Health Agency of Canada. WNV activity in North America, 2010. Map from Public Health Agency of Canada. Accessed September 13, 2010 at http://www.eidgis.com/wnvmonitor.
9. CDC. Locally acquired Dengue—Key West, Florida, 2009–2010. MMWR 2010;59(19):577–81.
10. Hotez PJ. Neglected infections of poverty among the indigenous peoples of the Arctic. PLoS Negl Trop Dis 2010;4(1):e606.
11. Bisno AL. Acute pharyngitis. N Engl J Med 2001;344(3):205–11.
12. Rosenfeld RM, Andes D, Bhattacharyya N, et al. Clinical practice guideline: adult sinusitis. Otolaryngol Head Neck Surgery 2007;137:S1–31.
13. Gwaltney JM Jr. Acute community-acquired sinusitis. Clin Infect Dis 1996;23(6):1209–23.
14. Jackson ML, Neuzil KM, Thompson WW, et al. The burden of community-acquired pneumonia in seniors: results of a population-based study. Clin Infect Dis 2004; 39:1642–50.
15. Foy HM, Cooney MK, Allan I, Kenny GE. Rates of pneumonia during influenza epidemics in Seattle, 1964–1975. JAMA 1979;241:253–8.
16. Oseasohn R, Skipper BE, Tempest B. Pneumonia in a Navajo community: a two-year experience. Am Rev Resp Dis 1978;117:1003–9.
17. Marston BJ, Plouffe JF, File TM, et al. Incidence of community-acquired pneumonia requiring hospitalization. Results of a population-based active surveillance study in Ohio. The community-based pneumonia incidence study group. Arch Int Med 1997;157:1709–18.
18. Fowler VG, Schelenz S, Bayer AS. Endocarditis and intravascular infections. In: Mandell GL, Bennett JE, Dolin R (eds). Mandell, Douglas, and Bennett's Principles and Practice of Infectious Disease, 6th edn. Philadelphia: Churchill Livingstone; 2005:975–1021.
19. Murdoch DR, Corey GR, Hoen B, et al. Clinical presentation, etiology and outcome of infective endocarditis in the 21st century. Arch Intern Med 2009;169(5):463–73.
20. Correa De Sa DD, Tleyjeh IM, Anavekar NS, et al. Epidemiological trends of infective endocarditis: a population-based study in Olmstead County, Minnesota. May Clin Proc 2010;85 (5):422–6.
21. CDC. Surveillance for acute viral hepatitis—United States, 2007. MMWR 2009;58(SS03): 1–27.
22. Osiowy C, Larke B, Giles E. Distinct geographical and demographic distribution of hepatitis B virus genotypes in the Canadian Arctic as revealed through an extensive molecular epidemiological survey. J Viral Hepat 2011 Apr;18(4):e11–9.
23. Teshale EH, Hu DJ, Holmberg SD. The two faces of hepatitis E virus. Clin Infect Dis 2010;51:328–34.
24. Minuk GY, Sun A, Sun DF, et al. Serological evidence of hepatitis E virus infection in an indigenous North American population. Can J Gastroenterol 2007;21(7):439–42.
25. Caldwell GG, Heath CW. Surveillance of infectious mononucleosis cases by use of existing data from state laboratories. Public Health Reports 1982;97(6):579–82.
26. Kim WR, Terrault NA, Pedersen RA, et al. Trends in waiting list registration for liver transplantation for viral hepatitis in the United States. Gastroenterology 2009;137(5):1680–6.
27. Foxman, B. Epidemiology of urinary tract infections: incidence, morbidity, and economic costs. Am J Med 2002;113(1A):5S–13S.
28. Foxman B, Brown P. Epidemiology of urinary tract infections transmission and risk factors, incidence, and costs. Infect Dis Clin North Am 2003;17:227–41.
29. CDC. Sexual and reproductive health of persons aged 10–24 years—United States, 2002–2007. MMWR 58(SS06):1–58.

30. CDC. Increases in gonorrhea—eight western states, 2000–2005. MMWR 2007;56(10):222–5.
31. CDC. Primary and secondary syphilis—United States, 2003–2004. MMWR 2006;55(10):269–73.
32. Hall HI, Song R, Rhodes P, et al. Estimation of HIV incidence in the United States. JAMA 2008;300(5):520–9.
33. Lipsky BA, Weigelt JA, Gupta V, et al. Skin, soft tissue, bone, and joint infections in hospitalized patients: epidemiology and microbiological, clinical, and economic outcomes. Infect Control Hosp Epi 2007;28(11):1290–8.
34. Bacon RM, Kugeler KJ, Mead PS; Centers for Disease Control and Prevention (CDC). Surveillance for lyme disease—United States, 1992–2006. MMWR 2008;57(SS10):1–9.
35. Townes JM. Reactive arthritis after enteric infections in the United States: the problem of definition. Clin Infect Dis 2010;50(2):247–54.
36. Kennedy ED, Hall RL, Montgomery SP, et al. Trichinellosis surveillance—United States, 2002–2007. MMWR 2009;58(SS9):1–7.
37. CDC. Trichinellosis associated with bear meat—New York and Tennessee, 2003. MMWR 2004;53(27):606–10.
38. Hotez PJ, Wilkins, PP. Toxocariasis: America's most common neglected infection of poverty and a helminthiasis of global importance? PLoS Negl Trop Dis 2009;3(3):e400.
39. CDC. *Baylisascaris procyonis* has caused eosinophilic encephalitis in Illinois and California. MMWR 2002;50(51):1153–5.
40. Richter SS, Heilmann KP, Beekmann SE, et al. Macrolide-resistant *Streptococcus pyogenes* in the United States 2002–2003. Clin Infect Dis 2005;41:599–608.
41. CDC. Active bacterial core surveillance report of Emerging Infections Program Network. Accessed June 8, 2010 at http://www.cdc.gov/abcs/reports-findings/survreports/spneu08.pdf.
42. Richter SS, Heilmann KP, Dohrn CL, et al. Changing epidemiology of antimicrobial-resistant *Streptococcus pneumoniae* in the United States, 2004–2005. Clin Infect Dis 2009;48:e233–33.
43. Hoban D, Waites K, Felmingham D. Antimicrobial susceptibility of community-acquired respiratory tract pathogens in North America in 1999–2000: findings of the PROTEKT surveillance study. Diagn Microbiol Infect Dis 2003;45:251–9.
44. CDC. Active bacterial core surveillance report of Emerging Infections Program Network. Accessed June 8, 2010 at http://www.cdc.gov/abcs/reports-findings/survreports/mrsa08.pdf.
45. Naseri I, Jerris RC, Sobol SE. Nationwide trends in pediatric *Staphylococcus aureus* head and neck infections. Arch Otolarygol Head Neck Surg 2009;135:14–16.
46. Brown SD, Rybak MJ. Antimicrobial susceptibility of *Streptococcus pneumoniae, Streptococcus pyogenes* and *Haemophilus influenzae* collected from patients across the USA, in 2001–2002, as part of the PROTEKT US study. J Antimicrob Chemother 2004;54(Suppl. 1):i7–15.
47. Peterson J, Kaul S, Khashab M, Fisher A, Kahn JB. Identification and pretherapy susceptibility of pathogens in patients with complicated urinary tract infection or acute pyelonephritis enrolled in a clinical study in the United States from November 2004 through April 2006. Clin Ther 2007;29:2215–21.
48. Migliori GB, Richardson MD, Sotgui G, Lange C. Multidrug resistant and extensively drug-resistant tuberculosis in the West. Europe and United States: epidemiology, surveillance, and control. Clin Chest Med 2009;30:637–65.
49. Hall-Baker PA, Nieves E, Jajosky RA, et al. Summary of notifiable diseases—United States, 2007. MMWR 2009;56:1–94.
50. Chen TH, Kutty P, Lowe LE, et al. Measles outbreak associated with an international youth sporting even in the United States, 2007. Pediatr Infect Dis J 2010;29:794–800.
51. Dayan GH, Quinlisk MP, Parker AA, et al. Recent resurgence of mumps in the United States. N Engl J Med 2008;358:1580–9.
52. Public Health Agency of Canada. Immunization schedules. Accessed June 6, 2010 at www.phac-aspc.gc.ca/im/is-cv/index-eng.php.
53. Center for Disease Control and Prevention. Vaccines and immunizations. Accessed June 6, 2010 at www.cdc.gov/vaccines/recs/schedules/child-schedule.htm.
54. Committee on Infectious Diseases. Policy statement—recommendations for the prevention of *Streptococcus pneumoniae* infections in infants and children: use of 13-valent pneumococcal conjugate vaccine (PCV13) and pneumococcal polysaccharide vaccine (PPSV23). Pediatrics 2010;126:186–90.

Chapter 24
Australia and New Zealand

Karin Leder,[1] Joseph Torresi[2] and Marc Shaw[3]

[1]School of Public Health and Preventive Medicine, Monash University and Victorian Infectious Disease Service, Royal Melbourne Hospital, Melbourne, Victoria, Australia
[2]Department of Infectious Diseases, Austin Hospital, Melbourne Australia
[3]School of Public Health, James Cook University, Townsville, Australia and WORLDWISE Travellers Health & Vaccination Centres, Auckland, New Zealand

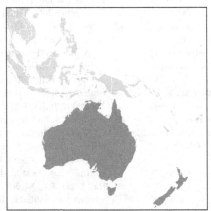

Australia
New Zealand

Australia has both temperate and tropical areas, the temperate areas being the southern and coastal regions, and the tropical areas being central and northern Australia. Temperate Australia and New Zealand have similar health services and diseases, with the risks of most common community illnesses (e.g., gastroenteritis, respiratory viruses) being similar to those in other developed countries globally. However, a number of diseases found in temperate Australia have never been reported from New Zealand, including Ross River virus (RRV), Murray valley encephalitis (MVE), Barmah Forest virus (BFV), Q fever, tick typhus, scrub typhus, Hendra virus, lyssavirus, and *Mycobacterium ulcerans*.

The tropical areas of Australia are sparsely populated, have relatively basic medical services, and have different disease patterns. Especially among Australian Aborigines, there are high rates of infections such as *Strongyloides stercoralis*, HTLV-1, rheumatic fever, trachoma, melioidosis, and scabies.

Infectious Diseases: A Geographic Guide, First Edition.
Edited by Eskild Petersen, Lin H. Chen & Patricia Schlagenhauf.
© 2011 John Wiley & Sons, Ltd. Published 2011 by John Wiley & Sons, Ltd.

Bacterial and mycobacterial infections

Brucellosis (due to *Brucella suis*) is uncommon and occurs almost exclusively in association with hunting feral pigs. The 2009 notification rate in Australia was 0.2/100,000 population with virtually all infections acquired in rural areas of Queensland followed by northern New South Wales (NSW) [1,2].

Melioidosis, caused by *Burkholderia pseudomallei*, is endemic in northern Australia (Northern Territory, Far North Queensland, and Western Australia) and the Torres Strait Islands. Melioidosis is the most common cause of fatal community-acquired pneumonia in Darwin. In the top end of the Northern Territory, cases most frequently occur during the summer monsoonal wet season (November through April) [3–6].

Bartonellosis (Cat scratch disease, caused by *Bartonella henselae*) is widespread throughout Australia and New Zealand. It is associated with bites/scratches from domestic cats.

The overall prevalence of tuberculosis in Australia and New Zealand is low (<10 cases per 100,000 population) [1]. *Mycobacterium tuberculosis* strains are usually sensitive to all major antituberculosis agents.

Mycobacterium ulcerans occurs almost entirely in southeastern Australia, especially in Victoria (Bairnsdale, Phillip Island, and Bellarine and Mornington Peninsulas). The incidence of infection is low: 78 cases were reported in Victoria between 2003 and 2005 [7]. Infections often occur in clusters, but the exact mode of *M. ulcerans* transmission is unknown.

Rickettsial infections have been reported from all states of Australia and occur in travelers to rural, forested and coastal areas of Australia [8]. Infections are divided into the spotted fever group that are spread by ticks and the typhus group, spread by fleas from mice and rats.

Spotted fever group: Queensland tick typhus is caused by *Rickettsia australis* and has been reported from Queensland, NSW, coastal areas of eastern Victoria, and Tasmania. Flinder's Island spotted fever, caused by *Rickettsia honei*, has been reported from Flinder's Island in southern Australia, Tasmania, and southeastern Australia.

Typhus group: Murine typhus, caused by *Rickettsia typhi*, is present in Queensland and Western Australia. Scrub typhus, caused by *Orientia tsutsugamushi*, occurs throughout coastal northern Queensland (north of Townsville) and tropical northern Australia, including the top end of the Northern Territory (in particular Litchfield Park south of Darwin) and the Kimberley region of Western Australia.

In Australia, the epidemiology of meningococcal disease follows the pattern seen in most other industrialized nations [9]. In 2000, the incidence of notified meningococcal disease reached about 3/100,000 [10]. Disease incidence has declined since the introduction of the meningococcal C conjugate vaccine, and in 2008 it was around 1.3/100,000. The case fatality is approximately 4% [1]. In contrast, New Zealand had high rates of meningococcal disease during the 1990s due to the emergence of a serogroup B clone, which by 2000 accounted for 85% of cases. Cases were disproportionately seen among Maori and Pacific Islands' children in the North Island of New Zealand, and infants <1 year had an age-specific rate of 124/100,000 in 2003 [11]. Mass vaccination with the MeNZB vaccine was introduced in mid-2004, and disease incidence subsequently declined to 2.6/100,000 in 2007.

Although overall rates of acute rheumatic fever (ARF) in Australia and New Zealand are low, the rates of ARF among indigenous people are among the highest in the world [12,13]. The annual incidence of confirmed ARF in aboriginal people aged 5–14 years in the top end of the Northern Territory is 254/100,000. In New Zealand, the incidence among Maoris is 8/100,000, 10 times higher than occurring among people of European descent [12].

Leptospirosis occurs in all parts of Australia, mainly as an occupational disease among livestock and agricultural workers. Most cases (>70%) occur in Queensland, with serovars Zanoni, Australis, and Hardjo accounting for most of the disease. Since 1999 in Australia there has been a downward trend in notifications of leptospirosis [14], which has been attributed to recent persistent drought conditions. In New Zealand, the incidence of the disease is reported as 2.1/100,000 population, with serovars Hardjo and Pomona being most common [14,15].

Viral infections

Australia and New Zealand have relatively small HIV epidemics. The adult HIV prevalence in the general population in these countries is about 0.2%. Transmission is primarily through sexual contact between men [16,17].

Australia is the only country in the world that has reported cases of Hendra virus. The natural reservoir for the Hendra virus is the fruit-eating bat. It can be transmitted to horses and has occasionally been reported among horses in Queensland and NSW. Illness has occurred in humans working with infected horses, mostly among veterinarians, leading to either an acute respiratory illness or a meningoencephalitis. The risk to travelers is extremely low.

Dengue virus is not endemic in Australia, but the presence of mosquito vectors in northern Australia has resulted in epidemics following the introduction of dengue virus by travelers returning from other endemic countries. Outbreaks of dengue fever are periodically reported from northern Queensland in the region extending from the Torres Strait south to Cairns, Townsville, and Charters Towers [2]. A major dengue outbreak occurred in the northern suburbs of Cairns between December 2008 and May 2009, causing more than 900 cases. Cases were also reported from Townsville, Port Douglas, Yarrabah, Injinoo, and Innisfail. In the rest of the country, dengue fever is predominantly a disease of returned travelers. In 2009 the Australian notification rate was 2.7/100,000 population [1].

RRV is the most common arboviral disease in Australia and is characterized by fever, rash, and arthralgias. RRV has become established in most parts of Australia and has resulted in several outbreaks [1,2]. The overall incidence of RRV disease in Australia is approximately 22/100,000/year [1], although this varies widely according to season and geographical regions (e.g., Queensland: average 61 (24–144) cases per 100,000/year; Northern Territory: 2–203/100,000/year) [1,2]. In May 2010 a fourfold increase in the number of RRV cases was reported from the Riverina Murray region in NSW, due to greater rain and a larger number of mosquitoes.

BFV is closely related to arbovirus that is spread by the same mosquito vectors and hence epidemics of mixed RRV and BFV infections have been reported. BFV is less common with an annual notification rate of about 6.5 (4.4–7.8)/100,000/year [1,2]. The incidence of BFV in the Northern Territory varies from 25 to 83/100,000/year, Queensland from 17 to 32/100,000/year, and in NSW from 6.6 to 10.6/100,000/year [1,2]. BFV also occurs in Western Australia (including the Kimberley, Pilbara, and Gascoyne regions). Incidence peaks between the months of February and May.

Murray valley encephalitis (MVE) is an infrequent disease. Over the last decade cases have been reported from the Northern Territory, South Australia, northwest Western Australia, outback Queensland, and outback NSW [1]. Two cases of MVE were reported in 2005, one from Normanton in Queensland and one from Arnhem land in the Northern Territory [2]. Two fatal cases of MVE were also reported from the Northern Territory in 2009. The risk period is maximal from February to early April in central Australia but can persist until June.

Kunjin virus infection is uncommon and only sporadic cases have been reported from Northern Territory, South and Western Australia, and Queensland [1,2]. The Australian notification rate is 0.1–0.4/100,000 population [1].

Japanese encephalitis (JE) is not endemic on mainland Australia but nine cases have been notified since 1995. Four of these were reported from Badu Island in the Torres Strait. One locally acquired case was reported in a resident of the Cape York Peninsula of Far North Queensland. The remaining four cases were reported in travelers who had acquired infection overseas [2].

Australia and New Zealand are rabies-free, but the Australian bat lyssavirus (ABL) has been isolated from insectivorous and fruit-eating bats in NSW, Northern Territory, Queensland, Victoria, and Western Australia, and has caused two human fatalities. Potential exposure is most likely among professional bat handlers, although inadvertent exposure following handling of bats by individuals in the general community has also been reported. There have been no reports of human ABL cases over the last 10 years [1,2].

Parasite infections

Infection with the dog hookworm, *Ancylostoma caninum*, has a worldwide distribution but so far the only reports of it also causing an eosinophilic infiltration of the gut wall have been from Australia.

Cases of *Angiostrongylus cantonensis*, the rat lungworm, have been reported from Australia, particularly from Queensland and NSW [18]. It is acquired by eating contaminated leafy vegetables (in salads), infected snails and slugs (often inadvertently), and land crabs. Symptoms include paraesthesia and eosinophilic meningitis.

High rates of *S. stercoralis* are found in some indigenous communities in central Australia. Complicated strongyloidiasis often occurs in association with HTLV-1 infection as these two infections are co-endemic.

Australia and New Zealand are free of endemic malaria and human schistosomiasis.

In addition to infectious outcomes listed in the following tables, travelers also need to be aware of the risks of toxins, envenomations, and bites (spiders and snakes).

CNS infections: meningitis, encephalitis, and other infections with neurological symptoms

Acute infections with less than 4 weeks of symptoms

Frequently found microorganisms	Rare microorganisms	Very rare microorganisms
Viral meningitis (enterovirus group)	*Listeria monocytogenes*	*Naegleria fowleri* and other free-living ameba including *Acanthamoeba* spp. and *Balamuthia mandrillaris*

(Continued)

Frequently found microorganisms	Rare microorganisms	Very rare microorganisms
Streptococcus pneumoniae (meningitis)	Treponema pallidum (neurosyphilis)	Influenza
Herpes virus (group I and II)	HIV	B. suis
Neisseria meningitides	MVE	B. pseudomallei
		Hendra virus
		ABL
		JE (Torres Strait Islands only)
		Kunjin virus
		A. cantonensis

CNS infections: meningitis and encephalitis with symptoms for more than 4 weeks and in the immunocompromised host

Microorganisms with symptoms for more than 4 weeks	Microorganisms in the immunocompromised host
HIV	Nocardia spp.
M. tuberculosis	Polyomavirus
Tropheryma whipplei	Cryptococcus spp.
	JC virus
	M. tuberculosis
	Toxoplasma gondii
	Acanthamoeba spp.

Consider noninfectious causes like vasculitis and lymphoma.

Ear, nose, and throat infections

Ear, nose, and throat infections with less than 4 weeks of symptoms

Frequently found microorganisms	Rare microorganisms and conditions	Very rare microorganisms
Group A streptococci (streptococcal throat infection)	Peritonsillar abscess[a]	Corynebacterium diphtheriae
Epstein–Barr virus (EBV)	M. tuberculosis	
Herpes simplex virus (type I and II)	Fusobacterium necrophorum (Lemierre's syndrome)	

[a]Requires acute ENT evaluation.

Ear, nose, and throat with symptoms for more than 4 weeks and in the immunocompromised host

Microorganisms with symptoms for more than 4 weeks	Microorganisms in the immunocompromised host
M. tuberculosis	*Candida* spp. Herpes simplex virus

Consider noninfectious causes like vasculitis and lymphoma.

Cardiopulmonary infections

Pneumonia with less than 4 weeks of symptoms

Frequently found microorganisms	Rare microorganisms and conditions	Very rare microorganisms
S. pneumoniae *Mycoplasma pneumoniae* *Chlamydia psittaci* *Legionella pneumophila* *Chlamydia pneumoniae*	*Coxiella burneti* (Q fever) Influenza virus Parainfluenza virus	*C. diphtheriae* *B. pseudomallei* Hendra virus

Endocarditis with less than 4 weeks of symptoms

Frequently found microorganisms	Rare microorganisms and conditions	Very rare microorganisms
Staphylococcus aureus Viridans group streptococci and *Streptococcus bovis* Coagulase-negative staphylococci (*Staphylococcus epidermidis*) *Enterococcus* spp.	*Neisseria gonorrhoeae* *C. burnetii*[a] *Propionebacterium* HACEK group *S. pneumoniae*	*Bartonella* spp. *Brucella* spp. *T. whipplei*

[a]Q fever has not been reported from New Zealand.

Pulmonary symptoms for more than 4 weeks and in the immunocompromised host

Microorganisms and diseases with symptoms for more than 4 weeks	Microorganisms in the immunocompromised host
M. tuberculosis *Bordetella pertussis* *Aspergillus* spp.	*Pneumocystis jirovecii* Cytomegalovirus (CMV) *Aspergillus* spp. *Candida* spp.

Consider noninfectious causes like lung cancer, autoimmune lung fibrosis, and Wegener's granulomatosis.

Endocarditis for more than 4 weeks and in the immunocompromised host

Microorganisms and diseases with symptoms for more than 4 weeks	Microorganisms in the immunocompromised host
Viridans group streptococci and *S. bovis* Coagulase-negative staphylococci (*S. epidermidis*) *C. burnetii*[a] *Bartonella* spp.	*Aspergillus* spp. *T. whipplei*

Consider noninfectious causes like sarcoidosis.
[a]Q fever has not been reported from New Zealand.

Gastrointestinal infections

Gastrointestinal infections with less than 4 weeks of symptoms

Frequently found microorganisms	Rare microorganisms and conditions	Very rare microorganisms
Norovirus, calicivirus, and rotavirus *Campylobacter* spp. Enteropathogenic *Escherichia coli* *Giardia intestinalis*[a] *Salmonella* spp. (nontyphi) *Enterobius vermicularis* (pinworm)	*Cryptosporidium* spp. *S. aureus* toxin *Bacillus cereus* toxin *Ascaris lumbricoides* *S. stercoralis* *A. caninum* *Shigella* spp. *Trichuris trichiuria* *Aeromonas* spp. *Entamoeba histolytica*	*M. tuberculosis* *T. whipplei*

Consider noninfectious causes like inflammatory bowel disease, and intestinal malignancies like colon cancer.
[a]*Giardia* intestinalis can occur throughout Australia and New Zealand, but it is particularly endemic in Tasmania.

Diarrhea is often associated with infections with bacteria, virus, and parasites. Repeated negative bacterial cultures and microscopy for parasites should lead to the consideration that the symptoms may not be caused by an infection. Inflammatory bowel diseases like ulcerative colitis and Crohn's disease are differential diagnosis, and malabsorption and celiac disease must also be considered.

Gastrointestinal infections with symptoms for more than 4 weeks and in the immunocompromised host

Microorganisms with symptoms for more than 4 weeks	Microorganisms in the immunocompromised host
M. tuberculosis *T. whipplei* *Blastocystis hominis*[a] *Dientamoeba fragilis*[a] *Echinococcus granulosis*	*Candida* spp. Herpes virus, CMV

Microorganisms with symptoms for more than 4 weeks	Microorganisms in the immunocompromised host
E. vermicularis *S. stercoralis*[b] *Ancylostoma duodenale* (hookworm)[b] *A. lumbricoides*[b] *T. trichiuria*[b]	

Consider noninfectious causes like inflammatory bowel disease, and intestinal malignancies like colon cancer, malabsorption, and celiac disease.

[a]Of uncertain pathogenicity in humans.

[b]Mainly occur in the tropical north of Australia.

Infections of liver, spleen, and peritoneum

Acute infections of liver, spleen, and peritoneum with less than 4 weeks of symptoms

Frequently found microorganisms	Rare microorganisms and conditions	Very rare microorganisms
Hepatitis A Hepatitis B Hepatitis C	*Entamoeba histolytica*	*Fasciola hepatica*

Chronic infections of liver, spleen, and peritoneum with more than 4 weeks of symptoms

Microorganisms with symptoms for more than 4 weeks	Microorganisms in the immunocompromised host
M. tuberculosis *T. whipplei*	*Mycobacterium avium complex*

Infections in the immunocompromised host are generally similar as the immunocompetent host.

Genitourinary infections

Cystitis, pyelonephritis, and nephritis with less than 4 weeks of symptoms

Frequently found microorganisms	Rare microorganisms and conditions	Very rare microorganisms
E. coli *Klebsiella pneumonia*		*M. tuberculosis*

Consider noninfectious causes especially malignancies like renal cell carcinoma.

Sexually transmitted infections with less than 4 weeks of symptoms

Frequently found microorganisms	Rare microorganisms and conditions	Very rare microorganisms
Chlamydia spp. *N. gonorrhoeae*		

Cystitis, pyelonephritis, and nephritis with symptoms for more than 4 weeks and in the immunocompromised host

Microorganisms with symptoms for more than 4 weeks	Microorganisms in the immunocompromised host
M. tuberculosis	*Candida* spp.

Consider noninfectious causes especially malignancies like renal cell carcinoma.

Sexually transmitted infections with symptoms for more than 4 weeks and in the immunocompromised host

Microorganisms with symptoms for more than 4 weeks	Microorganisms in the immunocompromised host
T. pallidum	

Joint, muscle, and soft tissue infections

Joint, muscle, and soft tissue infections with less than 4 weeks of symptoms

Frequently found microorganisms	Rare microorganisms and conditions	Very rare microorganisms and conditions
S. aureus *S. pneumoniae* RRV and BFV	Necrotizing fasciitis caused by group G streptococci Dengue	

Joint, muscle, and soft tissue infections with more than 4 weeks of symptoms and in the immunocompromised host

Microorganisms with symptoms for more than 4 weeks	Microorganisms in the immunocompromised host
M. tuberculosis	*Candida* spp.

Skin infections

Skin infections with less than 4 weeks of symptoms

Frequently found microorganisms	Rare microorganisms and conditions	Very rare microorganisms and conditions
Erysipelas (*Streptococcus pyogenes*) and *S. pneumoniae* *S. aureus*	Scabies Necrotizing fasciitis caused by group A streptococci	*Vibrio vulnificus*

We have not listed rashes due to viral infections as these are not limited to the skin.

Skin infections with more than 4 weeks of symptoms and in the immunocompromised host

Microorganisms with symptoms for more than 4 weeks	Microorganisms in the immunocompromised host
T. pallidum *M. tuberculosis* *M. ulcerans*[a]	*Candida* spp.

[a]*Mycobacterium ulcerans* has not been reported from New Zealand.

Adenopathy

Adenopathy of less than 4 weeks' duration

Frequently found microorganisms	Rare microorganisms and conditions	Very rare microorganisms and conditions
EBV CMV Parvovirus B19 *T. gondii* HIV	*B. henselae*	

Adenopathy of more than 4 weeks' duration and in the immunocompromised host

Microorganisms with symptoms for more than 4 weeks	Microorganisms in the immunocompromised host
T. gondii *M. tuberculosis* Nontuberculous mycobacteria	CMV *M. avium* complex

If the diagnosis is not made within a few weeks, biopsies should be performed to exclude malignancies like lymphoma and carcinomas.

Fever without focal symptoms

Fever for less than 4 weeks without focal symptoms

Frequently found microorganisms	Rare microorganisms and conditions	Very rare microorganisms and conditions
Endocarditis	*M. tuberculosis*	
EBV	*C. burnetii*[a]	
CMV	*B. henselae*	
Parvovirus B19	Leptospirosis	
T. gondii	*Rickettsia* spp.	
HIV	Dengue virus	
	B. suis	

[a]Q fever has not been reported from New Zealand.

Fever for more than 4 weeks without focal symptoms and in the immunocompromised host

Microorganisms with symptoms for more than 4 weeks	Microorganisms in the immunocompromised host
T. gondii	CMV
M. tuberculosis	

All patients with adenopathy should have a CT- or MR scan of the thorax and abdomen performed soon to determine the extent of the adenopathy and to enable decision of the best approach to biopsy.

PET-CT will provide clues for inflammatory foci and malignancies.

Noninfectious causes like lymphoma, other malignancies and autoimmune diseases should be considered early.

Eosinophilia and elevated IgE

Eosinophilia and elevated IgE less than 4 weeks of symptoms

Frequently found microorganisms	Rare microorganisms and conditions	Very rare microorganisms and conditions
	Toxocara spp.	*F. hepatica*
	A. lumbricoides, T. trichiuria, and hookworm	
	S. stercoralis	

Eosinophilia and elevated IgE for more than 4 weeks and in the immunocompromised host

Microorganisms with symptoms for more than 4 weeks	Microorganisms in the immunocompromised host
A. lumbricoides, T. trichiuria, and hookworm S. stercoralis	Toxocara spp.

Basic diagnostics in patients with eosinophilia and elevated IgE

Microorganisms	Diagnostics
A. lumbricoides, T. trichiuria, and hookworm	Fecal microscopy
Toxocara spp.	Serology
S. stercoralis	Fecal microscopy, serology
F. hepatica	Fecal microscopy, serology, and imaging

Antibiotic resistance

Community-acquired methicillin-resistant *Staphylococcus aureus* (CA-MRSA) is still a relatively rare cause of *S. aureus* infections in patients presenting to medical practitioners and hospitals. The spectrum of infections includes skin and soft tissue infections, bacteremia, and community-acquired pneumonia. The highest rates have been reported from Western Australia, the Northern Territory, and Queensland, but CA-MRSA skin infections have now also been reported from Brisbane, Sydney, Canberra, and Melbourne. In Western Australia the notification rate for CA-MRSA in the metropolitan areas of Perth is as high as 144/100,000 population. In Darwin, CA-MRSA has accounted for up to 20% of community-onset *S. aureus* bacteremias, with a substantial proportion of patients having infective endocarditis. National surveillance has shown that there has been a statistically significant increase in the proportion of CA-MRSA isolates from 4.7% in 2000 to 7.3% in 2004. The most frequent clonal isolates have included ST1-MRSA-IV (Western Australia, Northern Territory, and South Australia) followed by ST93-MRSA-IV (Queensland and NSW), and ST30-MRSA-IV (Northern Territory, Queensland, and NSW). ST129-MRSA-IV and ST5-MRSA-IV are most frequently encountered in Victoria, Tasmania, and Western Australia [19].

Although cases of high-level penicillin-resistant pneumococcus causing pneumonia or meningitis have been reported; they are infrequent (<5%). Extended-spectrum β-lactamases (ESBL) and metallo-β-lactamases (MBL) gram-negative infections are also uncommon and are seen almost exclusively as nosocomial infections or in travelers returning from areas such as South and Southeast Asia.

Vaccine-preventable diseases in children

Australia has a National Immunisation Program Schedule (funded by the Australian Government) which currently includes vaccines against a total of 16 diseases. There is also an Australian Childhood Immunisation Register (the ACIR), which aims to (i) provide an accurate measure of the immunization coverage of children in Australia under 7 years of age and (ii) provide an effective management tool for monitoring immunization coverage and service delivery. The childhood vaccination schedule consists of the vaccines listed below [20], and over 90% of children are fully vaccinated.

- Birth: Hepatitis B
- 2, 4, and 6 months: Diphtheria, tetanus, pertussis, polio, Hib, hepatitis B, pneumococcal, and rotavirus
- 12 months: Measles, mumps, rubella, Hib, and meningococcal C
- 18 months: Varicella
- 12–24 months: Hepatitis A and pneumococcal polysaccharide (23vPPV) (only for Aboriginal and Torres Strait Islander's children in high-risk areas)
- 4 years: Diphtheria, tetanus, pertussis, polio, measles, mumps, and rubella

The New Zealand National Immunisation Schedule [21,22] currently includes vaccines against a total of 12 diseases offered free to babies, children, adolescents, and adults. New Zealand also has a National Immunisation Register. Approximately 95% of children are fully immunized by 2 years of age (Dr Nikki Turner, Director of the Immunisation Advisory Centre (IMAC), personal communication).

- 6 weeks, 3 and 5 months: Diphtheria, tetanus, acellular pertussis, polio, *Haemophilus influenzae* type b, Hepatitis B
- 6 weeks, 3, 5, and 15 months: 7-valent pneumococcal conjugate vaccine
- 15 months: *H. influenzae* type b
- 15 months: Measles, mumps, and rubella
- 4 years: Measles, mumps, rubella, diphtheria, tetanus, and acellular pertussis
- 11 years: Diphtheria, tetanus, acellular pertussis
- 12 years (girls only): Human papillomavirus (3 doses)
- 45 and 65 years adult: Tetanus and diphtheria
- All adults 65 years and over and high-risk other groups: Seasonal influenza.

There are additional scheduled vaccines offered:

- BCG to babies who will be living in a household or family with a person with either current TB or a past history of TB, have one or both parents who are of Pacific ethnicity, have parents or household members who, within the past 5 years, lived for a period of 6 months or longer in a country with a high incidence of TB, during their first 5 years will be living for 3 months or longer in a country with a high incidence of TB.
- Babies of HBsAg-positive mothers need Hepatitis B immune globulin (HBIG) and hepatitis B vaccine at birth; then they continue with the usual schedule at 6 weeks, 3 and 5 months.
- Women of childbearing age who are nonimmune to rubella are offered the MMR vaccine.

Basic economic and demographic data

	GNI[a] per capita (USD)	Life expectancy at birth (total, years)	School enrollment, primary (% net)
Australia	40,350	81	97
New Zealand	27,940	80	99

World Bank (www.worldbank.org).
[a]Gross national income.

Courses of death in children under 5 years in Australia

	Australia
Neonatal causes	56
Pneumonia	1
Diarrheal diseases	0
Malaria	0
HIV/AIDS	0
Measles	0
Injuries	11
Others	

Most common causes of deaths all ages in Australia

	Australia (%)
Ischemic and hypertensive heart disease	20
Cerebrovascular disease	9
Lower respiratory infections	2
Perinatal conditions	NS
Tuberculosis	NS
Diarrheal disease	NS
Measles	NS
Chronic obstructive lung disease	4
Malnutrition	NS
Diabetes	3
Alzheimer and other dementias	3
Nephritis and nephrosis	NS
Cancers	14
Asthma	NS
Endocrine disorders	NS

WHO, 2006 (http://www.who.int/whosis/mort/profiles/en/#P).
NS, not stated.

References

1. Communicable Diseases Network, Australia New Zealand. Accessed at http://www9.health .gov.au/cda/Source/CDA-index.cfm.

2. Owen R, Roche PW, Hope K, et al. Australia's notifiable diseases status, 2005: annual report of the National Notifiable Diseases Surveillance System. Commun Dis Intell 2007;31: 1–70.

3. Currie BJ, Jacups SP, Cheng AC, et al. Melioidosis epidemiology and risk factors from a prospective whole-population study in northern Australia. Trop Med Int Health 2004;9: 1167–74.

4. Currie BJ. Melioidosis: an important cause of pneumonia in residents of and travellers returned from endemic regions. Eur Respir J 2003;22:542–50.

5. Cheng AC, Currie BJ. Melioidosis: epidemiology, pathophysiology, and management. Clin Microbiol Rev 2005;18:383–416.

6. Currie BJ, Dance DAB, Cheng AC. The global distribution of *Burkholderia pseudomallei* and

melioidosis: an update. Trans R Soc Trop Med Hyg 2008;102(Suppl. 1):S1–4.

7. Quek TYJ, Athan E, Henry MJ, et al. Risk factors for *Mycobacterium ulcerans* infection, southeastern Australia. Emerg Infect Dis 2007;13: 1661–6.

8. Graves S, Stenos J. Rickettsioses in Australia. Ann N Y Acad Sci 2009:151–5.

9. Harrison LH, Trotter CL, Ramsay ME. Global epidemiology of meningococcal disease. Vaccine 2009;27(Suppl. 2):B51–63.

10. Patel MS. Australia's century of meningococcal disease: development and the changing ecology of an accidental pathogen. Med J Aust 2007;186:136–41.

11. Baker MG, Martin DR, Kieft CEM, Lennon D. A 10-year serogroup B meningococcal disease epidemic in New Zealand: descriptive epidemiology, 1991–2000. J Paediatr Child Health 2001;37(5):S13–19.

12. Steer AC, Carapetis JR. Acute rheumatic fever and rheumatic heart disease in indigenous populations. Pediatr Clin North Am 2009; 56:1401–19.

13. White H, Walsh W, Brown A, et al. Rheumatic heart disease in indigenous populations. Heart Lung Circ 2010;19:273–81.

14. 2009 National Leptospirosis Surveillance Report by the WHO/FAO/OIE Collaborating Centre for Reference and Research on leptospirosis. Accessed September 21, 2010, at http://www.health.qld.gov.au/qhcss/lepto.asp.

15. Benschop J, Heuer C, Jaros P, Collins-Emerson J, Midwinter A, Wilson P. Sero-prevalence of leptospirosis in workers at a New Zealand slaughterhouse. N Z Med J 2009;122:39–47.

16. National Centre in HIV Epidemiology and Clinical Research. HIV/AIDS, viral hepatitis and sexually transmissible infections in Australia—Annual Surveillance Report. Accessed October 10, 2010, at http://www.nchecr.unsw.edu.au/NCHECRweb.nsf/resources/SurvReports_3/$file/ASR2009-updated-2.pdf.

17. World Health Organization. Epidemiological fact sheet on HIV and AIDS: core data on epidemiology and response, Australia, 2008. Accessed October 10, 2010, at http://apps.who.int/globalatlas/predefinedReports/EFS2008/full/EFS2008_au.pdf.

18. McDonald M, Richard M, Robers S. Potential health hazards in travelers to Australia, New Zealand, and the southwestern Pacific (Oceania). In:UpToDate, Basow, DS (Ed), UpToDate, Waltham, MA, 2011.

19. Nimmo GR, Coombs GW. Community-associated methicillin-resistant *Staphylococcus aureus* (MRSA) in Australia. Int J Antimicrob Agents 2008;31:401–10.

20. Australian Immunisation Handbook, 9th Edition. Australian Government Department of Health and Ageing, and the National Health and Medical Research Council, 2008.

21. New Zealand Ministry of Health. Immunisation Handbook 2006. Wellington: Ministry of Health, 2006.

22. 2008 National Immunisation Schedule Health Provider Booklet. New Zealand: Ministry of Health, 2008.

Chapter 25
Oceania

Karin Leder,[1,2] Joseph Torresi[3] and Marc Shaw[4,5]
[1]School of Public Health and Preventive Medicine, Monash University, Victoria, Australia
[2]Victorian Infectious Disease Service, Royal Melbourne Hospital, Melbourne, Victoria, Australia
[3]Department of Infectious Diseases, Austin Hospital, Melbourne, Australia
[4]School of Public Health, James Cook University, Townsville, Australia
[5]WORLDWISE Travellers' Health and Vaccination Centres, New Zealand

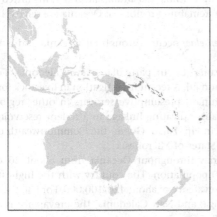

American Samoa
Cook Islands
Fiji
Guam
Kiribati
Marshall Islands
Micronesia
 (Federate States of)
Northern Mariana
 Islands
New Caledonia
Nauru
Niue

Palau
Papua New Guinea
Pitcairn
Samoa
Solomon Islands
Tahiti (French
 Polynesia)
Tonga
Tuvalu
Vanuatu

Oceania comprises over 20 countries with differing levels of health care, socioeconomics, disease surveillance, and intensity of various infections. Whereas some risks occur throughout the region, such as travelers' diarrhea, there is marked nonuniformity in the risks of other diseases. This is well highlighted by malaria: most Oceanic countries pose no malaria risk, but the Solomon Islands, Papua New Guinea (PNG), and Vanuatu have high intensity of both *Plasmodium falciparum* and *Plasmodium vivax* malaria. Information regarding which Oceanic countries report specific diseases has been summarized in the text and tables below to indicate where in the region infectious risks are likely to be greatest.

Infectious Diseases: A Geographic Guide, First Edition.
Edited by Eskild Petersen, Lin H. Chen & Patricia Schlagenhauf.
© 2011 John Wiley & Sons, Ltd. Published 2011 by John Wiley & Sons, Ltd.

Bacterial and mycobacterial infections

Travelers' diarrhea is a frequent problem for travelers to Oceania, often due to bacterial pathogens (enterotoxigenic *Escherichia coli*, *Campylobacter*, *Salmonella*, *Shigella*). Cholera is uncommon, but sporadic cases and outbreaks are reported. Typhoid fever also occurs; Fiji in particular has reported a significant number of typhoid cases in recent years.

Cases of yaws still occur in some parts of Oceania. Eradication campaigns have greatly reduced the geographic extension and global burden, with a few resisting foci of cases occurring in Papua New Guinea, Solomon Islands, and Vanuatu [1–3].

Melioidosis has been reported from the Western Province of PNG, with most cases occurring in children. Cases of melioidosis have also been recently reported from New Caledonia [4].

Rickettsial infections: Scrub typhus, caused by *Orientia tsutsugamushi* and transmitted by a chigger bite, has been reported from PNG. The remaining regions of Oceania are relatively free of rickettsial infections [5–7].

Cat scratch disease, caused by *Bartonella henselae*, occurs throughout Oceania and is transmitted by the bite or scratch of domestic cats.

Leptospirosis is endemic in much of Oceania [8]. In particular, New Caledonia, French Polynesia, and Papua have reported this infection [9]. A recent investigation in livestock found a dominance of serovar Hardjo, while the dominant presumptive serovars in other regions of Oceania were Icterohaemorrhagiae and Australis indicating linkage to a rodent reservoir [10]. Foci of leptospirosis have also been described in Fiji, Palau, Guam, the Commonwealth of the Northern Mariana Islands, and the Federated States of Micronesia.

The overall prevalence of tuberculosis varies throughout Oceania from about 20 cases/100,000 population to over 400 cases/100,000 population. The country with the highest case load in the region is PNG, with an estimated prevalence of about 420/100,000. For Fiji, the Cook Islands, Samoa, Guam, French Polynesia, Tonga, and New Caledonia, the prevalence is about 20–40/100,000 [11].

Leprosy is endemic in most countries within Oceania, although underreporting makes exact prevalence rates difficult. Reported rates are highest in PNG, Micronesia, Kiribati, and Marshall Islands [12].

In Oceania, *Mycobacterium ulcerans* infection is most commonly reported from Papua New Guinea. The majority of cases occur in children 15 years of age or younger and infection in travelers to these regions has been reported [13,14].

Acute rheumatic fever (ARF) continues to be a huge public health burden on many Pacific Island countries [15–18]. Prevalence rates of rheumatic heart disease (RHD) are high in Samoa (77.8/1,000), Tonga (30/1,000), the Cook Islands (18.5/1,000), and New Caledonia (10/1,000). Indigenous Fijians are also disproportionately affected. ARF incidence data suggest the following: 113–236/100,000 in French Polynesia, 98/100,000 in New Caledonia, and 206/100,000 in Samoan children. RHD causes around 115,000 deaths per year in the Western Pacific region [18].

Viral infections

Hepatitis A infections occur in the region, and outbreaks are intermittently reported. Hepatitis E may be endemic in some countries, but levels of endemicity are unknown. Hepatitis B is endemic throughout the Pacific region with HBsAg carrier rates above 8% for most countries and islands in the region [19]. However, chronic carrier rates have started to decline since the introduction of HBV vaccination programs.

It is estimated that 0.4% of the adult population of Oceania is living with human immuno-deficiency virus (HIV)/AIDS, with the highest incidence occurring in PNG (estimate of 2% of the adult population). Heterosexual transmission is the predominant means of infection [20].

Dengue is reported from most countries in Oceania, and the number of cases reported annually has been rising dramatically over recent years (approximately 1,500 cases in 2004 and 12,500 in 2009) [21]. Highest rates are reported from French Polynesia, Fiji, American Samoa, Cook Islands, PNG, New Caledonia, and Tonga. Outbreaks have also been reported from Kiribati, Micronesia, Nauru, Palau, Samoa, Solomon Islands, and Vanuatu. Given that reported cases are undoubtedly an underestimation of the true number of cases, travelers visiting Oceania are at risk of infection, especially during the rainy seasons.

Japanese encephalitis has been reported from Palau, Guam, and the Northern Mariana Islands since 1990 [22]. This zoonotic flavivirus has spread down through the Indonesian archipelago to PNG (as well as to the Torres Strait of northern Australia) [23].

Ross River virus is a mosquito-transmitted *Alphavirus* that is endemic and enzootic in Australia and PNG. It has also been reported to cause large epidemics in Fiji, New Caledonia, Samoa, and the Cook Islands in the South Pacific [24,25].

Murray Valley encephalitis (MVE) has been reported from PNG. The virus in PNG is closely related to MVE in Australia, although separate foci of MVE evolution and greater strain variation exist in PNG [26].

Zika virus is a flavivirus that was first isolated in 1947 from a rhesus monkey in the Zika forest near Entebbe, Uganda. No transmission of Zika virus had been reported outside of Africa and Asia until 2007 when physicians in the Federated States of Micronesia Island reported an outbreak of illness characterized by rash, conjunctivitis, subjective fever, arthralgia, and arthritis. The virus emerged unexpectedly on the island of Yap and adjoining islands of Ulithi, Fais, Earpik, Woleai, and Ifalik with over 150 cases [2]. It is transmitted to humans by infected Aedes mosquitoes [27,28].

All countries in Oceania are considered rabies free, although for many areas there is minimal surveillance.

Parasitic infections

The soil-transmitted helminths, hookworm, *Ascaris lumbricoides*, and *Trichuris trichiura*, are common and represent a significant public health problem in many countries of Oceania, particularly in rural and small village settings. Travelers who have walked barefoot may be at particular risk of infection. *Strongyloides stercoralis* infection is also endemic in many regions. Diarrhea secondary to *Entamoeba histolytica* and *Giardia* infections also occur.

Both falciparum malaria and vivax malaria are present in three Oceanic countries: PNG, Solomon Islands, and Vanuatu. In PNG, malaria occurs in areas below <1,800 m, and increased risk occurs along coastal areas and in the lowlands, especially during the wetter months (December through February). In the Solomon Islands and Vanuatu, malaria occurs country-wide, including urban areas. Vivax malaria from Oceania is becoming increasingly resistant to chloroquine, so chloroquine should not be used as first-line therapy for vivax malaria acquired in this region. Reduced susceptibility to primaquine is also common.

Lymphatic filariasis is a major public health problem in many countries in Oceania, caused by infection with either *Wuchereria bancrofti* or *Brugia malayi*. Adult worms develop in the lymphatic vessels, causing severe damage and swelling, and in late stages painful, disfiguring swelling of the legs and genital organs (elephantiasis). Countries endemic for filariasis include PNG, Niue, Tonga, Vanuatu, Fiji, French Polynesia, New Caledonia, Samoa, Cook Islands, American Samoa, Nauru, Tuvalu, Kiribati, and the Solomon Islands, with most of the people at risk being in PNG. In recent years, efforts to eliminate the disease through annual mass drug administration have been carried out in most endemic countries. Short term travelers are usually at very low risk of infection.

Infection due to *Angiostrongylus cantonensis*, the rat lungworm, occurs in Oceania, and has been particularly reported from PNG [29]. It is acquired by eating contaminated leafy vegetables (in salads), infected snails and slugs, and land crabs. Symptoms include paresthesia and eosinophilic meningitis.

Of note, Oceania is also free of human schistosomiasis.

In addition to specific infectious outcomes listed, travelers also need to be aware of the risks of toxins, envenomations, and bites (spiders and snakes). Safety of the blood supplies is not guaranteed.

CNS infections: meningitis, encephalitis, and other infections with neurological symptoms

Acute infections with less than 4 weeks of symptoms

Frequently found microorganisms	Rare microorganisms	Very rare microorganisms
Viral meningitis (enterovirus group)	*Listeria monocytogenes*	*Naegleria* and other free-living ameba
Pneumococcal meningitis	Neurosyphilis	Influenza
Herpes virus (group I and II)	HIV	*Burkholderia pseudomallei*
Neisseria meningitidis	MVE	Japanese encephalitis
		A. cantonensis

CNS infections: meningitis and encephalitis with symptoms for more than 4 weeks and in the immunocompromised host

Microorganisms with symptoms for more than 4 weeks	Microorganisms in the immunocompromised host
HIV	*Nocardia* spp.
Mycobacterium tuberculosis	Polyomavirus
	Cryptococcus spp.[a]
	JC virus

Consider noninfectious causes like vasculitis and lymphoma.

[a]In PNG, *Cryptococcus gattii* infection occurs relatively more frequent than *Cryptococcus neoformans*.

Ear, nose, and throat infections

Ear, nose, and throat infections with less than 4 weeks of symptoms

Frequently found microorganisms	Rare microorganisms and conditions	Very rare microorganisms
Streptococcal throat infection Epstein–Barr virus (EBV) Herpes virus (type I and II)	Peritonsillar abscess[a] Tuberculosis Diphtheria[b]	

[a]Requires acute ENT evaluation.
[b]PNG has more diphtheria cases than other countries in the region.

Ear, nose, and throat infections with symptoms for more than 4 weeks and in the immunocompromised host

Microorganisms with symptoms for more than 4 weeks	Microorganisms in the immunocompromised host
M. tuberculosis	*Candida spp.* Herpes simplex virus

Consider noninfectious causes like vasculitis and lymphoma.

Cardiopulmonary infections

Pneumonia with less than 4 weeks of symptoms

Frequently found microorganisms	Rare microorganisms and conditions	Very rare microorganisms
Streptococcus pneumoniae *Mycoplasma pneumoniae*	*Legionella* Influenza	*Corynebacterium diphtheriae* *B. pseudomallei* Tropical pulmonary eosinophilia

Endocarditis with less than 4 weeks of symptoms

Frequently found microorganisms	Rare microorganisms and conditions	Very rare microorganisms
Staphylococcus aureus Nonhemolytic streptococci	*Neisseria gonorrhoeae* *Coxiella burnetii*	*Bartonella spp.*

(Continued)

Frequently found microorganisms	Rare microorganisms and conditions	Very rare microorganisms
Coagulase-negative staphylococci (*Staphylococcus epidermidis*) S. pneumoniae *Enterococcus* spp.	*Propionibacterium* spp. HACEK group	

Pulmonary symptoms for more than 4 weeks and in the immunocompromised host

Microorganisms and diseases with symptoms for more than 4 weeks	Microorganisms in the immunocompromised host
M. tuberculosis *Aspergillus* spp.	*Pneumocystis jirovecii* Cytomegalovirus (CMV) *Aspergillus* spp., *Candida* spp.

Consider noninfectious causes like lung cancer, autoimmune lung fibrosis, and Wegener's granulomatosis.

Endocarditis for more than 4 weeks and in the immunocompromised host

Microorganisms and diseases with symptoms for more than 4 weeks	Microorganisms in the immunocompromised host
Coagulase-negative staphylococci (*S. epidermidis*) Nonhemolytic streptococci *C. burnetii* *Bartonella* spp.	*Aspergillus* spp.

Consider noninfectious causes like sarcoidosis.

Gastrointestinal infections

Gastrointestinal infections with less than 4 weeks of symptoms

Frequently found microorganisms	Rare microorganisms and conditions	Very rare microorganisms
Norovirus and calicivirus, rotavirus *Campylobacter*	*Cryptosporidium* spp. *S. aureus* toxin	*M. tuberculosis* Morbus Whipple

Frequently found microorganisms	Rare microorganisms and conditions	Very rare microorganisms
Enterotoxigenic *Escherichia coli* (ETEC) *Giardia intestinalis* *Salmonella* (nontyphi) *Salmonella typhi* *Shigella* Enteropathogenic *E. coli* *Enterobius vermicularis* *S. stercoralis* Hookworm *A. lumbricoides* *T. trichiura* *E. histolytica* Hepatitis A virus	*Bacillus cereus* toxin *Vibrio cholerae*	

Consider noninfectious causes like inflammatory bowel disease and intestinal malignancies like colon cancer.

Diarrhea is often associated with infections with bacteria, virus, and parasites. Repeated negative bacterial cultures and microscopy for parasites should lead to the consideration that the symptoms may not be caused by an infection. Inflammatory bowel diseases like ulcerative colitis and Crohn's disease are differential diagnosis and malabsorption and celiac disease must also be considered.

Gastrointestinal infections with symptoms for more than 4 weeks and in the immunocompromised host

Microorganisms with symptoms for more than 4 weeks	Microorganisms in the immunocompromised host
M. tuberculosis Morbus Whipple *Blastocystis hominis*[a] *Dientamoeba fragilis*[a] *E. histolytica* *E. vermicularis* *S. stercoralis* Hookworm *A. lumbricoides* *T. trichiura*	*Candida* Herpes virus *S. stercoralis*

Consider noninfectious causes like inflammatory bowel disease, intestinal malignancies like colon cancer, malabsorption, and celiac disease.
[a]Of uncertain pathogenicity in humans.

Infections of liver, spleen, and peritoneum

Acute infections of liver, spleen, and peritoneum with less than 4 weeks of symptoms

Frequently found microorganisms	Rare microorganisms and conditions	Very rare microorganisms
Hepatitis A	Hydatid infection due to *Echinococcus granulosus*	*Fasciola hepatica*
Hepatitis B		
Hepatitis C		
Hepatitis E[a]		
E. histolytica		

[a]Hepatitis E is probably present, but has not been reported so far.

Chronic infections of liver, spleen, and peritoneum with more than 4 weeks of symptoms

Microorganisms with symptoms for more than 4 weeks	Microorganisms in the immunocompromised host
M. tuberculosis	
Tropheryma whipplei	

Infections in the immunocompromised host are generally similar as the immunocompetent host.

Genitourinary infections

Cystitis, pyelonephritis, and nephritis with less than 4 weeks of symptoms

Frequently found microorganisms	Rare microorganisms and conditions	Very rare microorganisms
E. coli		*M. tuberculosis*
Klebsiella pneumoniae		

Consider noninfectious causes, especially malignancies like renal cell carcinoma.

Sexually transmitted infections with less than 4 weeks of symptoms

Frequently found microorganisms	Rare microorganisms and conditions	Very rare microorganisms
Chlamydia spp.	L-serovars of *Chlamydia trachomatis* (lymphogranuloma venereum)	
N. gonorrhoeae		

Cystitis, pyelonephritis, and nephritis with symptoms for more than 4 weeks and in the immunocompromised host

Microorganisms with symptoms for more than 4 weeks	Microorganisms in the immunocompromised host
Bacterial infections in patients with long-term catheters and renal stones *M. tuberculosis*	*Candida* spp.

Consider noninfectious causes, especially malignancies like renal cell carcinoma.

Sexually transmitted infections with symptoms for more than 4 weeks and in the immunocompromised host

Microorganisms with symptoms for more than 4 weeks	Microorganisms in the immunocompromised host
Treponema pallidum	

Joint, muscle, and soft tissue infections

Joint, muscle, and soft tissue infections with less than 4 weeks of symptoms

Frequently found microorganisms	Rare microorganisms and conditions	Very rare microorganisms and conditions
S. aureus	Necrotizing fasciitis	Fournier's gangrene (perineum and urogenital)
	Group G streptococci	
S. pneumoniae		
Ross River virus		*Trichinella* species (*Trichinella papuae*)[a]

[a]*T. papuae* is found in PNG in domestic and feral pigs and can cause human infection.

Joint, muscle, and soft tissue infections with more than 4 weeks of symptoms and in the immunocompromised host

Microorganisms with symptoms for more than 4 weeks	Microorganisms in the immunocompromised host
M. tuberculosis	*Candida* spp.

Skin infections

Skin infections with less than 4 weeks of symptoms

Frequently found microorganisms	Rare microorganisms and conditions	Very rare microorganisms and conditions
Erysipelas, *S. pneumoniae* *S. aureus*	Scabies Cutaneous larva migrans (CLM)	Cutaneous diphtheria

We have not listed rashes due to viral infections as these are not limited to the skin.

Skin infections with more than 4 weeks of symptoms and in the immunocompromised host

Microorganisms with symptoms for more than 4 weeks	Microorganisms in the immunocompromised host
T. pallidum *M. tuberculosis* *Mycobacterium leprae* *M. ulcerans* Yaws Dermatophytes	*Candida* spp.

Adenopathy

Adenopathy of less than 4 weeks duration

Frequently found microorganisms	Rare microorganisms and conditions	Very rare microorganisms and conditions
EBV CMV Parvovirus B19 *Toxoplasma gondii* HIV	*Bartonella*	

Adenopathy of more than 4 weeks duration and in the immunocompromised host

Microorganisms with symptoms for more than 4 weeks	Microorganisms in the immunocompromised host
T. gondii	CMV
Tuberculosis	Atypical mycobacteria
Lymphatic filariasis	

If the diagnosis is not made within a few weeks, biopsies should be performed to exclude malignancies like lymphoma and carcinomas.

Fever without focal symptoms

Fever for less than 4 weeks without focal symptoms

Frequently found microorganisms	Rare microorganisms and conditions	Very rare microorganisms and conditions
EBV	Tuberculosis	Zika virus
CMV	C. burnetii	
Parvovirus B19	Bartonella spp.	
T. gondii	Leptospirosis	
HIV	Rickettsia, Orientia	
Dengue virus	Hepatitis A	
Malaria	Amebic liver abscess	
Enteric fever		
Influenza virus		

Fever for more than 4 weeks without focal symptoms and in the immunocompromised host

Microorganisms with symptoms for more than 4 weeks	Microorganisms in the immunocompromised host
HIV	CMV
M. tuberculosis	

Noninfectious causes should be considered from the beginning including malignancies like lymphoma and autoimmune diseases.

Eosinophilia and elevated IgE

Eosinophilia and elevated IgE for less than 4 weeks

Frequently found microorganisms	Rare microorganisms and conditions	Very rare microorganisms and conditions
A. lumbricoides, T. trichiura, hookworm Filariasis, tropical pulmonary eosinophilia *S. stercoralis*	*Toxocara* spp.	*Trichinella spiralis*

Eosinophilia and elevated IgE for more than 4 weeks and in the immunocompromised host

Microorganisms with symptoms for more than 4 weeks	Microorganisms in the immunocompromised host
A. lumbricoides, T. trichiura, hookworm *S. stercoralis* Filariasis, tropical pulmonary eosinophilia	*Toxocara* spp.

Antibiotic resistance

Penicillin-resistant *S. pneumoniae* is prevalent in parts of Oceania, especially in PNG; this should be taken into account when travelers develop pneumonia or meningitis.

Vaccine-preventable diseases in children

Vaccine schedules for Oceania are similar for all countries in the region, with primary prevention against the following disease being a focus: tetanus, diphtheria, hepatitis B, *Haemophilus influenzae* B, pertussis, measles, mumps, rubella, polio, and tuberculosis. The data can be extracted from the World Health Organization Vaccine Preventable Diseases Monitoring System 2010 Global Summary. Last updated September 9, 2010, and is next to be updated in 2010. Available at: http://apps.who.int/immunization_monitoring/en/globalsummary/countryprofileselect.cfm (Accessed October 8, 2010).

Cook Island

Vaccine	Schedule
BCG	Birth
DT	11 years; from June 2009
DTwP	6, 10, 14 weeks; 5–6 years
DTwPHibHep	6 weeks; 3, 5 months; from June 2009

Vaccine	Schedule
HepB	Birth
MMR	15 months; 4 years
OPV	6, 10, 14 weeks
TT	4 weeks; 3, 5 months; 4, 11 years; pregnancy

Fiji

Vaccine	Schedule
BCG	Birth
DTaPHibHep	6, 10, 14 weeks
HepB	Birth
HPV	9–12 years
MR	12 months; 6 years
OPV	birth; 6, 10, 14 weeks
TT	1st contact; +1, +6 months; +1 year

Kiribati

Vaccine	Schedule
BCG	Birth
Dip	6 years
DTwPHibHep	6, 10, 14 weeks
HepB	Birth
MR	1, 6 years
OPV	6, 10, 14 weeks
TT	6, 13 years

Marshall Islands

Vaccine	Schedule
BCG	Birth
DTaP	2, 4, 6, 12 months
HepB	Birth; 2, 6 months (and adolescents)
Hib	2, 4, 12 months
HPV	11–12 years; +2, +6 months
Influenza	High risk populations
MMR	12, 13 months
OPV	2, 4, 6 months; 4-6 years
Pneumo_conj	2, 4, 6, 12 months

(Continued)

Vaccine	Schedule
Rotavirus	2, 4, 6 months
TT/Td	Adolescents and adults
Vitamin A	6–59 months

Federated States of Micronesia

Vaccine	Schedule
BCG	Birth
DTaP	2, 4, 6, 12 months; 4 years
HepB	Birth; 2, 6 months
Hib	2, 4, 12 months
MMR	12, 13 months
OPV	2, 4, 6, 12 months; 4 years
Pneumo_conj	2, 4, 6 months; 1, 4 years
Td	7, 9 years

Nauru

Vaccine	Schedule
BCG	Birth
DTwP	18 months; 4 years
DTwPHibHep	6, 10, 14 weeks
HepB	Birth
MR	12, 15 months
OPV	6, 10, 14 week; 18 months; 4 years
TT	1st visit; +4 weeks; pregnant women

Palau

Vaccine	Schedule
DTaP	15 months; 4–6 years
DTaPHepIPV	6 weeks; 4, 6 months
HepB	1 day
Hib	2, 4, 6, 12 months
HPV	
Influenza	>6 months
IPV	4–6 years
MMR	12, 15 months
Pneumo_conj	3, 5, 7, 15 months
Rotavirus	2, 4, 6 months

Papua New Guinea

Vaccine	Schedule
BCG	Birth
DTwPHibHepB	1, 2, 3 months
HepB	Birth
Measles	6, 9 months
OPV	4, 8, 12 weeks
TT	7, 13 years; pregnancy; +1, +6 months; +1 year
Vitamin	6, 12 months

Samoa

Vaccine	Schedule
BCG	Birth
DTaP	5 years
DTaPHibHep	6, 10, 14 weeks
HepB	Birth
MMR	12, 15 months
OPV	6, 10, 14 weeks
Td	1st visit; +4 weeks; +6 months; +1 year

Solomon Islands

Vaccine	Schedule
BCG	Birth
DTwPHibHep	6, 10, 14 weeks
HepB	Birth; 2, 4, 6 months
Measles	12 months
OPV	6, 10, 14 weeks; 5 years
TT	5 years

Tonga

Vaccine	Schedule
BCG	Birth
DTwP	18 months; 5–6 years
DTwPHib	6, 10, 14 weeks
HepB	Birth; 6, 10 weeks
MR	12, 18 months
OPV	6, 10, 14 weeks
Td	15–19 years; and pregnant women

Tuvalu

Vaccine	Schedule
BCG	Birth
DTwP	6, 10, 14 weeks
DTwPHibHep	6, 10, 14 weeks; from July 2009
HepB	Birth
MR	12, 18 months
OPV	6, 10, 14 weeks
TT	1st contact; +4 weeks; +6 months; +1 year

Vanuatu

Vaccine	Schedule
BCG	Birth
DTwP	6, 10, 14 weeks
DTwPHibHep	6, 10, 14 weeks
HepB	Birth; 6, 14 weeks
Measles	1 year
OPV	6, 10, 14 weeks; 6, 12 years
Td	6, 7 years
TT	1st contact; +1, +6 months; +1 year

Basic economic and demographic data

	GNI per capita (USD)	Life expectancy at birth (total, years)	School enrollment, primary (% net)
American Samoa	NA	NA	NA
Cook Islands	NA	NA	NA
Fiji	3,930	69	91
Guam	NA	76	NA
Kiribati	2,000	61	97
Marshall Islands	3,270	65	66
Federated States of Micronesia	2,340	69	NA
Nauru	NA	NA	NA
New Caledonia	14,020	76	NA
Niue	NA	NA	NA
Northern Mariana Islands	NA	NA	NA
Palau	8,650	69	96
PNG	1,010	57	NA
Pitcairn	NA	NA	NA
Samoa	2,780	72	90
Solomon Islands	1,180	64	62
Tahiti (French Polynesia)	NA	NA	NA

	GNI per capita (USD)	Life expectancy at birth (total, years)	School enrollment, primary (% net)
Tonga	2,560	72	96
Tuvalu	NA	NA	NA
Vanuatu	2,30	70	87

GNI, gross national income; NA, not available.
World Bank (www.worldbank.org).

Causes of death in children under 5 years in PNG and Fiji

	%	
	PNG	Fiji
Neonatal causes	35	41
Pneumonia	18	9
Diarrheal diseases	15	11
Malaria	1	0
HIV/AIDS	0	0
Measles	2	0
Injuries	2	3
Others	25	36

WHO, regional average, 2000–2003 (http://www.who.int/whosis/mort/profiles/en/#P).

Most common causes of death in all ages in PNG and Fiji

	PNG	Fiji
Ischemic and hypertensive heart disease	11	20
Cerebrovascular disease	4	13
Lower respiratory infections	8	5
Perinatal conditions	10	3
Tuberculosis	7	NS
Diarrheal disease	5	NS
Measles	2	NS
Chronic obstructive lung disease	2	2
Malnutrition	2	NS
Diabetes	NS	4
Alzheimer and other dementias	NS	NS
Nephritis and nephrosis	NS	4
Cancers	NS	NS
Asthma	NS	3
Endocrine disorders	NS	2

NS, not stated.

References

1. Walker SL, Hay RJ. Yaws—a review of the last 50 years. Int J Dermatol 2000;39: 258–60.
2. Fegan D, Glennon M, Macbride-Stewart G, Moore T. Yaws in the Solomon Islands. J Trop Med Hyg 1990;93:52–7.
3. Fegan D, Glennon MJ, Thami Y, Pakoa G. Resurgence of yaws in Tanna, Vanuatu: time for a new approach? Trop Doct 2010;40: 68–9.
4. Currie BJ, Dance DAB, Cheng AC. The global distribution of *Burkholderia pseudomallei* and melioidosis: an update. Trans R Soc Trop Med Hyg 2008;102 Suppl 1:S1–4.
5. Silpapojakul K. Scrub typhus in the western pacific region. Ann Acad Med Singapore 1997;26:794–800.
6. Jensenius M, Fournier PE, Raoult D. Rickettsioses and the international traveler. Clin Infect Dis 2004;39:1493–9.
7. Botelho-Nevers E, Raoult D. Fever of unknown origin due to rickettsioses. Infect Dis Clin North Am 2007;21:997–1011.
8. Daudens E, Frogier E, Mallet H-P. Recrudescence of leptospirosis in French Polynesia in early 2010. Inform Action 2010;32:3–6.
9. Berlioz-Arthaud A, Kiedrzynski T. Survey on leptospirosis in the Pacific. Inform Action 2003;16:5–8.
10. Victoriano AFB, Smythe LD, Gloriani-Barzaga N, et al. Leptospirosis in the Asia Pacific region. BMC Infect Dis 2009;9:147.
11. Tuberculosis Control in the Western Pacific Region, 2009 Report. World Health Organisation, 2009. Accessed October 10, 2010 at http://www.wpro.who.int/NR/rdonlyres/2894B832-5677-4BB1-B01F-1962551F9304/0/tbcontrol_2009.pdf.
12. Epidemiological Review of Leprosy in the Western Pacific Region 2007. World Health Organisation. Accessed October 10, 2010 at http://www.wpro.who.int/internet/resources.ashx/leprosy/2007_Leprosy_Review.pdf.
13. Walsh DS, Portaels F, Meyers WM. Buruli ulcer (*Mycobacterium ulcerans* infection). Trans R Soc Trop Med Hyg 2008;102:969–78.
14. Walsh DS, Portaels F, Meyers WM. Recent advances in leprosy and Buruli ulcer (*Mycobacterium ulcerans* infection). Curr Opin Infect Dis 2010;23:445–55.
15. Steer AC, Carapetis JR. Acute rheumatic fever and rheumatic heart disease in indigenous populations. Pediatr Clin North Am 2009; 56:1401–19.
16. Viali S. Rheumatic fever and rheumatic heart disease in Samoa. Pac Health Dialog 2006; 13:31–8.
17. Colquhoun SM, Carapetis JR, Kado JH, Steer AC. Rheumatic heart disease and its control in the Pacific. Expert Rev Cardiovasc Ther 2009; 7:1517–24.
18. Steer A, Colquhoun S, Noonan S, Kado J, Viale S, Carapetis J. Control of rheumatic heart disease in the Pacific region. Pac Health Dialog 2006; 13:49–55.
19. Gust ID. Epidemiology of hepatitis B infection in the Western Pacific and South East Asia. Gut 1996;38 Suppl 2:S18–23.
20. Health in Asia and the Pacific: Priority Communicable Diseases. World Health Organisation. Accessed October 10, 2010 at http://www.wpro.who.int/NR/rdonlyres/9A055F24-324C-483F-BD6D-1BCEAB633713/0/12_Chapter7Prioritycommunicablediseases.pdf.
21. Annual Dengue Data in the Western Pacific Region. World Health Organisation. Accessed July 27, 2010 at http://www.wpro.who.int/internet/resources.ashx/MVP/D2009_30.03.10.pdf.
22. Mitchell CJ, Savage HM, Smith GC, Flood SP, Castro LT, Roppul M. Japanese encephalitis on Saipan: a survey of suspected mosquito vectors. Am J Trop Med Hyg 1993;48: 585–90.
23. Japanese encephalitis on the Australian mainland. Commun Dis Intell 1998;22:60.
24. Harley D, Sleigh A, Ritchie S. Ross river virus transmission, infection, and disease: a cross-disciplinary review. Clin Microbiol Rev 2001;14:909–32.
25. Mackenzie JS, Chua KB, Daniels PW, et al. Emerging viral diseases of Southeast Asia and the Western Pacific. Emerg Infect Dis 2001; 7:497–504.
26. Lobigs M, Marshall ID, Weir RC, Dalgarno L. Murray Valley encephalitis virus field strains from Australia and Papua New Guinea: studies on the sequence of the major envelope protein gene and virulence for mice. Virology 1988;165:245–55.

27. Duffy MR, Chen TH, Hancock WT, et al. Zika virus outbreak on Yap Island, Federated States of Micronesia. N Engl J Med 2009;360: 2536–43.

28. MacKenzie JS, Williams DT. The zoonotic flaviviruses of southern, south-eastern and eastern Asia, and australasia: the potential for emergent viruses. Zoonoses Public Health 2009;56:338–56.

29. McDonald M, Richard M, Robers S. Potential health hazards in travelers to Australia, New Zealand, and the southwestern Pacific (Oceania). In:UpToDate, Basow, DS (Ed), UpToDate, Waltham, MA, 2011.

Chapter 26
Arctic and Antarctica

Anders Koch,[1,2] Michael G. Bruce[3] and Karin Ladefoged[4]

[1]Department of Epidemiology Research, Statens Serum Institut, Copenhagen, Denmark
[2]Department of Infectious Diseases, Copenhagen University Hospital, Copenhagen, Denmark
[3]Arctic Investigations Program, NCEZID, CDC, Anchorage, Alaska, USA
[4]Department of Internal Medicine, Queen Ingrids Hospital, Nuuk, Greenland

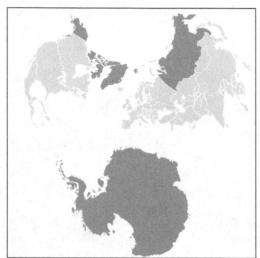

Alaska (United States)
Northern Canada
(Labrador, Nunavut,
Nunavik, Northwest
Territories, Yukon)
Greenland (Home Rule/Denmark)
Svalbard (Norway)
Siberia (Russian Federation)
Antarctica

Arctic parts of Russia (Siberia), Alaska, Canada, and Greenland are characterized by scarce and mostly native populations living wide apart and often under crowded conditions. Caucasians live in Svalbard and the Antarctic. The main infectious diseases that occur in excess numbers in indigenous population in the Arctic compared with Northern European/American populations include invasive disease caused by *Streptococcus pneumoniae* and *Haemophilus influenzae*, tuberculosis, chronic otitis media, respiratory tract infections including RSV and influenza, hepatitis B virus infection, sexually transmitted infections, *Helicobacter pylori* infection, parasitic infections, and bacterial zoonoses. Infectious disease patterns in people living in Svalbard and Antarctica mainly reflect those of their native countries.

Infectious Diseases: A Geographic Guide, First Edition.
Edited by Eskild Petersen, Lin H. Chen & Patricia Schlagenhauf.
© 2011 John Wiley & Sons, Ltd. Published 2011 by John Wiley & Sons, Ltd.

Introduction

The Arctic denotes the northern "top of the world." While no uniform definition of "Arctic" exists, the treeline, the 10° July isotherm, and the line of continuous permafrost have been used interchangeably to refer to this region. This covers most of Alaska, Northern Canada, Greenland, Svalbard, Siberia (denotes Arctic parts of Russian Federation), Iceland, and the northern parts of Sweden, Norway, and Finland.

The Arctic and Antarctic regions are dominated by sparse populations living far apart and often under crowded conditions. Arctic regions of Alaska, Canada (Nunavut, Nunavik, Northwest Territories, and Yukon), Siberia, and Greenland are populated by indigenous people and also Caucasians mostly originating from their southern counterparts (USA, Canada, Denmark, and Russia). Although regional differences exist, living conditions and disease patterns for these populations are relatively comparable. The population of Svalbard mainly consists of northern Europeans. Iceland and Northern portions of Sweden, Norway, and Finland are populated by Caucasians and health conditions are described in "Northern Europe" chapter. In the following, "Arctic" refers to Alaska, Northern Canada, Greenland, Svalbard, and Siberia.

Most health facilities in the Arctic (hospitals, etc.) are small, geographically separated by large distances, and often served by staff on short-term contracts. Diagnostic capacity is often lacking, and when laboratories are available, services are frequently limited to basic microbiology. Laboratories must also contend with long distances over which specimens must be transported which can result in poor survival of bacterial specimens, lower culture-positivity rates, and delayed reporting of results back to health care providers. Furthermore, the actual numbers of infectious disease cases across the Arctic are small relative to other regions of the world, in large part, due to limited populations. Health statistics from Arctic regions are often lacking or are very sparse when compared to their southern counterparts (e.g., Southern USA, Southern Canada, and Denmark for Greenland).

Scientific studies on infectious diseases in the Arctic are most often performed on diseases of high incidence. A number of infectious diseases, such as invasive disease caused by *Streptococcus pneumoniae* and *Haemophilus influenzae*, tuberculosis, chronic otitis media, hepatitis B virus, sexually transmitted infections (STIs), *Helicobacter pylori*, parasitic infections, and bacterial zoonoses, occur at higher rates in Arctic regions than in their southern counterparts. However, studies looking at infectious diseases of lower incidence are rare.

There is much travel between Northern Europe and Greenland, and between Arctic and subarctic areas in Alaska, Canada, and Siberia. Correspondingly, many pathogens that appear in Northern Europe exist in Arctic areas too.

This chapter describes infections with known (high) prevalence in the Arctic regions of Alaska, Canada, Greenland, and Siberia and should be viewed as supplementing the Northern Europe, Northern America, and Russian Federation chapters of this book. Among the Arctic countries, there is far more information on infectious diseases available for Alaska, Canada, and Greenland than for Siberia.

Knowledge of infectious diseases in the immunocompromised host and of infectious diseases of longer duration (lasting for more than 4 weeks) in Arctic populations is limited.

The infectious disease patterns for persons living in and traveling to Svalbard and the Antarctic reflect those of their corresponding populations (e.g., Norway and Russian Federation for Svalbard and countries of origin of persons traveling to the Antarctic). For these regions please see relevant chapters.

Diagnostic techniques for infectious diseases in Arctic regions are essentially identical to those of western countries; however, access to microbiological laboratories, X-ray equipment and other diagnostic facilities is limited due to long distances required for travel and fewer medical facilities. Therefore, diagnostic work up will not be described in this chapter.

Risk for travelers

There is virtually no information available regarding infectious disease risk in persons traveling to Arctic areas. Likewise, there are few prevention recommendations, although hepatitis A and B vaccination should be considered in persons traveling for extended periods of time to Arctic areas with intermediate to high prevalence of these infections.

Important infections in the Arctic [1]

Invasive disease and respiratory agents

Invasive pneumococcal disease (IPD) is a leading cause of pneumonia, septicemia, meningitis, and other invasive diseases (e.g., endocarditis, cellulitis, and septic arthritis) with incidence rates being higher among indigenous persons compared with nonindigenous persons [2,3]. In addition, otitis media that may be caused by *S. pneumoniae* is highly prevalent in Arctic indigenous populations [4]. Vaccine campaigns with the 7-valent pneumococcal conjugate vaccine have markedly reduced rates of vaccine-type IPD in Alaska and Canada, but an increase in invasive disease caused by nonvaccine serotypes has been observed [2], rendering *S. pneumoniae* a public health concern.

Rates of invasive disease caused by *H. influenzae* type B (Hib) among native populations of the Northern American Arctic were among the highest in the world, but decreased markedly after vaccine introduction in the 1980s and 1990s. However, serotype replacement with nontype B strains has resulted in epidemics of *H. influenzae* serotype A [5]. Common manifestations of invasive *H. influenzae* disease include meningitis, pneumonia, and septic arthritis.

Respiratory syncytial virus (RSV) infection is particularly incident among Canadian and Alaskan indigenous infants [6,7]. Alaskan indigenous people have an average of two- to three-fold higher mortality rates due to seasonal pneumonia and influenza than nonindigenous Alaskan persons [8]. Increased crowding, especially during colder fall and winter months, may facilitate transmission of respiratory pathogens [9]. Increased rates of 2009 pandemic influenza A H1N1 (pH1N1) were documented in indigenous populations of Canada and Alaska [10,11].

Tuberculosis

While tuberculosis in the first part of the twentieth century was the single major case of morbidity and mortality in Arctic regions [12], the incidence fell markedly following massive targeted efforts in Alaska, Arctic Canada, and Greenland; lowest incidence rates were reached in the 1980s. However, local outbreaks of tuberculosis occurred in the 1990s in Greenland resulting in a doubling of national tuberculosis rates to reach a stable level of 140/100,000 [13]. Today, rates of tuberculosis are markedly higher in Arctic areas than in their southern counterparts. In Alaska, tuberculosis incidence in the indigenous population is twice that of the national US incidence rate and mortality is five times the national average [14]. In Canada, the overall tuberculosis incidence rate among Inuit is 20 times higher than the national Canadian average [15]. Studies among school children in Greenland indicate high rates of ongoing transmission with a cumulative incidence of tuberculosis infection at the 18th birthday of 13.4% and an annual risk of tuberculosis infection of 0.87% among Inuit children and 0.02% in non-Inuit children [16]. In Siberia, incidence rates are similarly high as in Greenland, and drug-resistant tuberculosis is a considerable public health problem [17].

Viral hepatitis

Viral hepatitis is frequent in the Arctic. Hepatitis A virus (HAV) infection tends to occur in epidemics, the latest in Greenland in 1970–1974 with 11% of the population developing clinical hepatitis [18], and in Canada in 1991–1992 when 20% of children aged 2–20 years in affected communities developed clinical hepatitis [19]. Serosurveys show that 50–70% of Arctic indigenous populations have been exposed to HAV. In 1992, a vaccine campaign among young persons living in 1 of 25 Alaska villages was able to stop an epidemic within 3 weeks, and later introduction of HAV in the childhood vaccine program markedly reduced the incidence [20].

Hepatitis B virus (HBV) infection is endemic in Arctic populations. Serosurveys have shown rates of HBV exposure and chronic infection, respectively, of 42–75% and 7–20% of the population of Greenland 1965–2008, and of 25% and 5% of the population of Canada 1980–1999 [1]. Rates of chronic infection of 6–14% among Alaskan indigenous peoples led Alaska to introduce statewide vaccination programs that dramatically reduced the incidence of clinical hepatitis in affected populations [21]. In Alaska, HBV infection is associated with increased risk of cirrhosis and liver cancer. In Greenland, HBV infection is similarly associated with increased risk of these diseases but for unknown reasons at lower rates than expected. Superinfection with hepatitis D occurs in Greenland [22] and Siberia, but seldom in Canada and Alaska.

Hepatitis C virus (HCV) infection is rare in Greenland and Alaska (seroprevalence 0.5%), but higher in Canada (seroprevalence 1–18%). HCV infection is mainly associated with IV drug use and blood transfusion [23].

Human immunodeficiency virus

Human immunodeficiency virus (HIV) was suspected to reach alarmingly high levels in Arctic populations, but in Greenland the yearly incidence has remained stable at 10–12/100,000 with a decrease in recent years [13]. HIV rates are lower in Alaska than the national average, but slightly higher in indigenous than in nonindigenous peoples. In Greenland, transmission is mainly heterosexual (80%) and most patients are middle aged at the time of diagnosis. In contrast, men having sex with men accounted for 50% of infections in Alaska, while heterosexual contact and injection/drug users were responsible for 15% each.

Parasitic infections

With the strong hunting traditions of Northern indigenous populations, a range of parasitic and zoonotic diseases occur in humans residing in the Arctic, although at different rates by region [24]. Less reliance on hunting for and consumption of subsistence food may result in a lower incidence of such diseases, but present and future climate changes affecting temperature, humidity, flooding, and wildlife composition may increase the incidence of these infections in humans [25].

Protozoans: In Arctic Canada and Alaska the most frequent protozoan infections include toxoplasmosis and in lower numbers giardiasis [24]. As in other places of the world microsporidial species, *Cryptosporidium parvum* and *Pneumocystis jirovecii* are observed in immuno-compromised/HIV patients.

Helminths: Diphyllobothriasis include at least six species, with *Diphyllobothrium dendriticum* being particularly common, infecting 80% in some indigenous communities. Hydatid disease includes *Echinococcus granulosus* (cystic echinococcosis) and *Echinococcus multilocularis* (alveolar echinococcosis) and exists in Siberia, Alaska, and Arctic Canada with western Alaska being hyperendemic for *E. multilocularis* [26]. *E. granulosus* exists in two forms, the northern or cervid form that is widely distributed in northern regions and infecting a range of wild animals, and the European that is associated with husbandry [24]. *Trichinella nativa*, the freeze-resistant variant of *Trichinella*, is widespread in Arctic wildlife, mainly polar bear and walrus [24]. Clinical manifestations of trichinellosis in Arctic populations differ from those of other populations by the fact that the diarrheal phase which precedes the classical myopathic and fever phase is often the only sign, possibly because of repeated exposures to *Trichinella*. Other nematodes include *Toxocara canis*, Anisakidae, and *Enterobius vermicularis*. In addition, *Strongyloides* may be seen in the immunocompromised patient. In Siberia *Opisthorchis felineus* (mainly in Western Siberia) is frequent [24].

Bacterial zoonoses

Botulism is caused by ingestion of a neurotoxin produced by the anaerobic bacterium *Clostridium botulinum* that grows in meat and fish under special conditions. In the Arctic, traditional food preparation includes fermentation of meat and fish by anaerobic storage at low temperatures above freezing without salting, which may lead to outbreaks of botulism in Alaska, Canada, and Greenland. In recent years in Alaska, death rates from botulism have decreased, but incidence rates have increased. The latter may be caused by a shift from traditional fermenting techniques toward the use of plastic containers, which facilitates growth of anaerobic bacteria [27]. In Greenland, incidence rates decrease and cases have not been observed in recent years.

Seroprevalence studies have shown that seropositivity to *Leptospira* spp., *Coxiella burnetii*, and *Francisella tularensis* in Canada [28] and Arbovirus in Alaska [29] is not uncommon, although the extent of clinical disease from these organisms is unknown. *Brucella* has been observed in Siberia, Alaska, and Northern Canada [30].

CNS infections: meningitis, encephalitis, and other infections with neurological symptoms

A number of bacterial pathogens cause acute central nervous system (CNS) infections in Arctic areas (see table below). Some viral pathogens [e.g., cytomegalovirus (CMV), herpes simplex virus (HSV) 1 and 2, varicella zoster virus (VZV), and echovirus] are known to cause CNS infections in Arctic populations [31–33], but prevalence is unknown. Zoonotic infections with possible CNS symptoms exist (rabies, *Echinococcus*, *Toxoplasma*) [24,34].

Acute infections with less than 4 weeks of symptoms

Frequently found microorganisms	Rare microorganisms	Very rare microorganisms
S. pneumoniae	*Listeria monocytogenes*	Influenza
Neisseria meningitidis	*Escherichia coli*	HIV[a]
H. influenzae[b]	*Mycobacterium tuberculosis*	Streptococci
Herpes simplex	Botulism [35]	
Varicella zoster		

[a]HIV as cause of CNS symptoms is very rare in Greenland.
[b]Hib rare, other serotypes more frequent.

CNS infections: meningitis and encephalitis with symptoms for more than 4 weeks and in the immunocompromised host

Microorganisms with symptoms for more than 4 weeks	Microorganisms in the immunocompromised host
HIV and opportunistic infections *M. tuberculosis*	*M. tuberculosis* Polyomavirus (JC virus)

Ear, nose, and throat infections

Upper respiratory tract infections (bacterial and viral [4]) are highly prevalent in Arctic populations, in children mainly as common cold and chronic suppurative otitis media (CSOM) with cumulative incidence of CSOM up to 14% at age 4 [36]. Epstein–Barr virus (EBV) infects most children at a very young age and infectious mononucleosis is consequently rarely observed.

Ear, nose, and throat infections with less than 4 weeks of symptoms

Frequently found microorganisms	Rare microorganisms and conditions
Otitis media (acute and chronic) *S. pneumoniae* *Moraxella catarrhalis* *H. influenzae* Streptococci Respiratory virus (rhinovirus, enterovirus, adenovirus, influenza, parainfluenza, RSV, human metapneumovirus (hMPV), coronavirus, Epstein-Barr virus (EBV))[a]	*M. tuberculosis* *Staphylococcus aureus* Infectious mononucleosis *Chlamydia* *Neisseria gonorrhoeae*, HSV, human papillomavirus (HPV)

[a]EBV is highly prevalent, median age at infection is 3 years, but most often just symptoms of common cold. Mononucleosis is rare.

Cardiopulmonary infections

Arctic populations have high rates of lower respiratory tract infections, both hospitalization rates and community-based rates [37,38]. Main pathogens include both bacteria and virus, in particular *S. pneumoniae* and RSV.

Pneumonia with less than 4 weeks of symptoms

Frequently found microorganisms	Rare microorganisms
S. pneumoniae *H. influenzae*	*Bordetella pertussis* *Mycoplasma pneumoniae*

(Continued)

Frequently found microorganisms	Rare microorganisms
M. catarrhalis Respiratory virus (RSV, rhinovirus, enterovirus, adenovirus, influenza, parainfluenza, hMPV, coronavirus) *M. tuberculosis* *Pneumocystis jirovecii* (in immunocompromised host)	Streptococci *Klebsiella pneumoniae* Legionella Chlamydia S. aureus

Endocarditis with less than 4 weeks of symptoms

Compared with Caucasian populations, *S. pneumoniae* is a significantly more frequent cause of endocarditis in Inuit populations responsible for 16–24% of cases [39,40]. Clinical course and outcome of *S. pneumoniae* endocarditis is comparatively more severe than in Caucasian populations [40]. Pericarditis caused by *M. tuberculosis* is relatively frequent in Greenland.

Frequently found microorganisms	Rare microorganisms and conditions	Very rare microorganisms
S. pneumoniae *S. aureus* *Streptococcus viridans*	*E. coli* Coagulase-negative staphylococci Enterococci	*C. burnetii*

Gastrointestinal infections

Gastrointestinal infections with less than 4 weeks of symptoms

Gastrointestinal infections in Arctic areas may be caused by bacteria, virus, helminths, or protozoans. In Alaskan indigenous children, hospitalization rates for diarrheal diseases are comparable to those of US children, but outpatient rate visits are higher [41]. Of identified causes, most are rotavirus or unspecified virus, followed by unspecified bacterial and parasitic agents [41].

Frequently found microorganisms	Rare microorganisms and conditions
Rotavirus Noro virus Helminths (*Echinococcus*, anisakiasis, angiostrongyliasis, *Diphyllobothrium*, *Trichinella*) *E. vermicularis* *Clostridium difficile* *Salmonella*	*E. coli* *Shigella* *Campylobacter* Protozoans (*Giardia*, *Entamoeba*, *Cryptosporidium*, *Blastocystis hominis*) *Ascaris lumbricoides* Opisthorchiasis *Yersinia* Botulism

Gastrointestinal infections with more than 4 weeks of symptoms

Helicobacter pylori is prevalent in Arctic populations with age-specific seroprevalence patterns intermediate between developed and developing countries [42]. *H. pylori* may lead to chronic gastritis, peptic ulcer disease, and gastric cancer, and rates of gastric cancer are increasing in Arctic areas.

Infections of liver, spleen, and peritoneum

Acute infections of liver, spleen, and peritoneum with less than 4 weeks of symptoms

Frequently found microorganisms	Rare microorganisms and conditions
Gastrointestinal bacteria (including *E. coli, Clostridium perfringens*)	*Klebsiella*
Hepatitis B	*Pseudomonas aeruginosa*
Streptococci, including *S. pneumoniae*	*H. influenzae*
Staphylococci	*Candida*
M. tuberculosis	Hepatitis A
Hepatitis D	Hepatitis C
	Hepatitis E
	E. granulosus and *E. multilocularis*

Chronic infections of liver, spleen, and peritoneum with more than 4 weeks of symptoms

Main causes of chronic infections of the liver, spleen, and peritoneum include hepatitis B, and to a lesser degree hepatitis C and *Echinococcus*. Infections of the peritoneum and mesenteric glands are rather frequent manifestations of tuberculosis.

Genitourinary infections

Cystitis, pyelonephritis, and nephritis with less than 4 weeks of symptoms

Frequently found microorganisms	Rare microorganisms and conditions
E. coli	*M. tuberculosis*
Enterococci	
K. pneumoniae	

Sexually transmitted infections with less than 4 weeks of symptoms

Rates of STIs are high in Arctic populations, with Greenland having the highest rates [43]. Targeted efforts against gonorrhea and syphilis in the 1970s led to markedly lower rates of gonorrhea that have, however, stabilized in Greenland at about 1,000 cases per 100,000 through the last decade, and somewhat lower in Canada and Alaska. Syphilis is generally a very rare disease although seen in epidemics. Chlamydia remains the most prevalent STI with slightly increasing rates of 2,000 per 100,000 in Greenland since 1990, and somewhat lower, but also increasing rates in Canada and Alaska.

Frequently found microorganisms	Rare microorganisms and conditions
Chlamydia spp.	*Treponema pallidum*
N. gonorrhoeae	
Herpes simplex virus	
Human papillomavirus	
Trichomonas vaginalis	
Bacterial vaginosis	
Mycoplasma genitalium	
HIV	

Joint, muscle, and soft tissue infections

Joint, muscle, and soft tissue infections in Arctic populations are caused by many of the same bacterial pathogens as in Northern America and Europe, that is, *S. aureus*, *S. pneumoniae*, *H. influenzae*, and group A streptococci (GAS). Tuberculosis is frequent and may also cause such infections, both in immunocompromised and immunocompetent persons. A particular soft tissue infection is seal finger, an infection caused by accidental cutting with knives used for cutting seals, that progresses from a cellulitis to arthritis with eventual joint dissolution and healing by joint stiffness. The infection is believed to be caused by *Mycoplasma* spp. [44].

Skin infections

Skin infections of less than 4 weeks' duration such as cellulitis are frequent in Arctic indigenous populations [45], and may be caused by group A and group B streptococci and *S. aureus*. Methicillin-resistant *Staphylococcus aureus* (MRSA) and nonresistant *S. aureus* have caused skin abscesses (boils) in Alaskan indigenous peoples. Group A streptococci may, in many rare cases, cause necrotizing fasciitis. Skin infections with symptoms for more than 4 weeks include *M. tuberculosis* and *T. pallidum*.

Adenopathy

Adenopathy of less than 4 weeks' duration

Frequently found microorganisms	Rare microorganisms and conditions
EBV	Tularemia
CMV	*T. pallidum*
HIV	*Toxoplasma gondii*
M. tuberculosis	
Adenovirus	

Fever without focal symptoms

A range of bacteria may cause septicemia without known focus in Arctic populations, including *S. pneumoniae*, hemolytic streptococci, *S. aureus*, coagulase-negative staphylococci, *H. influenzae*, *N. meningitidis*, and gastrointestinal bacteria (*E. coli* and enterococci). In newborns, group B streptococci and *E. coli* may cause bacteremia.

Fever of unknown origin

Frequently found microorganisms	Rare microorganisms
EBV	*C. burnetii*
CMV	*M. tuberculosis*
HIV	*T. gondii*
	Brucella

Eosinophilia and elevated IgE

Main causes of eosinophilia include allergic diseases and parasitic diseases, mainly helminthic infections, although rarely found in Greenland.

Helminthic infections	
Diphyllobothriasis	*Toxocara* spp.
Trichinellosis	Opisthorchiasis
Anisakidae [*Anisachis simplex* (herring worm) and	*Strongyloides* (in immunocompromised host)
Pseudoterranova decipiens (cod worm)]	
E. granulosus and *E. multilocularis*	

Antibiotic resistance

Antimicrobial resistance patterns vary slightly in different Arctic areas. In Alaska, the percentage of invasive penicillin-resistant pneumococcal isolates increased from ~1% in 1993 to almost 15% in 2000, but diminished after the introduction of pneumococcal vaccination in the routine childhood immunization program in 2001 [1]. In Canada and Greenland rates are lower, around 3% and <1%. There has been considerable concern in Greenland over possible penicillin-resistant pneumococci due to high consumption of broad-spectrum antibiotics, but so far this has not occurred.

In Alaska and Canada, outbreaks of community-acquired MRSA occur in indigenous communities [1,46]. Across the United States, rates of MRSA increased from 1996–1998 to 2003–2005 to reach an age-adjusted rate of 58.8 hospitalizations per 100,000 among American Indians/Alaska Natives, compared with the 84.7 hospitalizations per 100,000 in the general US population [47]. In Greenland MRSA still only occurs sporadically.

High rates of antimicrobial resistance toward clarithromycin, metronidazole, and levo-floxacin are found in *H. pylori* isolates from Alaska [48,49], and toward metronidazole in Greenland.

Vaccine-preventable diseases in children

Childhood immunization programs in Alaska, Canada, and Greenland are fairly similar. In all countries, the program includes diphtheria, tetanus, pertussis, polio, *H. influenzae* type B (HIB), pneumococcal vaccine (PCV13), hepatitis B, measles, mumps, and rubella, besides varicella in Alaska and Canada. Meningococcal C vaccine is given in Canada, a quadrivalent meningococcal vaccine in Alaska, none in Greenland. Hepatitis A vaccination is given in Alaska and in some provinces in Canada, but not in Greenland. Rotavirus vaccine is given in Alaska. Human papillomavirus vaccine is given in Alaska, Greenland, and in some provinces of Canada. In Greenland, neonatal BCG vaccination (tuberculosis) was reinstalled in 1997 after having been halted in 1991.

On a national level 76% of US children and 85–90% of Canadian children at age 2 are fully vaccinated (see "Northern America" chapter). In Greenland, vaccination coverage at age 3–5 months is high, close to 100%, but somewhat lower at age 5 (~70%) [13].

In Alaska, vaccination coverage is greater than 85% for school-aged children, and greater than 90% among Alaskan indigenous children.

Vaccine introductions have had markedly beneficial effects in reducing targeted infections with few side effects. Hepatitis B vaccination has greatly reduced the incidence of clinical hepatitis B in Alaskan native people; 7-valent pneumococcal vaccination has reduced the incidence of targeted vaccine serotypes both in Canada and Alaska, and HIB vaccination has eradicated HIB in Greenland and reduced the incidence of HIB substantially in Alaska and Canada. However, replacement of vaccine serotypes with nonvaccine serotypes involved in IPD has been substantial in Alaska after vaccine introduction (113% in children <2 years of age) [2], and both in Alaska and Canada epidemics of invasive disease caused by non-B *H. influenzae* have been documented [5].

Demographic and health statistics

Statistical data for Arctic areas with indigenous populations are not readily available, but are in general included in national figures (e.g., national Canadian figures for Northern Canadian areas). There are no separate figures for Antarctica or Svalbard. The following tables show available key figures for Arctic areas with indigenous populations (causes of death <5 years of age not available).

Basic economic and demographic data

	GNI per capita (USD)[a]	Personal disposable income (USD)[b]	Life expectancy at birth (total, years)[b]	School enrollment, primary (% net)
Greenland	32,960	15,237	68	>96[c]
Canada	42,170	24,495	76	NA

	GNI per capita (USD)[a]	Personal disposable income (USD)[b]	Life expectancy at birth (total, years)[b]	School enrollment, primary (% net)
Alaska	51,054	32,811	77	NA
Siberia	9,370	10,772	64	NA

[a]Gross national income, national figures (http://data.worldbank.org/). No available figures specifically for Arctic areas except for Greenland.

[b]Figures for Arctic areas [50] [Canada: Labrador, Nunavut, Nunavik, Northwest Territories, Yukon; Siberia: Murmansk Oblast, Kareliya republic, Arkangelsk Oblast, Komi Republic, Yamalo-Nenets AO, Khanty-Mansi AO, Taymyr AO, Evenki AO, Sakha Republic, Magadan Oblast, Koryak AO, Chukotka AO (AO=autonomous okrug)].

[c]No separate figures for Greenland, but are expected to be similar to Denmark (http://data.worldbank.org/).

Most common causes of death in all ages in Greenland, Northern Canada, and Alaska natives [51]

	%			
Causes of death (ICD-10 codes)	Greenland	Canada	Alaska	Siberia[a]
Circulatory diseases (I00-I99)	29	27	24	53
Malignant neoplasms (C00-C97)	24	29	23	12
Accidents (V01-X59)	6	8	11	16[b]
Digestive and liver diseases (K00-K93)	5	2	6	3
Chronic lower respiratory diseases (J40-J47)	6	7	5	4[c]
Suicide (X60-X84)	6	4	4	
Influenza and pneumonia (J10-J18)	3	3	3	
Diseases of the nervous system (G00-H95)	1	2	2	
Infectious diseases (A00-B99)	3	2	2	1
Diabetes mellitus (E10-E14)	1	2	2	

Distribution of age-standardized mortality rates according to ICD10.

[a]Median figures for Murmansk Oblast, Kareliya republic, Arkangelsk Oblast, Komi Republic, Yamalo-Nenets AO, Khanty-Mansi AO, Taymyr AO, Evenki AO, Sakha Republic, Magadan Oblast, Koryak AO, Chukotka AO (AO=autonomous okrug).

[b]Injuries (accidents, suicide, assault, V01-Y89).

[c]Diseases of the respiratory system (J00-J99).

References

1. Koch A, Bruce M, Homøe P. Infectious diseases. In: Young TK, Bjerregaard P (eds). Health Transitions in Arctic Populations. Toronto, Buffalo, London: University of Toronto Press, 2008: 265–90.

2. Bruce MG, Deeks SL, Zulz T, et al. International Circumpolar Surveillance System for invasive pneumococcal disease, 1999–2005. Emerg Infect Dis 2008;14:25–33.

3. Christiansen J, Poulsen P, Ladefoged K. Invasive pneumococcal disease in Greenland. Scand J Infect Dis 2004;36:325–9.

4. Homøe P, Prag J, Farholt S, et al. High rate of nasopharyngeal carriage of potential pathogens among children in Greenland: results of a clinical survey of middle-ear disease. Clin Infect Dis 1996;23:1081–90.

5. Bruce MG, Deeks SL, Zulz T, et al. Epidemiology of *Haemophilus influenzae* serotype a, North American Arctic, 2000–2005. Emerg Infect Dis 2008;14:48–55.

6. Tam DY, Banerji A, Paes BA, Hui C, Tarride JE, Lanctot KL. The cost effectiveness of palivizumab in term Inuit infants in the Eastern Canadian Arctic. J Med Econ 2009;12:361–70.

7. Holman RC, Curns AT, Cheek JE, et al. Respiratory syncytial virus hospitalizations among American Indian and Alaska Native infants and the general United States infant population. Pediatrics 2004;114:e437–44.

8. State of Alaska BVS. Deaths in 2008. Accessed November 1, 2010 at http://www.hss.state.ak. us/dph/bvs/PDFs/2008/2008_Death_web.pdf.

9. Bulkow LR, Singleton RJ, Karron RA, Harrison LH. Risk factors for severe respiratory syncytial virus infection among Alaska native children. Pediatrics 2002;109:210–16.

10. Kumar A, Zarychanski R, Pinto R, et al. Critically ill patients with 2009 influenza A(H1N1) infection in Canada. JAMA 2009;302:1872–9.

11. Wenger JD, Castrodale L, Bruden D, et al. Pandemic influenza A H1N1 in Alaska: temporal and geographic characteristics of spread and increased risk of hospitalization among Alaska Native and Asian/Pacific Islander people. Clin Infect Dis 2011;52 Suppl. 1;S189–97.

12. Grzybowski S, Styblo K, Dorken E. Tuberculosis in Eskimos. Tubercle 1976;57:S1–58.

13. Landslægeembedet (Chief Medical Officer of Greenland). Årsberetning fra Landslægeembedet 2008 (Yearly Report from the Chief Medical Officer of Greenland 2008). Nuuk, Greenland. 2008:1–53.

14. Schneider E. Tuberculosis among American Indians and Alaska Natives in the United States, 1993–2002. Am J Public Health 2005; 95:873–80.

15. Nguyen D, Proulx JF, Westley J, Thibert L, Dery S, Behr MA. Tuberculosis in the Inuit community of Quebec, Canada. Am J Respir Crit Care Med 2003;168:1353–7.

16. Soborg B, Koch A, Thomsen VO, et al. Ongoing tuberculosis transmission to children in Greenland. Eur Respir J 2010;36:878–84.

17. Shin SS, Keshavjee S, Gelmanova IY, et al. Development of extensively drug-resistant tuberculosis during multidrug-resistant tuberculosis treatment. Am J Respir Crit Care Med 2010;182:426–32.

18. Skinhoj P, Mikkelsen F, Hollinger FB. Hepatitis A in Greenland: importance of specific antibody testing in epidemiologic surveillance. Am J Epidemiol 1977;105:140–7.

19. Pekeles G, McDonald J, Schreffler R, Allen R. Epidemic of hepatitis A in young Inuit associated with high incidence of fulminant hepatitis and renal insufficiency. Arctic Med Res 1994;53:635–8.

20. Singleton RJ, Hess S, Bulkow LR, Castrodale L, Provo G, McMahon BJ. Impact of a statewide childhood vaccine program in controlling hepatitis A virus infections in Alaska. Vaccine 2010;28:6298–304.

21. McMahon BJ, Rhoades ER, Heyward WL, Tower E, Ritter D, Lanier AP. A comprehensive programme to reduce the incidence of hepatitis B virus infection and its sequelae in Alaskan natives. Lancet 1987;2:1134–6.

22. Borresen ML, Olsen OR, Ladefoged K, et al. Hepatitis D outbreak among children in a hepatitis B hyper-endemic settlement in Greenland. J Viral Hepat 2010;17:162–70.

23. McMahon BJ, Hennessy TW, Christensen C, et al. Epidemiology and risk factors for hepatitis C in Alaska Natives. Hepatology 2004;39: 325–32.

24. Akuffo H, Ljungström I, Linder E, Wahlgren M (eds). Parasites of the Colder Climates. London, New York: Taylor and Francis, 2003;1–359.

25. Parkinson AJ, Butler JC. Potential impacts of climate change on infectious diseases in the Arctic. Int J Circumpolar Health 2005;64:478–86.

26. Rausch RL, Wilson JF, Schantz PM. A programme to reduce the risk of infection with *Echinococcus multilocularis*: the use of praziquantel to control the cestode in a village in the hyperendemic region of Alaska. Ann Trop Med Parasitol 1990;84:239–50.

27. Chiou LA, Hennessy TW, Horn A, Carter G, Butler JC. Botulism among Alaska natives in the Bristol Bay area of southwest Alaska: a survey of knowledge, attitudes, and practices related to fermented foods known to cause botulism. Int J Circumpolar Health 2002;61: 50–60.

28. Levesque B, Messier V, Bonnier-Viger Y, et al. Seroprevalence of zoonoses in a Cree community (Canada). Diagn Microbiol Infect Dis 2007;59:283–6.

29. Zarnke RL, Calisher CH, Kerschner J. Serologic evidence of arbovirus infections in humans and wild animals in Alaska. J Wildl Dis 1983;19:175–9.

30. Meyer ME. Identification and virulence studies of *Brucella* strains isolated from Eskimos and reindeer in Alaska, Canada, and Russia. Am J Vet Res 1966;27:353–8.

31. Zhu J, Davidson M, Leinonen M, et al. Prevalence and persistence of antibodies to herpes viruses, *Chlamydia pneumoniae* and *Helicobacter pylori* in Alaskan Eskimos: the GOCADAN Study. Clin Microbiol Infect 2006;12:118–22.

32. Gravelle CR, Noble GR, Feltz ET, Saslow AR, Clark PS, Chin TD. An epidemic of echovirus type 30 meningitis in an arctic community. Am J Epidemiol 1974;99:368–74.

33. Nicolle LE, Minuk GY, Postl B, Ling N, Madden DL, Hoofnagle JH. Cross-sectional seroepidemiologic study of the prevalence of cytomegalovirus and herpes simplex virus infection in a Canadian Inuit (Eskimo) community. Scand J Infect Dis 1986;18:19–23.

34. Messier V, Levesque B, Proulx JF, et al. Seroprevalence of *Toxoplasma gondii* among Nunavik Inuit (Canada). Zoonoses Public Health 2009;56:188–97.

35. McLaughlin JB. Botulism type E outbreak associated with eating a beached whale, Alaska. Emerg Infect Dis 2004;10:1685–7.

36. Koch A, Homoe P, Pipper C, Hjuler T, Melbye M. Chronic suppurative otitis media in a birth cohort of children in Greenland: population-based study of incidence and risk factors. Pediatr Infect Dis J 2010 aug 9 [EPUB ahead of print].

37. Peck AJ, Holman RC, Curns AT, et al. Lower respiratory tract infections among American Indian and Alaska Native children and the general population of U.S. children. Pediatr Infect Dis J 2005;24:342–51.

38. Koch A, Sørensen P, Homøe P, et al. Population-based study of acute respiratory infections in children, Greenland. Emerg Infect Dis 2002;8:586–93.

39. Finley JC, Davidson M, Parkinson AJ, Sullivan RW. Pneumococcal endocarditis in Alaska natives. A population-based experience, 1978 through 1990. Arch Intern Med 1992; 152:1641–5.

40. Madsen RG, Ladefoged K, Kjaergaard JJ, Andersen PS, Clemmesen C. Endocarditis in Greenland with special reference to endocarditis caused by *Streptococcus pneumoniae*. Int J Circumpolar Health 2009;68:347–53.

41. Singleton RJ, Holman RC, Yorita KL, et al. Diarrhea-associated hospitalizations and outpatient visits among American Indian and Alaska Native children younger than five years of age, 2000–2004. Pediatr Infect Dis J 2007;26: 1006–13.

42. Goodman KJ, Jacobson K, Veldhuyzen van ZS. *Helicobacter pylori* infection in Canadian and related Arctic Aboriginal populations. Can J Gastroenterol 2008;22:289–95.

43. Gesink LD, Rink E, Mulvad G, Koch A. Sexual health and sexually transmitted infections in the North American Arctic. Emerg Infect Dis 2008;14:4–9.

44. Hartley JW, Pitcher D. Seal finger—tetracycline is first line. J Infect 2002;45:71–5.

45. Holman RC, Curns AT, Singleton RJ, et al. Infectious disease hospitalizations among older American Indian and Alaska Native adults. Public Health Rep 2006;121:674–83.

46. Dalloo A, Sobol I, Palacios C, Mulvey M, Gravel D, Panaro L. Investigation of community-associated methicillin-resistant *Staphylococcus aureus* in a remote northern community, Nunavut, Canada. Can Commun Dis Rep 2008;34:1–7.

47. Byrd KK, Holman RC, Bruce MG, et al. Methicillin-resistant *Staphylococcus aureus*-associated hospitalizations among the American Indian and Alaska native population. Clin Infect Dis 2009;49:1009–15.

48. McMahon BJ, Hennessy TW, Bensler JM, et al. The relationship among previous antimicrobial use, antimicrobial resistance, and treatment outcomes for *Helicobacter pylori* infections. Ann Intern Med 2003;139:463–9.

49. Carothers JJ, Bruce M, Hennessy TW, et al. The relationship between previous fluoroquinolone use and levofloxacin resistance for *Helicobacter pylori* infections. Clin Infect Dis 2007;44:e5–8.

50. ECONOR II (2008). The economy of the North. In: Glomsrød S, Aslaksen I (eds). 1-102. 2009. Statistics Norway—Statistisk sentralbyrå. Available at http://portal.sdwg.org/media.php?mid=1069.

51. Young TK. Circumpolar health indicators: sources, data, and maps. In: Hassi J, Mäkinen T, Odland JO, Young TK (eds). Circumpolar Health Supplements (3). Oulu, Finland: International Association of Circumpolar Health Publishers, 2008:1–130.

Chapter 27
The immunosuppressed patient

Brian T. Montague, Terri L. Montague and Maria D. Mileno
Warren Alpert School of Medicine at Brown University, Providence, RI, USA

Immunocompromised patients present unique challenges for clinicians diagnosing and managing infectious diseases. A systematic approach to these patients emphasizing assessment of level of immune compromise, review of the use of prophylactic medications, a detailed history of potential exposures, and a thorough review of endemic risks in the region are key to obtaining a timely and accurate diagnosis. Given the atypical presentation and rapid progression of infections among the immunocompromised, early microbiologic diagnosis where feasible may be important to guide treatment. Where microbiologic diagnosis is not feasible, knowledge of the patients level of immune compromise and the epidemic and endemic risks is a critical guide to empiric therapy.

Introduction

Patients with immune deficiencies, whether primary or acquired, experience a broad spectrum of illness beyond than that seen in immunocompetent persons in a given region. Unique illnesses in the immunocompromised may result from abnormal responses to ordinarily nonpathogenic agents or atypical responses to typical pathogens. Though some localization of opportunistic infections has been described, many opportunistic infections are caused by agents that are ubiquitous and therefore represent important health concerns for the immunosuppressed across all regions of the world. This chapter discusses the basis for immune compromise, with definitions provided for minimal versus limited or severe immunodeficiency. Detailed discussion is presented related to infection risk and unique pathogens for persons with AIDS and recipients of organ transplants.

Approach to the patient

The assessment of illness after international travel requires prompt attention to fever, diarrhea, and skin lesions. Obtaining timely and accurate diagnoses of infections in the immunocompromised can be challenging. The differential diagnosis includes everything immunocompetent individuals may experience as well as the additional considerations addressed in this chapter [1]. Under the influence of immunosuppression, microorganisms may become opportunistic, commensal organisms may become pathogenic, normally poorly pathogenic organisms may become more aggressive, and patients may respond poorly to treatment. For these reasons, a systematic approach to diagnosis is required as described in Box 27.1.

Infectious Diseases: A Geographic Guide, First Edition.
Edited by Eskild Petersen, Lin H. Chen & Patricia Schlagenhauf.
© 2011 John Wiley & Sons, Ltd. Published 2011 by John Wiley & Sons, Ltd.

The assessment of the level of immune deficiency differs based on the underlying cause and may include white blood cell and CD4 cell counts as well as therapeutic drug monitoring for those on immunosuppressant medications. Well-defined protocols exist for prophylaxis against opportunistic infections for people with significant immune compromise due to HIV, immunosuppressive medications, and other causes. In evaluating an immunocompromised person with concern for infection, if the recommended prophylactic regimens have not been maintained, the opportunistic infections the medications target should become key considerations in the differential diagnosis.

Based on the assessed risk for opportunistic infections, the epidemiology of the region should be reviewed including both typical infections and opportunistic infections. Targeted testing should then be performed based on the resulting differential diagnosis. Peripheral blood smears should be considered for malaria. A focused assessment for common symptoms will guide testing which may include complete blood counts, liver function tests, urinalysis, cultures of blood, stool, and urine, and chest X-rays as well as specific testing for respiratory, urinary, and diarrhea pathogens. Knowledge of the typical incubation periods for considered differentials can be helpful to rule out a particular cause of infection or to prompt specific serologic assays for infections such as dengue or other arboviral diseases, rickettsiae, schistosomiasis, leptospirosis, and HIV. Because signs and symptoms of infection are often diminished in immunosuppressed patients, early microbial diagnosis which may require invasive diagnostic procedures is often essential to guide treatment.

Box 27.1 Approach to assessing the immunocompromised patient

1. Assess level of immunosuppression
2. Review antibiotic prophylaxis history
3. Evaluate risk of opportunistic infections
4. Review of epidemiology of region and exposure history
5. Targeted testing based on clinical syndrome and endemic risks

---

Aspects of immunodeficiency

The immune response represents the coordinated activity of multiple humoral and cytological factors. Specific deficiencies have been described at all levels, each conferring increased risk of different types of diseases. These deficiencies can be primary or acquired. In addition to primary immune deficiencies, a wide spectrum of acquired and induced immunodeficiency states exist with varying conferred infection risks.

Categories of immunodeficiency and conferred disease susceptibility

Functional deficiency	Disease susceptibility
Immunoglobulin deficiency	Increased susceptibility to bacterial infections
Defects in cell-mediated immunity	Increased risk of viruses, fungal, and protozoan infections
Inability to opsonize/ complement deficiency	Increased risk of infections by encapsulated organisms
Phagocytosis defects	Increased susceptibility to disease caused by catalase-positive bacterial pathogens, aspergillus, and intracellular organisms

Immunodeficiency types leading to increased risk of opportunistic infections

Cause	Immune dysfunction
Primary immunodeficiency syndromes	Various
Diabetes mellitus	Circulatory dysfunction due to microvascular and macrovascular disease, hyperglycemia induced phagocytic defects
Cirrhosis, nephrotic syndrome	Loss of immunoregulatory and immune system effector proteins
Asplenia from splenectomy or sickle cell disease	Inability to clear encapsulated organisms, increased susceptibility to intraerythrocytic infections
HIV	Dysregulation of B-cell function, impairment of cell-mediated immunity
Medication-induced immunosuppression	Multiple, cell-mediated immunity principle target

Though the pathophysiology of immune dysfunction related to these factors has been well described, no adequate assays exist to assess the relative degree of immune dysfunction associated with each. The risk is assessed principally through the sum experience of clinical infections seen associated with each risk factor, combined with the impact of these factors on the serologic response to immunizations. The CDC Yellow book for travel medicine offers a rough framework for assessing the functional level of immunosuppression as it relates to infection risk [2].

Levels of immune compromise

Immune compromise	Due To	Condition
Minimal	Disease	HIV CD4 >500
		Bone marrow transplant patients >2 years posttransplant off medication, without graft-versus-host disease
		Autoimmune disease not on immunosuppressive therapy
	Medications	Low-dose steroids (<20 mg daily or qod dosing, steroid inhalers, topical or intra-articular injections) or duration since last dose >1 month
		Chemotherapy last use 3 months ago or greater
		Immunosuppresive medications last use 1 month ago or greater
Limited immunosuppression	Disease	Asplenia (encapsulated organisms, malaria, *Babesia*, *Capnocytophaga*)
		Chronic renal disease
		Chronic liver disease (including chronic hepatitis C)
		Diabetes mellitus
		Complement deficiencies (meningococcal infection)
Severe immune deficiency	Disease	Active leukemia or lymphoma
		Generalized malignancy
		Aplastic anemia
		Graft-versus-host disease
		Congenital immunodeficiency

Immune compromise	Due To	Condition
		HIV, CD4 count less than 200
		Persons who have received current or recent radiation therapy or bone marrow transplant recipients within 2 years of transplantation
	Medications	High-dose corticosteroids (either >2 mg/kg of body weight or ≥20 mg/day of prednisone or equivalent in persons who weigh >10 kg, when administered for ≥2 weeks)
		Alkylating agents (e.g., cyclophosphamide)
		Antimetabolites (e.g., azathioprine, 6-mercaptopurine)
		Transplant-related immunosuppressive drugs (e.g., cyclosporine, tacrolimus, sirolimus, and mycophenolate mofetil) and mitoxantrone (used in multiple sclerosis)
		Cancer chemotherapeutic agents (excluding tamoxifen)
		Methotrexate, including low-dose weekly regimens, is classified as severely immunosuppressive
		Tumor necrosis factor (TNF)-blocking agents, IL6 antagonists (intracellular microorganisms, fungi), and other rheumatologic disease modifying agents

Organ transplantation

Potent immunosuppressive medications dramatically reduce the incidence of rejection of transplanted organs, yet increase patient susceptibility to opportunistic infections [3]. In addition to contracting infections through receipt of blood products, organ transplant recipients may acquire significant tropical diseases in four ways [4]:

Infectious mechanism	Example
Transmission with the graft	Human T-cell lymphotropic virus 1 (HTLV-1)
De novo infection	Visceral leishmaniasis
Reactivation of dormant infection	Histoplasmosis
Reinfection/reactivation in a healthy graft	Chagas' disease

The clinician should assess risk by considering the intensity of immunosuppression, the use of prophylactic medications, and the recipients' likely exposures based on results of both donor and recipient serological testing and epidemiologic history.

The level of immunosuppression is determined by the dose and duration of immunosuppressive therapies. The addition of the more potent antilymphocyte medications such as antithymocyte globulins (ATG), OKT3, and alemtuzumab which are used for induction or treatment of rejection also greatly enhances this risk. These medications lead to depletion of T cells and their effects persist for several months after treatment. ATG and OKT3 have been associated with increased rate of cytomegalovirus (CMV) (if prophylaxis is not used), fungal infections, as well as posttransplant lymphoproliferative disorder (PTLD) [5]. ATG is also associated with increased risk for BK nephropathy [6]. Non-T-lymphocyte-depleting agents such as the interleukin-2 receptor antagonists, such as daclizumab and basiliximab, seem to have a lower rate of infectious complications compared with the other induction therapies. Rituximab is a humanized chimeric monoclonal antibody directed against CD 20, a transmembrane protein located on pre-B and mature B cells used in induction regimens. Skin and soft tissue infections as well as blood stream infections may be increased with its use [7].

The typical timeframe for transplant-related infections relative to initiation of immunosuppression is described in the table below [3]. The timing of infection risk may be altered by subsequent intensification of immunosuppression. In the first month following transplantation, most of the infections were donor-derived, recipient-derived, or associated with complications from surgery. These infections included infection with antimicrobial resistant species such as methicillin-resistant *Staphylococcus aureus* (MRSA), vancomycin-resistant enterococcus (VRE), *Candida* species, aspiration, cathether or wound infection, or *Clostridium difficile* colitis. Donor-derived infections although uncommon included herpes simplex virus (HSV), lymphocytic choriomeningitis virus (LCMV), rhabdovirus (rabies), West Nile virus, HIV, and *Trypanosoma cruzi*. Recipient-derived infections occurring mostly through colonization included *Aspergillus* and *Pseudomonas*. Opportunistic infections are generally absent during the 1st month as the full effect of immunosuppression is not yet achieved.

In months 1–6 following transplantation, viruses account for the majority of infectious episodes. Infections include pneumocystis, infection with herpes viruses (HSV, VZV, CMV, and EBV), hepatitis B, *Listeria*, *Nocardia*, *Toxoplasma*, *Strongyloides*, Leishmania, and *T. cruzi*. This has changed with prophylactic medications. Trimethoprim–sulfamethoxazole generally prevents most urinary tract infections and opportunistic infections such as pneumocystis pneumonia, *Listeria monocytogenes*, *Toxoplasma gondii*, and susceptible *Nocardia* species. Herpes infections are also uncommon with routine antiviral prophylaxis, but other viral pathogens such as polyomavirus (BK), adenovirus, recurrent HCV have emerged. Infections due to ubiquitous fungi such as *Aspergillus*, *Cryptococcus*, as well as infections with *T. cruzi* or *Strongyloides* may occur which again highlights the usefulness of assays for detection of these pathogens.

Infectious disease risk decreases 6 months following transplantation correlating with the tapering of immunosuppressive medications in recipients with good allograft function. Recipients remain at risk however for community-acquired pathogens causing pneumonia or urinary tract infections. Some patients despite immunosuppression minimization may develop opportunistic infections from *Listeria* or *Nocardia* species, invasive fungal pathogens such as *Aspergillus*, atypical mold, or *Mucor* species.

Timeline of infection after transplantation (Adapted from Fishman NEJM 2007) [3]

Time period	Infectious risks
<1 Month	Antimicrobial resistant species, aspiration, line and wound infections, *C. difficile*
	Donor-derived infection (HSV, LCMV, rhabdovirus (rabies), West Nile virus, HIV, *T. cruzi*)
	Recipient-derived infection: *Aspergillus*, *Pseudomonas*
1–6 Months	With PCP and antiviral prophylaxis (CMV<HBV):
	Polyomavirus BK infection, nephrophathy
	C. difficile
	Hepatitis C virus
	Adenovirus infection, influenza

Time period	Infectious risks
>6 Months	*Cryptococcus neoformans* *Mycobacterium tuberculosis* Without PCP and antiviral prophylaxis (CMV<HBV): Pneumocystis Infection with herpes viruses (HSV, VZV, CMV, EBV) Hepatitis B virus *Listeria, Nocardia, Toxoplasma, Strongyloides, Leishmania, T. cruzi* Community-acquired pneumonia Urinary tract infection *Aspergillus*, atypical molds, *Mucor* species Infection with *Nocardia, Rhodococcus* species CMV infection (colitis and retinitis) Hepatitis (HBV, HCV) HSV encephalitis Community-acquired viral infections (SARS, West Nile virus infection) JC polyomavirus infection (progressive multifocal leukoencephalopathy) Skin cancer, lymphoma (posttransplant lymphoproliferative disease)

HIV and risk of opportunistic infections

HIV infection is now endemic throughout all areas of the world with the greatest burden of disease in sub-Saharan Africa and south and southeast Asia. HIV disease results in progressive immune dysfunction associated with disregulated B-cell function and progressive CD4 T-cell deficiency, TH2 polarization, and a resulting decline in cell-mediated immunity. The specific manifestations of HIV disease vary by CD4 count. The incidence of opportunistic infections is significantly impacted by availability of testing programs to permit the early diagnosis of HIV, the use of prophylactic medications, and the availability of and clinical practices related to antiretroviral therapy.

A portion of patients with markedly suppressed immune function indicated by a CD4 <100 cells/mm^3 prior to the initiation of HAART may experience an inflammatory syndrome known as IRIS (immune reconstitution inflammatory syndrome) with the recovery of their immune function. This is thought to represent the development of an immune response to previously tolerated infections or exogenous antigens. Though many opportunistic infections may be associated with IRIS, these events are particularly frequent in association with underlying mycobacterial infections such as tuberculosis, cryptococcosis, and other viral infections such as hepatitis B [8].

Relationship between CD4 and complications of HIV disease (Reproduced from Cecil's Essentials of Medicine, 7th edn) [9]

CD4 Range	Manifestations	Frequency
>500	Herpes zoster, polydermatomal	5–10%
200–500	*M. tuberculosis* infection and disease	4–20
	Bacteria pneumonia, recurrent	15–20
	Kaposi's sarcoma, mucocutaneous	15–25 (M)

(Continued)

CD4 Range	Manifestations	Frequency
	Oral hairy leukoplakia	25–40
	Candida pharyngitis (thrush)	20–35
	Cervical neoplasia	1–2 (F)
100–200	*Pneumocystis jirovecii* pneumonia	20–60
	Histoplasma capsulatum, disseminated	0–20
	Kaposi's sarcoma, visceral	3–8 (M)
	Lymphoma, non-Hodgkin's	3–5
	Progressive multifocal leukoencephalopathy	2–3
≤100	Candida esophagitis	15–20
	CMV retinitis, esophagitis, or colitis	10–20
	Mycobacterium avium-intracellulare, disseminated	20–35
	T. gondii encephalitis	5–25
	C. neoformans meningitis	10–20
	H. capsulatum, disseminated	2–20
	Cryptosporidium parvum enteritis	2–8
	Mucocutaneous herpes simplex ulcers, extensive	4–8
	Lymphoma, CNS	3–6

Studies regarding the impact of tropical diseases on HIV progression have shown mixed results. Coinfections with other agents have the potential to increase HIV viral replication through the release of proinflammatory cytokines and CD4 activation [10]. In settings with a high burden of acute and chronic infections, this process could contribute to an acceleration of HIV disease progression. Clinical studies have provided mixed results depending on both the infection studied and the phase of illness [10–13]. The clinical relevance of these interactions and their acute impacts as well as long term effects on HIV disease progression, remains unclear. It is clear, though, that HIV can exert a significant impact on the incidence, presentation, and severity of many tropical diseases and this will be described in more detail below.

Geographic distribution of opportunistic infections

The majority of pathogens associated with opportunistic among patients with HIV and other states of immunocompromise are thought to be ubiquitous. Only limited surveys exist, however, with regard to the distribution of these infectious agents. Even in regions where infectious agents are uniformly present, there exists the possibility that clustering of disease may occur based on other associated risk factors such as sanitation. This is particularly a concern with regard to illnesses such as infectious diarrhea and parasitic infections transmitted through the fecal oral route. Our ability to assess the potential for significant geographic localization of disease is further limited by the lack of access to comprehensive medical diagnostic services in the areas most impacted by the epidemic of HIV. Similarly, the lack of transplant registries in resource-limited settings makes assessment of the risk of transplant-related infections much more difficult. As a result, it is difficult to draw definite conclusions regarding the geographic distribution of many of these infections.

The localization of opportunistic infections based on available case reports and surveys is presented in the table below. Protozoan and fungal infections comprise the majority of localized opportunistic infections. Though not strictly opportunistic infections, infections such as malaria and schistosomiasis which are highly localized and the course of which may be impacted by immunocompromise are presented as well. The localization and unique clinical aspects of these infections in immunocompromised patients will be discussed in more detail below.

Geographically localized infections

Category	Organism	North America	Central/ South America	Northern Europe/Asia	Middle East	South and Southeast Asia	Africa
Protozoan	*Acanthamoeba* and *Balamuthia*	X	X	?	?	?	?
	Malaria[a]	X[b]	X		X	X	X
	Schistosomiasis[a]					X	X
	Trypanosomiasis[a]		X				X
	Babesiosis[a]	X		X			
Fungi	*Penicillium marneffei*					X	
	Coccidioides	X	X				
	Paracoccidioides brasiliensis		X				
	Histoplasma	X					X
	Sporothrix	X	X				
Viruses	HTLV 1,2	X	X	X	X	X	X

[a]Infection occurs in immunocompetent patients but course duration, morbidity, and/or mortality impacted by immunocompromised.
[b]Limited case reports of malaria have been reported in the North America in nontravelers.

Opportunistic infections and unusual presentations of common pathogens in immunocompromised patients

The impact of immune compromise on infection can be seen at multiple levels. Immunocompromised patients may have a higher susceptibility to infection leading to an increase in the incidence and/or prevalence of disease. Secondly, immunocompromised persons may present with higher burdens of the pathogenic organism leading to increased transmissibility. Finally, the inability to mount an effective immune response may lead to impaired clearance of infection with subsequent increases in both morbidity and mortality of disease. The majority of available research regarding the impact of immunosuppression on tropical diseases and geographically localized infections consists of case reports, most commonly associated with HIV [12][13a]. More limited data is available regarding the impact of immunosuppressive medications and other causes of immune deficiency on these infections. These correlations will be highlighted where available.

Bacteria

Increased frequency and severity of typical bacterial infections are noted both in transplant recipients and among persons with HIV and CD4 counts less than 350 cells/mm^3. The infections observed correlate with the infections commonly observed in the community with upper respiratory and sinus infections, pneumonias being most common and, less commonly, urinary tract infections. *Streptococcus pneumoniae, Haemophilus influenzae,* and *S. aureus* infections are commonly described [14]. Staphylococcal and pseudomonas infections may become more common with markedly depressed CD4 counts. Necrotizing pneumonia with abscess formation due to *Legionella* has been described in patients with HIV as well as among transplant recipients. Infections with less common pathogens such as *Listeria*, *Nocardia*, and *Rhodococcus* have been described in immunocompromised patients with high associated levels of morbidity and mortality.

The coepidemics of HIV and TB represent the most profound impact of HIV on endemic bacterial infections. Tuberculosis occurs with much greater frequency among persons with HIV, independent of CD4 count and accounts for a substantial portion of the mortality associated with HIV worldwide [15]. Disseminated and extrapulmonary TB become increasingly common as the CD4 count declines [16]. Though the patients typically present with more advanced disease, transmissibility, the impact of HIV on the risk of transmission of tuberculosis has been controversial [17–19]. In particular for individuals with marked immunosuppression, the increased frequency of extrapulmonary and sputum-negative pulmonary tuberculosis may lead to a reduced risk of transmission to close contacts [16].

Parasites

Information regarding the influence of immunosuppression and HIV on parasitic infections is more limited. Among patients with neurocysticercosis, cyst size in one series was shown to be greater in patients with HIV [13]. There is additionally a case report of a fatal abdominal mass attributed to an uncharacterized cestode [13]. Though hyperinfection with *Strongyloides* has been described in association with corticosteroids and other immunosuppressant use, there is no clear indication of an increased risk among patients with HIV [20,21]. Paradoxically, patients with HIV seem to have a reduction in the burden of infectious forms in the gut decreasing the extent of autoinfection [22].

Geographically localized parasitic infections

Schistosomiasis Studies have suggested that HIV may reduce the transmission of schistosomiasis, however, the epidemiologic significance of this is unclear [23,24]. Immunosuppression and HIV have not been shown to significantly alter the clinical course or response to treatment of patients with schistosomiasis [24–26]. The possibility of IRISs has been raised but no definitive cases have been identified [27–29].

Filariasis Lymphatic filariasis has also been shown to be more common in patients with HIV, however, the clinical course of infection has not been shown to be significantly altered [30,31].

Chagas' disease Reactivation Chagas' disease is a well-documented opportunistic infection among persons with AIDS, with CNS lesions being the most common presentation [12,32,33]. Patients typically present with multiple brain lesions, often with necrosis, hemorrhage, and inflammatory infiltrates. Clinically silent myocarditis is a common autopsy finding in persons who have died of meningoencephalitis [34]. When symptomatic, patients may present with arrhythmias or congestive heart failure. Parasite burdens in patients with HIV are significantly higher, whether presenting with chronic or reactivation disease. Reactivation Chagas' disease has been described among recipients of organ transplantation including detected parasitemia on surveillance and clinical cases of encephalitis, myocarditis, esophagitis, and cutaneous lesions [35–38].

African trypanosomiasis It is unclear whether HIV infection alters the epidemiology or clinical course of either West or East African trypanosomiasis [12]. Case series have suggested that mortality from trypanosomiasis may be higher among HIV-infected persons. There have additionally been case reports of disease among patients with HIV caused by normally nonpathogenic, lower trypanosomatids. Though risk of transmission of trypanosomiasis with organ transplantation has been described, the impact of immunosuppressive medications on the course of disease is not known.

Protozoa

Toxoplasmosis Toxoplasmosis is a common cause of opportunistic encephalitis in persons with HIV disease. Among those with HIV, disease is typically seen in persons with CD4 counts less than 100. Transmission of toxoplasmosis through organ transplantation has been well described, and there have been multiple reported cases of disseminated fatal toxoplasmosis in this context [39–41].

Cryptococcus Cryptococcal infections occur worldwide and are important causes of morbidity and mortality among transplant recipients and persons with HIV and low CD4 counts [42,43]. Meningitis and meningoencephalitis are the most commonly described presentations, but pulmonary disease, cutaneous infections, myositis, and disseminated infections have also been well described [44–48].

Leishmaniasis After toxoplasmosis, leishmaniasis is the most common tissue protozoan opportunistic infection in persons with AIDS. Though the bulk of the reported data involves visceral leishmaniasis (VL) due to *Leishmania infantum* in the Mediterranean region, there are increasing reports of HIV-related VL due to *Leishmania donovani* in southern Asia and Africa and to *Leishmania chagasi* in South America [12]. Though most clinical manifestations are the same as seen in non-HIV-infected patients, increased peripheral parasitemia and clinically evident ectopic parasites are more common in those HIV. Prolonged subclinical courses and delayed diagnoses have been described in case series of recipients of organ transplantation with leishmaniasis, with significant mortality [49–51]. Leishmaniasis can itself result in immunosuppression in otherwise immunocompetent hosts and case reports of coincident opportunistic infections have been described [52].

Babesiosis The majority of cases of human disease are attributable to *Babesia divergens* or *Babesia microti* species complex. Infections may be subclinical or more severe with fever and anorexia progressing to the acute respiratory distress syndrome, disseminated intravascular coagulation, congestive heart failure, and renal failure. More severe forms of the disease with prolonged courses have been reported in patients with HIV, including a malaria-like syndrome caused by temperate species of *Babesia* [12,53]. Longer duration of therapy may be required with the possible need for combination therapy. Similar prolonged courses have been described among those on immunosuppressive medications [53]. Fatal cases of babesiosis have been described among asplenic patients [54,55].

Ehrlichiosis Ehrlichiosis can be caused by a number species of coccobacilli in the genera *Anaplasma* or *Neorickettsia*. Species are found worldwide. Though the spectrum of illness in many series of immunocompromised patients has been similar to that in the general population, case reports of severe and at times fatal ehrlichiosis with multiorgan failure have been described among recipients of lung transplant and HIV patients with significantly impaired T-cell function [56–58].

Malaria Malaria is among the leading causes of morbidity and mortality worldwide. Immunosuppression from HIV appears to mitigate the acquired immunity usually seen in persons from endemic areas leading to both increased frequency of disease and increased incidence of severe malaria in these populations [59,60]. Cases of malaria transmission with organ transplantation have been well described and atypical clinical presentations in transplant recipients including lack of periodicity of fevers and clinical symptoms have been described [61,62]. More severe disease is seen in asplenic patients due to the inability to clear the parasite.

Free-living amoebae   *Acanthamoeba* and *Balamuthia* species appear to be rare causes of opportunistic encephalitis, sinusitis, and cutaneous disease in patients with late-stage AIDS [63–68]. Most case reports have been from the United States, but the worldwide distribution of these ubiquitous protozoa suggests that underdiagnosis is widespread in the tropics. Granulomatous amebic encephalitis is a subacute to chronic disease of immunocompromised hosts, generally causing death in weeks to months [12]. In patients with AIDS, the course of granulomatous amebic encephalitis may be more rapid and pathology often shows a paucity of well-formed granulomas. Patients with cerebral disease usually present with fever, headache, focal neurologic deficits, and mental status changes. Similar cases of disseminated infection have been described in recipients of organ transplantation [66,69].

Fungi

Aspergillus and zygomycetes   Invasive fungal infections are an important cause of morbidity and mortality among transplant patients, with mucormycosis being the most common in a recent large case series [70]. Invasive *Aspergillus* has been estimated to occur in between 1% and 14% of transplant recipients, with high morbidity and mortality [71]. Though it may occur in association with HIV disease in those with low CD4 counts, the association is much less pronounced [72]. Infections by zygomycetes among those with HIV are less common and typically seen in patients with simultaneous neutropenia from other causes [72].

Geographically localized fungal infections

Histoplasmosis   *Histoplasma capsulatum* var. *duboisii* is localized to western and central Africa and to Madagascar. *H. capsulatum* is endemic in the Mississippi and Ohio River valleys, Central America, and certain areas of Southeast Asia and the Mediterranean basin. In HIV-uninfected persons, the pathogen tends to cause chronic necrotizing cutaneous and skeletal infections. In patients with HIV, atypical and disseminated cases have been commonly described [73–75]. In transplant-associated cases described in the literature, symptoms started a median of 1 year after organ transplantation, and the majority of cases occurred in the first 18 months [13]. The majority of infections are thought to be due to new acquisition in an endemic area, though reactivation disease is possible. Rarely, histoplasmosis in transplant patients may be transmitted through an infected allograft from a patient with unrecognized histoplasmosis.

Penicillium marneffei   It is an endemic mycosis in southeast Asia and China seen among those with HIV. The disease is typically characterized by papular skin eruptions, but systemic disease has been described and is considered uniformly fatal if untreated [76]. Cases of disseminated infection have also been described among bone marrow and organ transplant recipients [77,78].

Paracoccidioides brasiliensis   The adult form of the disease accounts for the vast majority of cases in immunocompetent patients. A juvenile form is characterized by a rapid course with disseminated involvement of macrophages and lymphoid tissue and severe suppression of cellular immunity. Disseminated disease similar to the juvenile pattern is more common in the immunosuppressed [79,80].

Sporothrix schenckii   Described cases have been from tropical and subtropical areas of the Americas. Although cutaneous and lymphocutaneous disease are most common, extracutaneous involvement has been described in both immunosufficient and immunocompromised hosts [81]. *Sporothrix* is a dimorphic fungus that most commonly infects the skin. Disseminated disease with involvement of the joints and central nervous system also occurs and is more common among those with underlying immune deficiencies [82]. IRISs associated with sporotrichosis have been described [83].

Coccidioides immitis It is a dimorphic yeast found in semiarid to arid life zones, principally in the southwestern United States and northern Mexico. It is also found in parts of Argentina, Brazil, Colombia, Guatemala, Honduras, Nicaragua, Paraguay, and Venezuela [13]. During transplantation, possible routes of transmission include (i) reactivation of latent infection, (ii) posttransplant de novo infection of recipients who live or travel to areas of endemicity, and (iii) transmission secondary to transplantation of organs from an infected donor. Posttransplant reactivation of coccidioidomycosis has been most frequently described though in a few cases, brief visits to areas of endemicity have been sufficient for the infection to be acquired. Dissemination is common in transplant recipients, occurring in up to 75% in some series, with or without concurrent pulmonary involvement [13]. Disseminated disease has been similarly described for persons coinfected with HIV but has become less common in the era of HAART [84].

Viral infections

Influenza virus Cases have been documented among both transplant recipients and AIDS patients. AIDS patients have significant excess mortality due to pneumonia and influenza during flu season. Data have been less clear regarding the impact of transplant related immunosuppression on the course or severity of influenza [85,86].

Measles virus Measles virus is associated with an annual mortality rate in the tropics that far exceeds the annual mortality rate associated with "traditional" tropical disease viruses [13]. Measles is itself exacerbated in the presence of HIV coinfection and coinfected patients have a higher risk for prolonged shedding of measles virus [87]. Failure to develop or maintain protective immunity leading to recurrent infections has also been described in persons with HIV [88].

Herpes viruses Recurrent outbreaks of herpetic lesions including those of herpes simplex and herpes zoster are common among persons with immunosuppression. Atypical presentations become more common with severe immunodeficiency, whether from HIV or from immunosuppressive medications used following organ transplantation [89,90]. Epstein–Barr virus (EBV) activation in the immunocompromised is associated with a number of opportunistic and nonopportunistic malignancies including primary CNS lymphoma among those with HIV, posttransplant lymphoproliferative syndromes, Burkitt's lymphoma, and nasopharyngeal carcinoma [91–95]. CMV disease is a common cause of morbidity in the posttransplant population, most commonly colitis and pneumonitis. CMV disease, particularly retinitis, has been similarly described in persons with HIV with extremely low CD4 counts (<50). Because diagnosis requires tissue biopsy and detailed pathologic review, many cases of CMV disease likely go undiagnosed outside specialty referral centers.

Polyomaviruses JC virus activation in the central nervous system is associated with the development of progressive multifocal leukoencephalopathy. Though cases have been described in those without clear immunodeficiency states, this condition is most commonly seen in person with significant immune deficiency, frequently those with HIV with CD4 counts less than 200. BK virus is a cause of hemorrhagic cystitis and renal dysfunction among the transplant population [96]. Similar to JC virus, in patients with HIV and low CD4 counts, BK virus can cause a severe form of meningoencephalitis [97–99].

Other viral infections   Adenovirus is a well-described cause of hemorrhagic cystitis among transplant recipients [100]. Systemic illnesses involving central nervous system, respiratory system, hepatitis, and gastroenteritis have also been described among the immunocompromised with high morbidity and mortality [101,102]. Parvovirus has been well described as a cause of anemia and other hematologic abnormalities among transplant patients and parvovirus encephalitis has also been described [103–105].

Geographically localized viral infections

West Nile virus   Naturally acquired West Nile virus has been described in patients with HIV as well as in transplant recipients. The spectrum of illness appears to be similar to that seen in immunocompetent patients; however, some studies have suggested that the resulting morbidity may be higher [106–108]. Though the virus originated in Africa, its distribution has spread to include Europe, the Middle East, Asia, Oceania, and North America.

HTLV   HTLV is a viral infection that causes a less severe form of immunosuppression than that seen with HIV. Two strains have been identified. HTLV-1 has been localized to Japan, Carribean, and sub-Saharan Africa. HTLV-2 is principally seen among IVDU and sexual contacts in Americas, Europe, and Vietnam. Coinfection has been well described and may have some negative impact on HIV disease progression [109,110]. HTLV-3 and HTLV-4 have recently been described in Africa, but clinical data is limited at this time [111].

Illustrative case

A 25-year-old HIV-positive woman, 6 months pregnant, presented with an acute and painful red eye, and a visual acuity of count fingers in the right eye (RE) [112]. There was no history of rural activities. On ophthalmologic examination, she was found to have unilateral right-eye severe iridocyclitis, severe vitritis, and a granulomatous chorioretinal lesion adjacent to and involving the optic nerve. The left eye was uninvolved. After 1 week, the patient showed iris neovascularization, neovascular glaucoma (intraocular pressure, 50 mm Hg), and retinal detachment. The patient was inconsistently adherent to her antiretroviral medication regimen. Serologies for syphilis, toxoplasmosis (IgG/IgM), CMV, EBV, and herpes virus were negative; CD4 count was 25 cells/mm^3, and the viral load 30,000 copies/dL. The chest X-ray was normal. A cranial MRI examination showed a focal hypodense, ring enhancing lesion in the brain. Neurologic examination and cerebrospinal fluid evaluation were normal. Ultrasonography revealed CNS microcalcifications in the fetus. An aqueous and vitreous biopsy was performed. The sample was tested by polymerase chain reaction, and *T. gondii* DNA was found in the vitreous. Despite the negative serologies, specific therapy for toxoplasmosis (combination of sulfadiazine and pyrimethamine) and oral prednisone were initiated. The patient responded partially to the treatment, and the intraocular inflammatory reaction decreased and the CNS microcalcifications in the fetus on ultrasound resolved. One month later, the patient presented with seizures and delivered a premature newborn, who had no sign of clinical or ophthalmologic disease. Follow-up MRI showed a slight reduction in the size of the ring enhancing lesion. Two months after initial presentation, the patient had intolerable pain and complete loss of light perception in the right eye. Ocular ultrasonography disclosed total retinal detachment. An oropharyngeal lesion and lymph node enlargement were noted. The right eye was enucleated, and the oral lesion was biopsied. Macroscopic study of the enucleated eye showed a total retinal detachment with subretinal exudate and a white mass in the vitreous cavity displacing the lens to the anterior chamber. The histopathologic examination of the enucleated eye, as well as the oral lesion biopsy, revealed a chronic granulomatous inflammation with epithelioid cells, multinucleated giant cells, and several round yeasts with "ship's wheel" external budding that

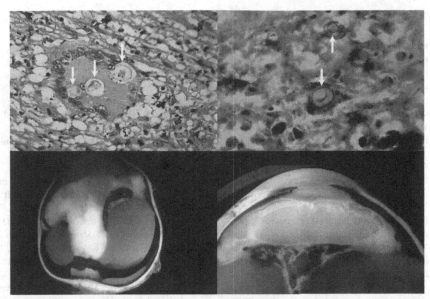

Fig. 27.1 (Top left, arrows) Granulomatous inflammation with multinucleated giant cells containing the yeasts (Hematoxylin and eosin stain, ×400). (Top right, arrows) Several round yeasts with external budding, typical of *Paracoccidioides brasiliensis* (Grocott's methenamine silver, ×400). (Bottom left and right) Macroscopic view of the enucleated eye with a total retinal detachment, subretinal exudate, and a white mass in the vitreous cavity.

stained best with periodic acid Schiff (PAS) and Grocott's methenamine silver, typical of *P. brasiliensis* (Figure 27.1). This case demonstrates an atypical presentation of an opportunistic infection in a patient with HIV with severe immunocompromise. The non-specific nature of the clinical findings highlights the importance of microbiologic diagnosis.

Summary

Immunocompromised patients present unique challenges for clinicians diagnosing and managing infectious diseases. A systematic approach to these patients emphasizing assessment of level of immune compromise, review of the use of prophylactic medications, a detailed history of potential exposures, and a thorough review of endemic risks in the region are key to obtaining a timely and accurate diagnosis. Given the atypical presentation and rapid progression of infections among the immunocompromised, early microbiologic diagnosis where feasible may be important to guide treatment. Where microbiologic diagnosis is not feasible, knowledge of the patients level of immune compromise and the epidemic and endemic risks is a critical guide to empiric therapy.

Acknowledgment

The authors would like to acknowledge the review and comments of Majid Sadigh, MD, and Frank Bia, MD, in the formulation of this chapter.

References

1. Ryan ET, Wilson ME, Kain KC. Illness after International Travel. N Engl J Med 2009;347 (7):505–16.
2. Jong E, Freedman D. Approach to the immunocompromised traveler. In: Brunette G (ed). CDC Health Information for International Travel 2010. Atlanta: U.S. Department of Health and Human Services, Public Health Service, 2010.
3. Fishman JA, Issa NC. Infection in organ transplantation: risk factors and evolving patterns of infection. Infect Dis Clin North Am 2010;24(2):273–83.
4. Franco-Paredes C, Jacob JT, Hidron A, Rodriguez-Morales AJ, Kuhar D, Caliendo AM. Transplantation and tropical infectious diseases. Int J Infect Dis 2010;14(3):e189–96.
5. Issa NC, Fishman JA. Infectious complications of antilymphocyte therapies in solid organ transplantation. Clin Infect Dis 2009;48(6): 772–86.
6. Dadhania D, Snopkowski C, Ding R, et al. Epidemiology of BK virus in renal allograft recipients: independent risk factors for BK virus replication. Transplantation 2008;86(4): 521–8.
7. Grim SA, Pham T, Thielke J, et al. Infectious complications associated with the use of rituximab for ABO-incompatible and positive cross-match renal transplant recipients. Clin Transplant 2007;21(5):628–32.
8. French MA. HIV/AIDS: immune reconstitution inflammatory syndrome: a reappraisal. Clin Infect Dis 2009;48(1):101–7.
9. Carpenter C, Beckwith C, Rodriguez B, Leventhal JS. Human immunodeficiency virus infection and acquired immunodeficiency syndrome. In: Andreoli T, Carpenter C, Griggs R, Benjamin I (eds). Cecil Essentials of Medicine, 7th edn. Philadelphia: Saunders/Elsevier, 2009: 989–1008.
10. Harms G, Feldmeier H. The impact of HIV infection on tropical diseases. Infect Dis Clin North Am 2005;19(1):121–35.
11. Karp CL, Neva FA. Tropical infectious diseases in human immunodeficiency virus-infected patients. Clin Infect Dis 1999;28(5):947–63.
12. Karp CL, Auwaerter PG. Coinfection with HIV and tropical infectious diseases. I. Protozoal pathogens. Clin Infect Dis 2007;45(9):1208–13.
13. Karp CL, Auwaerter PG. Coinfection with HIV and tropical infectious diseases. II. Helminthic,

fungal, bacterial, and viral pathogens. Clin Infect Dis 2007;45(9):1214–20.
13a. Mileno M & Bia FJ. The Compromised Traveler. Infectious Disease Clinics of North America. 1998;12(2):369–412.
14. Gilks CF. Acute bacterial infections and HIV disease. Br Med Bull 1998;54(2):383–93.
15. Dye C. Global epidemiology of tuberculosis. Lancet 2006;367(9514):938–40.
16. Sterling TR, Pham PA, Chaisson RE. HIV infection-related tuberculosis: clinical manifestations and treatment. Clin Infect Dis 2010;50:223–30.
17. Kenyon TA, Creek T, Laserson K, et al. Risk factors for transmission of *Mycobacterium tuberculosis* from HIV-infected tuberculosis patients, Botswana. Int J Tuberc Lung Dis 2002;6(10):843–50.
18. Cauthen GM, Dooley SW, Onorato IM, et al. Transmission of *Mycobacterium tuberculosis* from tuberculosis patients with HIV infection or AIDS. Am J Epidemiol 1996;144(1):69–77.
19. Carvalho AC, DeRiemer K, Nunes ZB, et al. Transmission of *Mycobacterium tuberculosis* to contacts of HIV-infected tuberculosis patients. Am J Respir Crit Care Med 2001;164(12): 2166–71.
20. Feely NM, Waghorn DJ, Dexter T, Gallen I, Chiodini P. *Strongyloides stercoralis* hyperinfection: difficulties in diagnosis and treatment. Anaesthesia 2010;65(3):298–301.
21. Roxby AC, Gottlieb GS, Limaye AP. Strongyloidiasis in transplant patients. Clin Infect Dis 2009;49(9):1411–23.
22. Viney ME, Brown M, Omoding NE, et al. Why does HIV infection not lead to disseminated strongyloidiasis? J Infect Dis 2004; 190(12):2175–80.
23. Ganley-Leal LM, Mwinzi PN, Cetre-Sossah CB, et al. Correlation between eosinophils and protection against reinfection with *Schistosoma mansoni* and the effect of human immunodeficiency virus type 1 coinfection in humans. Infect Immun 2006;74(4):2169–76.
24. Secor WE. Interactions between schistosomiasis and infection with HIV-1. Parasite Immunol 2006;28(11):597–603.
25. Mwanakasale V, Vounatsou P, Sukwa TY, Ziba M, Ernest A, Tanner M. Interactions between *Schistosoma haematobium* and human immunodeficiency virus type 1: the effects of coinfection on treatment outcomes in rural Zambia. Am J Trop Med Hyg 2003;69(4):420–8.

26. Secor WE, Karanja DM, Colley DG. Interactions between schistosomiasis and human immunodeficiency virus in Western Kenya. Mem Inst Oswaldo Cruz 2004;99(5, Suppl. 1):93–5.

27. Dautremer J, Pacanowski J, Girard PM, Lalande V, Sivignon F, Meynard JL. A new presentation of immune reconstitution inflammatory syndrome followed by a severe paradoxical reaction in an HIV-1-infected patient with tuberculous meningitis. AIDS 2007;21(3):381–2.

28. Fernando R, Miller R. Immune reconstitution eosinophilia due to schistosomiasis. Sex Transm Infect 2002;78(1):76.

29. Lawn SD. Schistosomiasis and immune reconstitution disease. AIDS 2007;21(14):1986–7.

30. Talaat KR, Kumarasamy N, Swaminathan S, Gopinath R, Nutman TB. Filarial/human immunodeficiency virus coinfection in urban southern India. Am J Trop Med Hyg 2008;79 (4):558–60.

31. Nielsen NO, Simonsen PE, Magnussen P, Magesa S, Friis H. Cross-sectional relationship between HIV, lymphatic filariasis and other parasitic infections in adults in coastal northeastern Tanzania. Trans R Soc Trop Med Hyg 2006;100(6):543–50.

32. Diazgranados CA, Saavedra-Trujillo CH, Mantilla M, Valderrama SL, Alquichire C, Franco-Paredes C. Chagasic encephalitis in HIV patients: common presentation of an evolving epidemiological and clinical association. Lancet Infect Dis 2009;9(5):324–30.

33. Sartori AM, Ibrahim KY, Nunes Westphalen EV, et al. Manifestations of Chagas disease (American trypanosomiasis) in patients with HIV/AIDS. Ann Trop Med Parasitol 2007;101 (1):31–50.

34. Rocha A, de Meneses AC, da Silva AM, et al. Pathology of patients with Chagas' disease and acquired immunodeficiency syndrome. Am J Trop Med Hyg 1994;50(3):261–8.

35. Gallerano V, Consigli J, Pereyra S, et al. Chagas' disease reactivation with skin symptoms in a patient with kidney transplant. Int J Dermatol 2007;46(6):607–10.

36. Riarte A, Luna C, Sabatiello R, et al. Chagas' disease in patients with kidney transplants: 7 years of experience 1989–1996. Clin Infect Dis 1999;29(3):561–7.

37. Di Lorenzo GA, Pagano MA, Taratuto AL, Garau ML, Meli FJ, Pomsztein MD. Chagasic granulomatous encephalitis in immunosuppressed patients. Computed tomography and magnetic resonance imaging findings. J Neuroimaging 1996;6(2):94–7.

38. Simoes MV, Soares FA, Marin-Neto JA. Severe myocarditis and esophagitis during reversible long standing Chagas' disease recrudescence in immunocompromised host. Int J Cardiol 1995;49(3):271–3.

39. Edvinsson B, Lappalainen M, Anttila VJ, Paetau A, Evengard B. Toxoplasmosis in immunocompromised patients. Scand J Infect Dis 2009;41(5):368–71.

40. Castagnini M, Bernazzali S, Ginanneschi C, et al. Fatal disseminated toxoplasmosis in a cardiac transplantation with seropositive match for *Toxoplasma*: Should prophylaxis be extended? Transplant Immunol 2007;18(2):193–7.

41. Wendum D, Carbonell N, Svrcek M, Chazouilleres O, Flejou JF. Fatal disseminated toxoplasmosis in a toxoplasma seropositive liver transplant recipient. J Clin Pathol 2002; 55(8):637.

42. Park BJ, Wannemuehler KA, Marston BJ, Govender N, Pappas PG, Chiller TM. Estimation of the current global burden of cryptococcal meningitis among persons living with HIV/AIDS. AIDS 2009;23(4):525–30.

43. Singh N, Forrest G; AST Infectious Diseases Community of Practice. Cryptococcosis in solid organ transplant recipients. Am J Transplant 2009;9(Suppl. 4):S192–8.

44. Shirley RM, Baddley JW. Cryptococcal lung disease. Curr Opin Pulm Med 2009;15(3):254–60.

45. Gave AA, Torres R, Kaplan L. Cryptococcal myositis and vasculitis: an unusual necrotizing soft tissue infection. Surg Infect 2004;5(3): 309–13.

46. Basaran O, Emiroglu R, Arikan U, Karakayali H, Haberal M. Cryptococcal necrotizing fasciitis with multiple sites of involvement in the lower extremities. Dermatol Surg 2003;29(11): 1158–60.

47. Lee YA, Kim HJ, Lee TW, et al. First report of *Cryptococcus albidus*—induced disseminated cryptococcosis in a renal transplant recipient. Korean J Intern Med 2004;19(1):53–7.

48. Romano C, Taddeucci P, Donati D, Miracco C, Massai L. Primary cutaneous cryptococcosis due to *Cryptococcus neoformans* in a woman with non-Hodgkin's lymphoma. Acta Derm Venereol 2001;81(3):220–1.

49. Antinori S, Cascio A, Parravicini C, Bianchi R, Corbellino M. Leishmaniasis among organ transplant recipients. Lancet Infect Dis 2008;8 (3):191–9.

50. Campos-Varela I, Len O, Castells L, et al. Visceral leishmaniasis among liver transplant recipients: an overview. Liver Transplant 2008;14(12):1816–19.

51. Oliveira CM, Oliveira ML, Andrade SC, et al. Visceral leishmaniasis in renal transplant recipients: clinical aspects, diagnostic problems, and response to treatment. Transplant Proc 2008;40(3):755–60.

52. Toledo AC Jr, de Castro MR. *Pneumocystis carinii* pneumonia, pulmonary tuberculosis and visceral leishmaniasis in an adult HIV negative patient. Braz J Infect Dis 2001;5(3):154–7.

53. Krause PJ, Gewurz BE, Hill D, et al. Persistent and relapsing babesiosis in immunocompromised patients. Clin Infect Dis 2008;46 (3):370–6.

54. Browne S, Ryan Y, Goodyer M, Gilligan O. Fatal babesiosis in an asplenic patient. Br J Haematol 2010;148(4):494.

55. Berman KH, Blue DE, Smith DS, Kwo PY, Liangpunsakul S. Fatal case of babesiosis in postliver transplant patient. Transplantation 2015;87(3):452–3.

56. Safdar N, Love RB, Maki DG. Severe *Ehrlichia chaffeensis* infection in a lung transplant recipient: a review of ehrlichiosis in the immunocompromised patient. Emerg Infect Dis 2002;8(3):320–3.

57. Paddock CD, Folk SM, Shore GM, et al. Infections with *Ehrlichia chaffeensis* and *Ehrlichia ewingii* in persons coinfected with human immunodeficiency virus. Clin Infect Dis 2001;33(9):1586–94.

58. Lawrence KL, Morrell MR, Storch GA, Hachem RR, Trulock EP. Clinical outcomes of solid organ transplant recipients with ehrlichiosis. Transplant Infect Dis 2009;11(3):203–10.

59. Slutsker L, Marston BJ. HIV and malaria: interactions and implications. Curr Opin Infect Dis 2007;20(1):3–10.

60. Skinner-Adams TS, McCarthy JS, Gardiner DL, Andrews KT. HIV and malaria co-infection: interactions and consequences of chemotherapy. Trends Parasitol 2008;24(6):264–71.

61. Martin-Davila P, Fortun J, Lopez-Velez R, et al. Transmission of tropical and geographically restricted infections during solid-organ transplantation. Clin Microbiol Rev 2008;21(1): 60–96.

62. Machado CM, Martins TC, Colturato I, et al. Epidemiology of neglected tropical diseases in transplant recipients. Review of the literature and experience of a Brazilian HSCT center. Rev Inst Med Trop Sao Paulo 2009;51(6):309–24.

63. Barete S, Combes A, de Jonckheere JF, et al. Fatal disseminated *Acanthamoeba lenticulata* infection in a heart transplant patient. Emerg Infect Dis 2007;13(5):736–8.

64. Mutreja D, Jalpota Y, Madan R, Tewari V. Disseminated acanthamoeba infection in a renal transplant recipient: a case report. Indian J Pathol Microbiol 2007;50(2):346–8.

65. Kumar M, Jain R, Tripathi K, et al. Acanthamoebae presenting as primary meningoencephalitis in AIDS. Indian J Pathol Microbiol 2007;50(4):928–30.

66. Duarte AG, Sattar F, Granwehr B, Aronson JF, Wang Z, Lick S. Disseminated acanthamoebiasis after lung transplantation. J Heart Lung Transplant 2006;25(2):237–40.

67. Paltiel M, Powell E, Lynch J, Baranowski B, Martins C. Disseminated cutaneous acanthamebiasis: a case report and review of the literature. Cutis 2004;73(4):241–8.

68. Marciano-Cabral F, Puffenbarger R, Cabral GA. The increasing importance of *Acanthamoeba* infections. J Eukaryot Microbiol 2000;47(1): 29–36.

69. Steinberg JP, Galindo RL, Kraus ES, Ghanem KG. Disseminated acanthamebiasis in a renal transplant recipient with osteomyelitis and cutaneous lesions: case report and literature review. Clin Infect Dis 2002;35(5): e43–9.

70. Einollahi B, Lessan-Pezeshki M, Pourfarziani V, et al. Invasive fungal infections following renal transplantation: a review of 2410 recipients. Ann Transplant 2008;13(4):55–8.

71. Singh N, Husain S; AST Infectious Diseases Community of Practice. Invasive aspergillosis in solid organ transplant recipients. Am J Transplant 2009;9(Suppl. 4):S180–91.

72. Sanchez MR, Ponge-Wilson I, Moy JA, Rosenthal S. Zygomycosis and HIV infection. J Am Acad Dermatol 1994;30(5, Part 2):904–8.

73. Bonifaz A, Chang P, Moreno K, et al. Disseminated cutaneous histoplasmosis in acquired immunodeficiency syndrome: report of 23 cases. Clin Exp Dermatol 2009;34(4):481–6.

74. Tobon AM, Agudelo CA, Rosero DS, et al. Disseminated histoplasmosis: a comparative study between patients with acquired immunodeficiency syndrome and non-human immunodeficiency virus-infected individuals. Am J Trop Med Hyg 2005;73(3):576–82.

75. Assi M, McKinsey DS, Driks MR, et al. Gastro-intestinal histoplasmosis in the acquired immunodeficiency syndrome: report of 18 cases and literature review. Diagn Microbiol Infect Dis 2006;55(3):195–201.
76. Ustianowski AP, Sieu TP, Day JN. *Penicillium marneffei* infection in HIV. Curr Opin Infect Dis 2008;21(1):31–6.
77. Wang JL, Hung CC, Chang SC, Chueh SC, La MK. Disseminated *Penicillium marneffei* infection in a renal-transplant recipient successfully treated with liposomal amphotericin B. Transplantation 2003;76(7):1136–7.
78. de la CR, Pinilla I, Munoz E, Buendia B, Steegmann JL, Fernandez-Ranada JM. *Penicillium brevicompactum* as the cause of a necrotic lung ball in an allogeneic bone marrow transplant recipient. Bone Marrow Transplant 1996;18(6):1189–93.
79. Paniago AM, de Freitas AC, Aguiar ES, et al. Paracoccidioidomycosis in patients with human immunodeficiency virus: review of 12 cases observed in an endemic region in Brazil. J Infect 2005;51(3):248–52.
80. Silva-Vergara ML, Teixeira AC, Curi VG, et al. Paracoccidioidomycosis associated with human immunodeficiency virus infection. Report of 10 cases. Med Mycol 2003;41(3):259–63.
81. Yelverton CB, Stetson CL, Bang RH, Clark JW, Butler DF. Fatal sporotrichosis. Cutis 2006;78 (4):253–6.
82. Shaw JC, Levinson W, Montanaro A. Sporotrichosis in the acquired immunodeficiency syndrome. J Am Acad Dermatol 1989;21(5, Part 2):1145–7.
83. Galhardo MC, Silva MT, Lima MA, et al. *Sporothrix schenckii* meningitis in AIDS during immune reconstitution syndrome. J Neurol Neurosurg Psychiatry 2010;81(6):696–9.
84. Masannat FY, Ampel NM. Coccidioidomycosis in patients with HIV-1 infection in the era of potent antiretroviral therapy. Clin Infect Dis 2010;50(1):1–7.
85. Ljungman P, Andersson J, Aschan J, et al. Influenza A in immunocompromised patients. Clin Infect Dis 1993;17(2):244–7.
86. Lin J & Nichol KL. Arch Intern Med 2001; 161:441–446.
87. Scott S, Mossong J, Moss WJ, Cutts FT, Cousens S. Predicted impact of the HIV-1 epidemic on measles in developing countries: results from a dynamic age-structured model. Int J Epidemiol 2008;37(2):356–67.
88. Permar SR, Griffin DE, Letvin NL. Immune containment and consequences of measles virus infection in healthy and immunocompromised individuals. Clin Vaccine Immunol 2006;13(4):437–43.
89. Patel AB, Rosen T. Herpes vegetans as a sign of HIV infection. Dermatol Online J 2008;14(4):6.
90. Dinotta F, De PR, Nasca MR, Tedeschi A, Micali G. Disseminated herpes simplex infection in a HIV+ patient. G Ital Dermatol Venereol 2009;144(2):205–9.
91. Yoon TY, Yang TH, Hahn YS, Huh JR, Soo Y. Epstein–Barr virus-associated recurrent necrotic papulovesicles with repeated bacterial infections ending in sepsis and death: consideration of the relationship between Epstein–Barr virus infection and immune defect. J Dermatol 2001;28(8):442–7.
92. Murata T, Nakamura S, Kato H, et al. Epstein–Barr virus-related Hodgkin's disease showing B cell lineage in an immunosuppressive patient seropositive for HTLV-I. Pathol Int 1997;47 (11):801–5.
93. Boman F, Gultekin H, Dickman PS. Latent Epstein–Barr virus infection demonstrated in low-grade leiomyosarcomas of adults with acquired immunodeficiency syndrome, but not in adjacent Kaposi's lesion or smooth muscle tumors in immunocompetent patients. Arch Pathol Lab Med 1997;121(8):834–8.
94. Sung L, Dix D, Allen U, Weitzman S, Cutz E, Malkin D. Epstein–Barr virus-associated lymphoproliferative disorder in a child undergoing therapy for localized rhabdomyosarcoma. Med Pediatr Oncol 2000;34(5):358–60.
95. Yu L, Aldave AJ, Glasgow BJ. Epstein–Barr virus-associated smooth muscle tumor of the iris in a patient with transplant: a case report and review of the literature. Arch Pathol Lab Med 2009;133(8):1238–41.
96. Hirsch HH, Randhawa P; AST Infectious Diseases Community of Practice. BK virus in solid organ transplant recipients. Am J Transplant 2009;9(Suppl. 4):S136–46.
97. Vidal J, Fink M, Cedeno-Laurent F, et al. BK virus associated meningoencephalitis in an AIDS patient treated with HAART. AIDS Res Ther 2007;4(1):13.
98. Vallbracht A, Lohler J, Gossmann J, et al. Disseminated BK type polyomavirus infection in an AIDS patient associated with central nervous system disease. Am J Pathol 1993;143 (1):29–39.

99. Bratt G, Hammarin AL, Grandien M, et al. BK virus as the cause of meningoencephalitis, retinitis and nephritis in a patient with AIDS. AIDS 1999;13(9):1071–5.

100. Ison MG, Green M; AST Infectious Diseases Community of Practice. Adenovirus in solid organ transplant recipients. Am J Transplant 2009;9(Suppl. 4):S161–5.

101. Tebruegge M, Curtis N. Adenovirus infection in the immunocompromised host. Adv Exp Med Biol 2010;659:153–74.

102. Hoffman JA. Adenovirus infections in solid organ transplant recipients. Curr Opin Organ Transplant 2009;14(6):625–33.

103. Eid AJ, Posfay-Barbe KM; AST Infectious Diseases Community of Practice. Parvovirus B19 in solid organ transplant recipients. Am J Transplant 2009;9(Suppl. 4):S147–50.

104. Shekar K, Hopkins PM, Kermeen FD, Dunning JJ, McNeil KD. Unexplained chronic anemia and leukopenia in lung transplant recipients secondary to parvovirus B19 infection. J Heart Lung Transplant 2008;27 (7):808–11.

105. Laurenz M, Winkelmann B, Roigas J, Zimmering M, Querfeld U, Muller D. Severe parvovirus B19 encephalitis after renal transplantation. Pediatric Transplant 2006;10 (8):978–81.

106. Torno M, Vollmer M, Beck CK. West Nile virus infection presenting as acute flaccid paralysis in an HIV-infected patient: a case report and review of the literature. Neurology 2007;68(7):E5–7.

107. Kleinschmidt-Demasters BK, Marder BA, Levi ME, et al. Naturally acquired West Nile virus encephalomyelitis in transplant recipients: clinical, laboratory, diagnostic, and neuropathological features. Arch Neurol 2004;61(8):1210–20.

108. Ravindra KV, Freifeld AG, Kalil AC, et al. West Nile virus-associated encephalitis in recipients of renal and pancreas transplants: case series and literature review. Clin Infect Dis 2004;38(9):1257–60.

109. Bassani S, Lopez M, Toro C, et al. Influence of human T cell lymphotropic virus type 2 coinfection on virological and immunological parameters in HIV type 1-infected patients. Clin Infect Dis 2007;44(1):105–10.

110. Brites C, Sampalo J, Oliveira A. HIV/human T-cell lymphotropic virus coinfection revisited: impact on AIDS progression. AIDS Rev 2009;11(1):8–16.

111. Mahieux R, Gessain A. The human HTLV-3 and HTLV-4 retroviruses: new members of the HTLV family. Pathol Biol 2009;57 (2):161–6.

112. Finamor LP, Muccioli C, Martins MC, Rizzo LV, Belfort R Jr. Ocular and central nervous system paracoccidioidomycosis in a pregnant woman with acquired immunodeficiency syndrome. Am J Ophthalmol 2002; 134(3):456–9.

Chapter 28
Emerging infections

Mary Elizabeth Wilson
Harvard School of Public Health, Department of Global Health and Population, Harvard University, Boston, MA, USA

Infectious diseases are dynamic and can be expected to continue to change in the foreseeable future. Characteristics of the world today including extensive interconnections via travel, trade, and migration; human population size, density, and location; expansion of food animal populations and increasing contact with wild animal populations; changes in the environment, land use, and climate; and poverty and lack of infrastructure to provide adequate food, clean water, and sanitation all contribute to the opportunity for new and changed microbes to emerge and spread. Microbes, because of their resilience, variety, abundance, short generation time, and capacity to change through a variety of maneuvers, can flourish in new settings. Several examples of diseases illustrate how multiple factors typically converge to contribute to disease emergence.

Infectious diseases in humans are dynamic. Infections have changed in distribution, intensity, and type in the past and will continue to change in the future. Infectious diseases have shaped human history, and they remain a reason for concern, research, and surveillance. The dynamic nature of human infections means that any attempt to capture where they exist and display this on a map will never be completely up to date for many diseases. Familiar, extensively studied infections, such as tuberculosis and staphylococcal infection, can change in virulence and resistance patterns. Infections that are new or newly recognized, such those caused by the Nipah and SARS viruses, appear and spread; their epidemiology is influenced by the biological characteristics of the viruses, their origins, and routes of spread.

The types of changes that can occur in known infections are several and include:
• Change in the distribution (expansion, contraction, or appearance in entirely new area or population); this may be the result of a new route of transmission.
• Increase in resistance to treatment.
• Increase in virulence or transmissibility of a pathogen, leading to infection that is more widespread, more severe, or both.
• Change in clinical expression because of host factors (e.g., Kaposi's sarcoma and other unusual expressions of common infections in individuals with AIDS).

Listed at the end of this section are examples of these types of changes, illustrating the wide range of contributing factors that can lead to change in a disease.

In addition to changes in familiar pathogens, in recent years, we have seen the appearance of infections in the human population which were previously absent or not recognized. It is

Infectious Diseases: A Geographic Guide, First Edition.
Edited by Eskild Petersen, Lin H. Chen & Patricia Schlagenhauf.
© 2011 John Wiley & Sons, Ltd. Published 2011 by John Wiley & Sons, Ltd.

notable that many of these infections are zoonoses and have crossed the species barrier from animals to humans, and some are now well adapted to person-to-person spread (e.g., HIV). Among these, viruses, especially RNA viruses, predominate. Multiple different routes of transmission characterize these infections, including transmission via mosquitoes and other arthropod vectors and via medical procedures.

Many factors can contribute to the emergence of new microbial threats [1], often working synergistically. This chapter will explore some of these major factors and will give examples to illustrate them. The main focus will be on infections that are new or newly recognized in the human population. The characteristics of microbes—abundant, diverse, ubiquitous, resilient, able to survive in extreme environments (extremophiles), capacity to change rapidly in response to an altered environment (mutation, acquisition of new genetic material, recombination, and other molecular maneuvers), and multiple survival mechanisms (e.g., spores, latency, and dormancy)—mean that microbes are well suited to occupying new niches provided for them [2]. They are simply trying to survive.

The factors in emergence defined in the 2003 IOM report [1] remain relevant today.
- Microbial adaptation and change
- Human susceptibility to infection
- Climate and weather
- Changing ecosystems
- Economic development and land use
- Human demography and behavior
- Technology and industry
- International travel and commerce
- Breakdown in public health measures
- Poverty and social inequality
- War and famine
- Lack of political will
- Intent to harm

Major global trends

Several major global trends should be highlighted because they provide the milieu in which infections are changing. Key ones include population size, density, location, and mobility [3]. Climate change, which can also influence infectious diseases, is covered in a separate chapter. The size of the human population is larger than ever in human history—a larger substrate for replication events in microbes. The same can be said for the population of food animals. The increasing affluence in China and other countries and the desire for more animal protein has resulted in major increases in the food animals. In China, for example, between 1968 and 2005, while the number of humans increased less than twofold, the pig population increased more than 100-fold and the poultry population more than 1,000-fold [4]. Commercial farms that are raising wild animals for human use (e.g., food, traditional medicines, pets, decoration, and souvenirs) have increased dramatically, especially in East and Southeast Asia, in the past two decades [5]. Among destinations for the animals are upscale urban wild meat restaurants. Animals raised on the farms are varied, and include sika deer, bears, tigers, crocodiles, turtles, Burmese pythons, field crickets, Chinese cobras, wild pigs, and many species of birds. These farms and the harvesting, preparation, and trade in these animals and their parts serve to expand the wild animal–human interface and allow the juxtaposition of species (microbial and other) that have never before been in contact. Live animals and their parts enter legal and illegal markets and are dispersed widely within and outside the region. In an analysis of 335 emerging infectious disease events reported between 1940 and 2004, researchers found that 60.3% of emerging infections were considered to be zoonoses, the majority (71.8%) originating from wildlife [6].

More than half of the global population now lives in urban areas, and the percentage of the population living in urban areas is expected to continue to increase. This means that more people are living in dense settlements, settings where infections can easily reach large, susceptible populations. Most of the population growth today is occurring in urban areas of developing countries, and much of it occurring in areas without adequate infrastructure. Many residents lack clean water and sanitary facilities and live in poorly constructed structures that permit contact with rodents and other animals, mosquito, and other arthropod vectors—factors that also place them at risk for infections.

In 2008 the majority of the 25 largest megacities (cities with more than 10 million inhabitants) were located in tropical and subtropical areas; only four were in temperate areas [7]. This is in contrast to the location of the world's largest cities in 1900, when they were located primarily in temperate zones. Most of the recent and projected population growth is also taking place in tropical and subtropical areas. It has been observed that the greatest species diversity (including pathogens) exists at the equator; species diversity declines at higher latitudes, something called the species latitudinal gradient [8]. Many low latitude cities today have vast slum areas and are poorly equipped to provide diagnosis, treatment, surveillance, and control of infectious diseases. These are areas where new infections may emerge and spread.

Travel, trade, and migration

The enormous volume of trade and travel in today's world is a key contributor to the movement of pathogenic microbes around the world—the old and the new [3,9]. In 2008, for example, international tourist arrivals reached 922 million, with 52% of the travel by air [10]. Infections that are carried by humans and spread from person to person, such as SARS, tuberculosis, HIV/AIDS, and influenza, can be easily transported to any part of the world by traveling humans [11]. Humans also transport resistance genes in pathogens and also as part of their commensal flora. Receiving medical care in India, often as part of so-called medical tourism, for example, was identified as a common factor in patients infected with *Enterobacteriaceae* carrying a resistance gene (New Delhi metallo-B-latamase-1) that confers resistance to all or most antimicrobial agents [12]. Bacteria carrying this resistance mechanism have now been found in many areas, including countries in Europe plus North America, and Australia.

The ease and speed of spread of an infection varies depending on the characteristics of the pathogen, route of spread, the population groups affected, and their travel and behavioral patterns. The influenza H1N1 virus that emerged in 2009, with genes from pigs, humans, and avian species, was easily transmissible from person to person and spread rapidly globally [13]. In contrast, the highly pathogenic avian-origin H5N1 virus that was first recognized in humans more than a decade ago is found widely in avian populations in Asia and has also appeared in Europe and Africa (see Figure 28.1—photo of smuggled birds) [14], but the majority of human cases have resulted from contact with infected wild or domestic poultry populations, and multiple chains of person-to-person transmission have not been established to date [15]. The SARS coronavirus that was first identified in humans in 2003 was carried by air travelers to multiple continents. Only because of the characteristics of the pathogen, that is, fever began before humans transmitted the virus—and there was no chronic carrier state, it was possible to halt the spread of this virus with intensive use of quarantine and isolation (see later) [16]. In contrast, the human immunodeficiency virus (HIV) epidemic and pandemic unfolded slowly, over years and decades. Because early symptoms may be mild, nonspecific, or absent, and

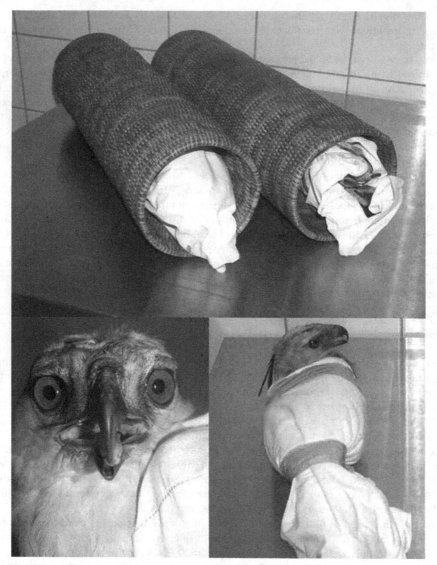

Fig. 28.1 Thai eagles infected with H5N1 smuggled into Brussels in hand luggage and were confiscated at the Brussels International Airport. (Reproduced from Van Borm et al. [14]) Photo Credit: U.S. Centers for Disease Control and Prevention.

infection is typically followed by prolonged asymptomatic infection during which the virus can be transmitted through sexual activity, needle sharing, from mother to infant, and other exposures to infected fluids or tissues, the virus was able to gain a foothold in all regions of the world before its clinical course and epidemiology were well understood. The factors that make it more likely that an introduced infection can be controlled are discussed in a paper by Fraser and colleagues [17] who point out the importance of the duration of the period of asymptomatic infection during which transmission can occur. Because influenza has a short incubation period and shedding can start before symptoms begin, spread occurs rapidly.

One of the factors that allows new infections to be transmitted and to become established in a new geographic area is the presence of competent arthropod vectors. Global trade has played a key role in the establishment of vectors in new geographic areas [18].

West Nile virus, which emerged in the United States starting in 1999, has now swept across the country and into Canada, Mexico, and other parts of Latin America. In this instance, competent mosquito vectors and susceptible avian species were already in place. The introduction of the virus—in a mosquito, animal, or person—allowed the virus to gain a foothold and move across the country over a several year period [19]. The virus is now established in animal/bird and mosquito populations and will not be eliminated. This summer outbreaks of West Nile virus infection were documented in humans for the first time in Greece [20], with neuroinvasive disease occurring primarily in older individuals.

Examples that follow demonstrate the range of factors and show that typically several factors act together to allow emergence and spread. A single factor is usually not sufficient.

SARS

The severe acute respiratory syndrome (SARS) was caused by a novel coronavirus (SARS-CoV) that was first identified in 2003. In retrospect, cases had occurred in China in late 2002 and a major outbreak in Guangzhou in January 2003. In February 2003, however, the virus spread to multiple countries and gained worldwide attention [21]. The virus spread to at least 28 countries. In the United States, cases were reported from 41 states, 97% of them following international travel. Collaborative research led to the rapid identification of the virus in 2003, and intensive control efforts globally were successful in interrupting spread. More than 8,000 cases were identified, almost 800 of them being fatal. The populations most affected were health care workers and their contacts. In Singapore, for example, 76% of the cases were nosocomial. The virus was carried by humans, and international travel allowed the virus to be dispersed to multiple countries over a period of weeks. Transmission probably occurred on airplanes (4/35 flights with travelers with SARS) and involved 27 travelers, including four flight attendants.

The proximate source was found to be masked palm civets, which were sold in live animal markets in Guangdong Province, China. They were culled after the SARS outbreaks. One study found that 14% of animal traders had IgG antibody to SARS Co-V, and 72.5% (16/22) of those who traded primarily with palm civets were antibody positive [22]. Subsequent studies of wild and farmed civets found no widespread infection of this species with SARS-CoV. Researchers subsequently found SARS-like coronaviruses in bats in China. Among groups of bats tested, 28–71% had antibodies to SARS-CoV, and fecal samples were PCR-positive for the virus [23]. This established bats as the likely natural reservoir host. Bats can be found in live animal markets in China, where it appears that the virus was able to enter the susceptible civet population, from which humans first acquired infection.

Other features of the SARS epidemic are notable. Marked differences occurred in the number of secondary cases generated by each infected individual. Although overall the basic reproductive rate (number of secondary cases generated by a single infectious case in a susceptible population) for SARS was about 3 [24], some individuals, sometimes called superspreaders, generated dozens of secondary cases. For example, in Singapore, five individuals were the source of infection for 103 of the first 201 cases (see Figure 28.2) [25]. Superspreading has also been noted as a feature in other emerging infectious diseases [26].

Because of the biological characteristics of the SARS Co-V, it was possible to contain the virus [17]. With SARS, infection almost always caused acute symptoms, and fever was virtually always present before the onset of transmissibility. This meant that by closely monitoring potentially

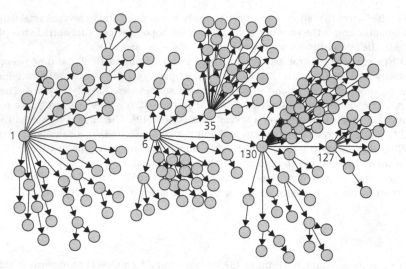

Fig. 28.2 Probable cases of SARS by reported source of infection (Singapore February 25 to April 30, 2003). (Reproduced from MMWR [25], with permission from CDC.)

exposed persons for the presence of fever and isolating those with fever, it was possible to interrupt spread. Unfortunately, with other infections, such as influenza and HIV infections, some or much of the transmission occurs before the onset of symptoms and during asymptomatic infection. This makes it extremely difficult to control the spread of infection in a susceptible population. Many of the early cases that spread from China occurred in cities (e.g., Hong Kong, Singapore, and Toronto) with excellent medical facilities and strong public health infrastructure, which also aided in the control of transmission.

One dramatic transmission event took place at the Amoy Gardens, a multibuilding apartment complex in Hong Kong. More than 300 residents of this complex became infected in the spring of 2003. A careful investigation was carried out by epidemiologists and engineers who could map the spatial distribution of the first 187 cases in that outbreak. They concluded that airborne transmission had occurred within the apartment complex, and the pattern of spread was consistent with virus-laden aerosols (generated from an index case with high concentrations of SARS-Co-V in feces and urine in drainage from a toilet). Spread was consistent with an aerosol carried by a rising plume of warm air in the air shaft between buildings. The contaminated plume entered other apartments through open windows [27]. They concluded that dried-up seals of floor drains allowed contamination to occur. Fortunately, interventions were available to halt the outbreak, but had it had occurred in a location with limited resources, control of the epidemic might have been slowed or impossible.

Monkeypox

Monkeypox is caused by a zoonotic orthopoxvirus first identified in 1970. Cases were first described in remote villages in central and western Africa rainforest countries. The majority of reported cases have been from the Democratic Republic of the Congo (DRC). The disease resembles smallpox, though lymphadenopathy is more prominent. Case fatality rate ranges from 1% to 14% in children not vaccinated against smallpox. The infection, acquired from direct contact with infected animals, can also spread from person to person. The longest chain of transmission was seven generations, but transmission usually does not extend beyond a second generation. A number of African rodents have been implicated as a source of the virus. Smallpox vaccination provides partial protection against infection. In the DRC smallpox vaccination was officially discontinued in 1980.

A recent study documented a major increase in human monkeypox incidence, which has coincided with the end of smallpox vaccination programs and the growing size of the unvaccinated population. Researchers assessed the number of cases of human monkeypox between 2005 and 2007 and compared data with those from population-based surveillance carried out in similar regions from 1981 to 1986 [28]. Overall they found an average annual cumulative incidence across zones of 5.5 per 10,000. Comparison with data from the 1980s suggested a 20-fold increase in human monkeypox incidence. Those who had been vaccinated against smallpox had a 5.2-fold lower risk of infection. As the proportion of the population that is unvaccinated expands, person-to-person transmission may become more common. Also, the expansion of the HIV-infected population means that infection in that immunocompromised population may be more severe and duration of viral shedding may be longer, providing opportunity for the virus to acquire mutations that could improve its fitness as a human pathogen.

Although the virus is found in squirrels and several other rodent species, its geographic habitat is Africa. In 2003, however, a human outbreak occurred for the first time in the Western Hemisphere, in the midwestern United States. The multistate outbreak was traced to imported African rodents that had been housed with prairie dogs from the United States which were being sold as pets [29]. The prairie dogs, which are not normal hosts for the virus, developed disease and were the source of infection in humans who handled them. There was no secondary person-to-person spread. There has been no evidence that new animal populations have become infected with the virus, but many animal species are susceptible to infection, including the American ground squirrels. This is a reminder of the important wildlife reservoirs for many infections and the multiple routes by which infections potentially can be established in a new geographic region.

Chikungunya virus

Vector-borne infections are also among those that can change rapidly in distribution. A competent vector must be present to allow the introduction of the infection into a new geographic area. One striking example has been the emergence and spread of chikungunya virus infection since 2004 outside its endemic zone in parts of West Africa, where the virus appears to be maintained in a cycle involving humans, *Aedes* mosquitoes, primates, and perhaps other animals [30].

Chikungunya is an RNA virus in the family Togaviridae, genus *Alphavirus*, and an arbovirus (arthropod-borne virus). The virus was first identified during an outbreak in East Africa in the early 1950s. A massive outbreak in Lamu, an island off the coast of Kenya, in 2004 was estimated (based on a serosurvey) to have affected 75% of the island's population of 18,000. Massive outbreaks followed in the Indian Ocean islands and infection subsequently spread to India, Sri Lanka, Indonesia, Malaysia, and Thailand. In India the epidemic was estimated to affect >1.5 million individuals between October 2005 and July 2009, and it spread to at least 17 states/union territories [31].

Many imported cases have been reported in travelers to areas experiencing outbreaks. Although chikungunya infection has been considered a tropical disease, in the summer of 2007 an outbreak occurred in two villages in northern Italy with 175 of the cases being laboratory confirmed. An investigation implicated a visitor from India as the index case [32]. The outbreak took place during the hottest months of the year and transmission stopped with arrival of cooler weather. No cases have subsequently been detected in this region. A 2010 report from ProMED describes two cases of locally acquired chikungunya infection in southern France in the summer of 2010 [33].

Key factors that have contributed to the recent spread of chikungunya include a mutation in a gene encoding the envelope protein of the virus [34,35]. This mutation has been associated with enhanced susceptibility of Aedes albopictus to infection with chikungunya virus and with more rapid viral dissemination to the mosquito salivary glands. This means that a mosquito can become infected when exposed to a lower level of virus in the bloodstream of the host. The mutant virus may have enhanced survival capacity.

The mosquito vector, Ae. albopictus (the Asian tiger mosquito) has also become widely distributed globally, moved largely by ships and often in used tires which provide an ideal way to transport mosquitoes or their eggs or larvae to new locations [18,36]. The mosquito is now found in many parts of Europe [37], the Americas, and Africa, having expanded from its original distribution in Asia. Laboratory studies of mosquitoes Aedes aegypti and Ae. albopictus strains from Florida revealed that these mosquito strains could be infected with a chikungunya isolate from the Reunion outbreak, and were capable of transmitting infection [38]. The other conditions that must be met for the virus to be introduced into a new area are infected humans who are viremic when they reach an area infested with Aedes mosquitoes, and environmental temperatures that are sufficiently warm to allow the virus to disseminate to the mosquito salivary glands. The infected mosquito must survive long enough to bite a susceptible human host. Warmer temperatures shorten the extrinsic incubation period of the virus in mosquitoes. The huge volume of global traffic today makes it easy for the chikungunya, similar to the dengue virus, to easily reach new populations. Dengue fever, also spread by Aedes mosquitoes, has also increased in number of cases and number of countries affected [30]. Recent transmission of dengue virus was also documented in southeastern France, where Ae. albopictus, a competent vector, is established [39].

Changes continue to occur in old diseases, such as tuberculosis, which has increasingly become resistant to treatment. Many social factors and interaction with HIV/AIDS have made it a formidable foe. Influenza, another old disease, continues to change in ways that have not been predictable. Highly pathogenic H5N1 emerged initially in poultry in 1996, caused a few human cases in 1997, appeared to have been halted, and then resurged in humans starting in 2003. The virus is now distributed in avian populations in Asia and parts of Africa. More than 500 human cases have been documented, more than half of them being fatal. Although to date the virus has been able to transmit easily from person to person, the virus continues to evolve. Recent studies in Indonesia show that pigs can become infected from adjacent chicken flocks, and do not show signs of influenza-like illness. Pigs have sometimes been called mixing vessels for avian and human influenza viruses. Studies of receptor specificity in these isolates from pigs in Indonesia revealed that one had acquired the ability to recognize a human-type receptor [40].

The above examples illustrate the complexity of disease emergence and some of the reasons why the global community must expect and prepare for the continued emergence of old and new microbial threats.

Examples of the dynamic nature of known infections

Observation	Infection	Event	Contributors	Consequences
Expansion of distribution	Dengue fever	Increase in number of countries with outbreaks Increase in severity with circulation of multiple serotypes	Increase in international travel Increase in urbanization and population growth, especially in tropical and subtropical areas Inadequate vector control programs Spread of *Aedes* vector Ecoclimatic conditions	Increase in cases and deaths Economic consequences because of loss of time in school and at work Decrease in illness and death
Contraction of distribution	Measles	Elimination of indigenous transmission of measles in the Americas	Availability and wide use of measles vaccine	Infections and small outbreaks occur related to travel Objections to use of vaccine in some groups
Increasing resistance to treatment	Tuberculosis	Appearance of MDR and XDR tuberculosis with spread to multiple countries and populations	Inappropriate use of anti-TB drugs Evolutionary potential of microbes Lack of access to appropriate anti-TB drugs Lack of laboratory capacity to diagnose TB and test drug susceptibility testing Increased susceptibility because of HIV infection Expanding populations infected with HIV Crowded housing facilities; clinics with patients and HIV and TB Congregate settings that favor transmission (e.g., prisons, hospital, and underground mines) Increase in international travel Evolutionary potential of microbes	Increase in disease and death Marked increase in cost of treatment for infections Need to treat with multiple drugs with significant toxicity No effective drugs available for some infections
Increase in virulence or transmissibility	*Clostridium difficile* colitis	Appearance and spread of strain that produces more toxin	Extensive use of antimicrobials in hospitals and chronic facilities Movement of patients and staff between acute and chronic care facilities	Increase in hospitalizations and deaths Appearance of community-acquired *C. difficile* colitis Change in the epidemiology

References

1. Smolinski MS, Hamburg MA, Lederberg J (eds). Microbial Threats to Health: Emergence, Detection, and Response. Washington, DC: The National Academy Press, 2003.
2. Wilson ME. Infectious diseases: an ecological perspective. BMJ 1995;311:1681–4.
3. Wilson ME. Global travel and emerging infections. In: Infectious Disease Movement in a Borderless World. Microbial Threats Forum, Institute of Medicine. Workshop Summary. Washington, DC: The National Academies Press, 2010:90–104, 126–9.
4. Osterholm MT. Preparing for the next pandemic. N Engl J Med 2005;352:1839–42.
5. Wildlife Conservation Society (WCS). Commercial Wildlife Farms in Vietnam: A Problem or Solution for Conservation? Hanoi, Vietnam: WCS, 2008. Technical report. Copies available from owstons@fpt.vn or wildlife@fpt.vn.
6. Jones KE, Patel NG, Levy MA, et al. Global trends in emerging infectious diseases. Nature 2008;45(7181):990–3.
7. Wilson ME. Megacities and emerging infections: case study of Rio de Janeiro, Brazil. In: Kahn O, Pappas G (eds). Megacities and Health. Washington, DC: American Public Health Association. Chapter 5 (in press).
8. Guernier V, Hockberg ME, Guegan JE. Ecology drives the worldwide distribution of human diseases. PLoS Biol 2004;2(6):740–6.
9. Wilson ME. Travel and the emergence of infectious diseases. Emerg Infect Dis 1995;1:39–46.
10. World Tourism Organization. UNWTO Tourism Highlights, 2009 edition. Available from http://www.unwto.org/facts/eng/pdf/highlights/UNWTO_Highlights09_en_LR.pdf.
11. Wilson ME. The traveller and emerging infections: sentinel, courier, transmitter. J Appl Microbiol 2003;94:1S–11S.
12. Kumarasamy KK, Toleman MA, Walsh TR, et al. Emergence of a new antibiotic resistance mechanism in India, Pakistan, and the UK: a molecular, biological, and epidemiological study. Lancet Infect Dis 2010;10:597–602.
13. Smith GJ, Vijaykrishna D, Bahl J, et al. Origins and evolutionary genomics of the 2009 swine-origin H1N1 influenza A epidemic. Nature 2009;459:1122–5.
14. Van Borm S, Thomas I, Hanquet G, et al. Highly pathogenic H5N1 influenza virus in smuggled Thai eagles, Belgium. Emerg Infect Dis 2005;11:702–5.
15. Li KS, Guan Y, Wang J, et al. Genesis of a highly pathogenic and potentially pandemic H5N1 influenza virus in eastern Asia. Nature 2004;430:209–13.
16. Riley S, Fraser C, Donnelly CA, et al. Transmission dynamics of the etiological agent of SARS in Hong Kong: impact of public health interventions. Science 2003;300:1961–6.
17. Fraser C, Riley S, Anderson RM, Ferguson NM. Factors that make an infectious disease outbreak controllable. Proc Natl Acad Sci USA 2004;101:6146–51.
18. Tatem AJ, Hay SI, Rogers DJ. Global traffic and disease vector dispersal. Proc Natl Acad Sci USA 2006;103:6242–7.
19. Petersen LR, Hayes EB. West Nile virus in the Americas. Med Clin North Am 2008;92:1307–22.
20. Papa A, Danis K, Baka A, et al. Ongoing outbreak of West Nile virus infections in humans in Greece, July–August 2010. Euro Sruveill 2010;15(34):pii=19644. Available online: http://www.eurosurveillance.org/ViewArticle.aspx?Articleid=19644.
21. World Health Organization. Consensus document on the epidemiology of severe acute respiratory syndrome (SARS). WHO/CDS/SCR/GAR/2003. Monograph on the Internet. Available from http://www.who.int/csr/sars/en/WHOconsensus.pdf.
22. Yu D, Li H, Xu R, et al. Prevalence of IgG antibody to SARS-associated coronavirus in animal traders—Guangdong Province, China, 2003. Centers for Disease Control and Prevention. MMWR Morb Mortal Wkly Rep 2003;52(41):986–7.
23. Li W, Shi Z, Yu M, et al. Bats are natural reservoirs of SARS-like coronaviruses. Science 2005;310:676–9.
24. Lipsitch M, Cohen C, Cooper B, et al. Transmission dynamics and control of severe acute respiratory syndrome. Science 2003;300:166–170.
25. Centers for Disease Control and Prevention. Severe acute respiratory syndrome—Singapore, 2003. MMWR Morb Mortal Wkly Rep 2003;52(18):405–11.
26. Lloyd-Smith JO, Schreiber SJ, Kopp PE, Getz WM. Superspreading and the effect of individual variation on disease emergence. Nature 2005;438:355–9.

27. Yu ITS, Li Y, Wong TW, et al. Evidence of airborne transmission of the severe acute respiratory syndrome virus. N Engl J Med 2004;355(17):1731–9.
28. Rimion AW, Mulembakani PM, Johnston SC, et al. Major increase in human monkeypox 30 years after smallpox vaccination campaigns cease in the Democratic Republic of Congo. Proc Natl Acad Sci USA 2010;107(37):16262–7.
29. Reed KD, Melski JW, Graham MB, et al. The detection of monkeypox in humans in the Western Hemisphere. N Engl J Med 2004; 350:342–50.
30. Chen LH, Wilson ME. Dengue and chikungunya infections in travelers. Curr Opin Infect Dis 2010;23:438–44.
31. Manimunda S, Sugunan AP, Rai SK, et al. Short report: outbreak of chikungunya fever, Dakshina Kannada district, south India, 2008. Am J Trop Med Hyg 2010;84(4):751–4.
32. Rezza GL, Nicoletti R, Angelini R, et al. Infection with chikungunya virus in Italy: an outbreak in a temperate region. Lancet 2007;370:1840–6.
33. ProMED-mail post. Chikungunya—France (03): Alpes-Maritimes, September 2010. Available from http://www.promedmail.org.
34. Schuffenecker I, Iteman I, Michault A, et al. Genome microevolution of chikungunya viruses causing the Indian Ocean outbreak. PLoS Med 2006;3:1058–71.
35. Tsetsarkin KA, Vanlandingham DL, McGee CE, Higgs S. A single mutation in chikungunya virus affects vector specificity and epidemic potential. PLoS Pathog 2007;3(12):1895–1906.
36. Reiter P, Fontenille D, Paupy C. *Aedes albopictus* as an epidemic vector of chikungunya virus: another emerging problem? Lancet Infect Dis 2006;6:463–4.
37. ECDC Technical Report. Development of *Aedes albopictus* risk maps. Stockholm, May 2009. Accessed April 5, 2010 at http://ecdc.europa.eu/en/activities/pages/programme_on_emerging_and_vector-borne_diseases_maps.aspx.
38. Reiskind MH, Pesko K, Westbrook Cj, Mores CN. Susceptibility of Florida mosquitoes in infection with chikungunya virus. Am J Trop Med Hyg 2008;78(3):422–5.
39. LaRuche G, Souares Y, Armengaud A, et al. First two autochthonous dengue virus infections in metropolitan France, September 2010. Euro Surveill 2010;15(39):pii19676. Available online: http://www.eurosurveillance.org/ViewArticle.aspx?ArticleId=19676.
40. Nidom CA, Takano R, Yamada S, et al. Influenza A (H5N1) viruses from pigs, Indonesia. Emerg Infect Dis 2010;16(10):1515–23.

Chapter 29
Migration and the geography of disease

Rogelio López-Vélez, Francesca F. Norman and José-Antonio Pérez-Molina

Tropical Medicine & Clinical Parasitology, Infectious Diseases Department, Ramón y Cajal Hospital, Madrid, Spain

The total number of international migrants has increased over the last 10 years to 214 million persons today. Most migrants are healthy, young adults, but they often bear a disproportionate burden of infectious diseases that can be classified as common infections, vaccine-preventable diseases, worldwide transmissible infections, and tropical diseases. The incidence of such diseases is related to the geographical origin of the immigrants, such as Chagas' disease in Latin Americans.

Migration and infectious diseases

Mobile populations are increasing worldwide. Migrants are a heterogeneous population which includes internally displaced persons, temporary migrants and workers, students, conventional travelers, VFR (visiting friends and relatives) travelers, immigrants, refugees and adoptees. Each of these groups will present distinct challenges regarding public health issues and possible interventions. The total number of international migrants has increased over the last 10 years to 214 million persons today. The number of refugees has remained stable at 15 million in 2009 and the number of internally displaced people has grown from 21 million in 2000 to 27 million at the end of 2009 [1].

The health of migrants has social and economic consequences for host countries as well as for individuals and their families. A variety of factors may influence immigrants' health, and these include biological factors, exposure to endemic diseases in their countries of origin, migration routes, overcrowding, and occupational hazards [2].

Noncommunicable diseases associated with migration include genetic diseases such as hemoglobinopathies, autoimmune diseases, psychological or psychiatric problems, and nutritional deficiencies. Certain tumors may also be included, such as cervical and hepatocellular carcinoma, associated with higher prevalences of human papillomavirus (HPV) and hepatitis B virus (HBV) infection, respectively, and gastric and esophageal cancer linked to specific dietary habits.

Communicable diseases and infectious diseases in immigrants can be classified as common infections (such as respiratory infections and vaccine-preventable diseases); transmissible infections (HIV, TB, syphilis), and infections which are more typical of tropical areas, such as typhoid fever (more frequent in immigrants from the Indian subcontinent), malaria (in refugees from Southeast Asia), schistosomiasis and filariasis (in West Africans), and cysticercosis and

Infectious Diseases: A Geographic Guide, First Edition.
Edited by Eskild Petersen, Lin H. Chen & Patricia Schlagenhauf.
© 2011 John Wiley & Sons, Ltd. Published 2011 by John Wiley & Sons, Ltd.

Chagas' disease (in Latin Americans) [3,4]. Most migrants are healthy, young adults, but they often bear a disproportionate burden of infectious diseases [5].

Measles

According to WHO data, more than 20 million people are affected by measles each year and more than 95% of deaths occur in countries with low per capita incomes. Even though measles vaccination has led to a decrease in measles cases and deaths worldwide, outbreaks have recently occurred even in developed countries following conventional travel (tourism) and travel for international adoption, in unvaccinated students returning from developing countries, and in specific migrant populations [6]. Recent data from the WHO European region reflect how national vaccination programs have led to interruption of several indigenous chains of transmission. However, cases have also been associated with virus importation from other continents where measles is highly endemic and this may lead to prolonged circulation and spread after introduction into high-risk unvaccinated mobile populations [7]. A measles outbreak with >20,000 reported cases has been ongoing since 2009 in Bulgaria, and clusters of cases have been reported from several other European countries such as Poland, Slovenia, Ireland, Italy, Germany, and Greece [8]. Many of these cases have occurred in members of the migrant Roma population where vaccination coverage is low, highlighting the need for specific initiatives focusing on members of the community who are currently hard to reach due to their mobile nature.

Rubella

The number of countries using rubella vaccine in their national immunization system has risen from 83 in 1996 to 127 in 2008 (WHO). However, adults born before the start of routine immunization may remain susceptible and there are regions where vaccination is still not included in programs, as occurs in most African countries. Rubella infection remains endemic in many areas of the world such as Latin America where vaccination was only introduced in the late 1990s. Many adult immigrants from Latin American countries to western countries will therefore not be immunized. These circumstances may lead to outbreaks as occurred in 2003, 2004, and 2005 in Madrid, Spain, mainly involving nonvaccinated populations from Latin America as well as Spanish males born before the introduction of universal measles–mumps–rubella vaccination in the early 1980s [9]. Studies of specific outbreaks are essential in order to obtain accurate data on the distribution of different rubella genotypes worldwide which may allow better management and monitoring of epidemics.

Hepatitis A

Even though hepatitis A virus (HAV) has a worldwide distribution, HAV seroprevalence is highest in less developed countries of Central and South America, Africa and Asia. As health standards improve in certain areas, a decrease in seroprevalence may be observed. Importation of HAV by immigrant VFR children and subsequent transmission to the general population in the host country has been demonstrated [10]. However, even though vaccination is recommended for at risk travelers to areas of high endemicity, enhanced vaccination programs for immigrant children to reduce importation and secondary HAV infections may only partially contribute to a decline in HAV incidence. A study carried out in the Netherlands assessing the effects of enhanced vaccination programs for HAV in migrant children concluded that causes other than vaccination could have contributed to the decline in HAV incidence seen in the Netherlands which coincided with that observed for the rest of Europe [11].

Hepatitis B

Although by the year 2006, 164 countries were vaccinating infants against hepatitis B during national immunization programs as compared with 31 countries in 1992 (WHO); prevalence of HBV infection among certain immigrant groups may be high. Although rates may vary according to country/area of origin, observed rates particularly in Asian and sub-Saharan immigrant groups are generally higher than those found in the general population in host countries of the western world. Further, several studies have shown that low-income immigrant populations may receive insufficient evaluation of their chronic hepatitis B infection and they may be undertreated [12]. Studies have also shown evidence for both vertical/perinatal and horizontal transmission of HBV infection in children born in the western world to refugee or immigrant parents from countries of high endemicity, as illustrated in studies carried out in US-born children of Hmong refugees [13]. This supports the need for specific surveillance systems in risk groups and systems to ensure adequate vaccination protocols.

Human papillomavirus

Cervical cancer is caused by persistent infection with certain high-risk oncogenic types of HPVs. This type of cancer is a major cause of morbidity and mortality worldwide, and 80% of this burden has been estimated to occur among women residing in less developed countries (PAHO). With the recent development of new vaccines for some types of HPV, immunization strategies may need to be developed in the near future to specifically include high-risk groups such as immigrant women from resource-poor countries.

Other vaccine-preventable infections such as *meningococcal disease, polio, mumps*, and *influenza* have been transmitted and imported into different areas by different types of mobile populations. Practitioners attending special risk groups should be aware of the detailed and updated information regarding the geographic distribution and prevalence of vaccine-preventable diseases in order to implement adequate and targeted control measures.

Tuberculosis

Tuberculosis (TB) remains a leading cause of morbidity and mortality worldwide. The African continent with a prevalence of 480 cases per 100,000 inhabitants is by far the most affected, followed by Southeast Asia (220 cases/100,000 inhabitants) and the Eastern Mediterranean region (150 cases/100,000 inhabitants) [14].

Migration from less developed areas of the world has led to a progressive increase in the number of cases of TB among the foreign-born population in the western world. In some countries, these cases now account for the majority of new diagnoses of TB. The risk of developing active TB is greater in patients from highly endemic countries, and reactivation is commonest in the first 2 years following migration [15]. In the United States, the proportion of total cases occurring in foreign-born persons has been increasing since 1993. In 2008, the case rate in foreign-born patients was approximately 10 times higher than among the US-born population [16].

The rate of TB among foreigners in Western Europe in 2006 was 20%. Data showed significant geographic differences, ranging from more than 50% in Iceland, Sweden, Denmark, Norway, United Kingdom, Switzerland, and the Netherlands, to less than 20% in Finland, Estonia, Latvia, Portugal, and Spain [17]. Overall, 35% of cases in foreign-born patients were from Asia, 32% from Africa, 20% from another country in Western Europe or the Balkans, and 7% from former Soviet Union countries.

In recent years, another concern has been the spread of multidrug-resistant and extensively drug-resistant tuberculosis (MDR-TB and XDR-TB), partly as a consequence of the mismanagement of infectious cases and lack of adequate prevention. In 2008, an estimated 440,000 cases of MDR-TB emerged globally resulting in 150,000 deaths (53,000 of them in HIV-infected individuals). Worldwide, 3.6% of TB cases are estimated to have MDR-TB, and around 50% of them appear to have originated from China and India. The overall proportion of MDR-TB cases with XDR-TB is estimated to be 5.4% [18].

Data estimating the impact of the migrant population on MDR-TB in western countries are scarce, but migration appears to have a clear influence on the spread of MDR-TB. A study of TB cases during 1993–1999 found 2.0% of people born outside the United Kingdom (mainly from Africa and India) had an MDR-TB isolate compared with 1.0% of those born in the United Kingdom (OR 1.97; $p<0.001$) [19]. In another study, MDR-TB and XDR-TB among foreign-born patients in California accounted for 84.6% and 83.3%, respectively, of all cases of resistant TB diagnosed during the period 1993–2006 [20] (Figure 29.1).

HIV infection

Since the HIV epidemic was first described in 1981, millions have become infected and have died worldwide. This virus, originating from Equatorial Africa, has now spread extensively in all continents, and although the rate of new cases of HIV infection has stabilized in some parts of the developed world, in other areas, especially in sub-Saharan Africa, Southeast Asia, and Eastern Europe, the number of newly infected individuals continues to rise. The introduction of highly active antiretroviral therapy (HAART) in the mid-1990s led to a dramatic decrease in mortality rates and new AIDS diagnoses in many countries. Albeit at a slower rate, the benefits of treatment are now spreading to less developed areas such as sub-Saharan Africa. The number of people living with HIV worldwide continued to grow in 2008, reaching an estimated 33.4 million. More than 50% of these cases occurred in women and children below 15 years of age accounted for 2.1 million cases. However, the epidemic affects the developing world disproportionately and sub-Saharan Africa bears the greatest burden of the disease. In 2008, this region accounted for 67% of HIV infections worldwide, 68% of new HIV infections among adults, 91% of new HIV infections among children, and 72% of the world's AIDS-related deaths. The prevalence rates in south and southeast Asia are much lower than in Africa (5.2% vs. 0.3%). However, given that 60% of the world's population lives in this region, this represents a substantial proportion of the HIV-infected population. In the year 2008, approximately 140,000 newly diagnosed HIV cases were reported from Europe. Most of them were from Eastern Europe and Central Asia (110,000) where the prevalence of HIV infection is estimated to be 0.7%, as compared to 0.3% in Western and Central Europe. In the year 2008, the number of new cases of HIV infection in North America was 55,000 (0.6% prevalence). In Latin America, the epidemic remains stable with a regional HIV prevalence of 0.6% and 170,000 new cases. Prevalence is higher in the Caribbean area (1.0%) [21–23].

Migrants from HIV-endemic countries comprise a substantial proportion of all HIV patients in western countries. They are typically younger than local HIV-infected individuals, with a greater proportion of females, and heterosexual contact is the main mode of transmission. Data on the prevalence of HIV among immigrants is scarce and the majority of studies focus on high-risk groups. In Europe, overall prevalence among immigrants is estimated to be 0.6–1% [24], accounting for 21–37% of cases. The main areas of origin for this population are sub-Saharan Africa, the Caribbean, and Latin America [25–27]. In the United States, data regarding HIV infection among the immigrant population are reported as CDC surveillance data according to race and ethnicity, rather than by country of origin. Many come from regions with high rates of HIV infection, such as Africa, Asia, and Eastern Europe. Of note, some ethnic groups, such as Hispanics and African Americans, are disproportionately affected [28,29].

Some migrant and ethnic minority populations are especially vulnerable to the harmful impact of the HIV/AIDS epidemic. Language barriers, social exclusion, and cultural and socio-economic factors can act as barriers to prompt medical attention and early diagnosis. Moreover,

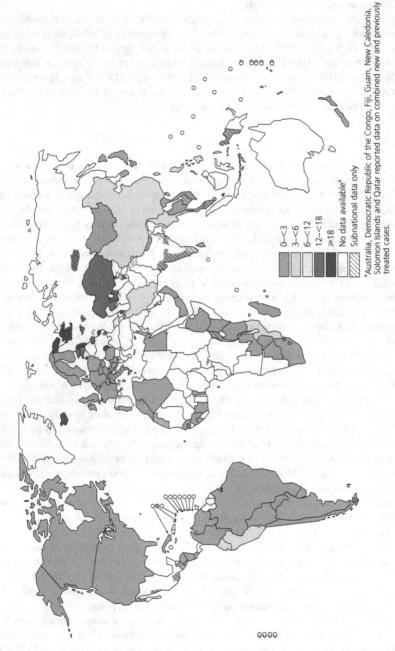

Fig. 29.1 Distribution of proportion of MDR-TB among new TB cases, 1994–2009. (Reproduced from World Health Organization [18], with permission from WHO.)

0–<3
3–<6
6–<12
12–<18
≥18
No data available[a]
Subnational data only

[a] Australia, Democratic Republic of the Congo, Fiji, Guam, New Caledonia, Solomon Islands and Qatar reported data on combined new and previously treated cases.

HIV infection in immigrants may present certain features that should be borne in mind by health-care professionals. These include the higher prevalence of non-B subtypes, different reference ranges for laboratory tests, concomitant imported infections, different AIDS-defining illnesses, different patterns of HBV/HCV coinfection, slower disease progression, differential response to antiretrovirals, and different tolerance to antiretroviral drug adverse effects and HIV-associated symptoms [30–32].

Chagas' disease (American trypanosomiasis)

Chagas' disease results from infection with the protozoan parasite *Trypanosoma cruzi*. The parasite is mainly transmitted to humans through the infected feces of triatomine bugs (vectorial transmission) and less frequently through vertical transmission, transfusion, or organ transplantation from an infected donor, and more rarely through oral contamination and laboratory accidents.

After infection, the acute phase is usually asymptomatic and rarely presents with severe disease (myocarditis or encephalomyelitis with 5–10% mortality without treatment). Infected individuals then enter an asymptomatic chronic phase, with positive serology and fluctuating parasitemia. The majority of patients are in this phase and may transmit the disease. After 10–30 years, around 20–35% of patients develop symptoms, mainly characterized by cardiac (20–30%) and/or gastrointestinal (10%) involvement. Clinical follow-up requires chest X-ray, electrocardiogram, echocardiogram, barium enema or barium swallow, and repeated serology and *T. cruzi*-PCR. Some patients will require pacemakers, defibrillators, and even heart transplantation. Treatment with benznidazole (or nifurtimox) has been shown to be effective in infants and in the acute phase of the disease, but the efficacy declines with the duration of infection. Treatment in the late chronic phase remains controversial as tolerance is poor and about 30% abandon treatment due to adverse reactions. Based on nonrandomized trials demonstrating a significant decrease in disease progression and mortality in treated adults, there is an increasing tendency to offer treatment with benznidazole to every patient under age 50 years, without severe cardiac involvement, who has not previously received a correct treatment course. A multicenter, randomized, placebo-controlled trial in patients with early Chagas' heart disease is currently under way (BENEFIT study) [33].

Chagas' disease is endemic in countries of the American continent from Mexico to the north of Argentina and Chile, and affects 8–10 million, the majority in rural areas. Bolivia, with a population of 9 million, has the highest prevalence of the disease, with more than 180,000 cases annually [34].

From the 1960s to the 1980s, there was a large flux of immigrants from Latin America to North America, Australia, and Japan. However, from the 1990s, there has been a dramatic increase in immigration to Western Europe. Due to international migration, Chagas' disease is no longer limited to the Latin American continent and has emerged in North America, in the Western Pacific (Australia and Japan) and in Western Europe (mainly in Spain) (Figure 29.2). Those who migrate seeking work opportunities and wanting to improve their quality of life are usually healthy and younger than the general population. Most Latin Americans will have been infected with *T. cruzi* during childhood and therefore, based on the natural course of the disease, these migrants would now be at an age when the first manifestations of cardiac involvement may be expected to appear.

The number of infected immigrants may be inferred from national infection rates for each country of origin. Up to 20% of patients with Chagas' disease will have clinical manifestations and may require health assistance. Taking these figures into account the burden of Chagas' disease in the main host countries may be estimated [35].

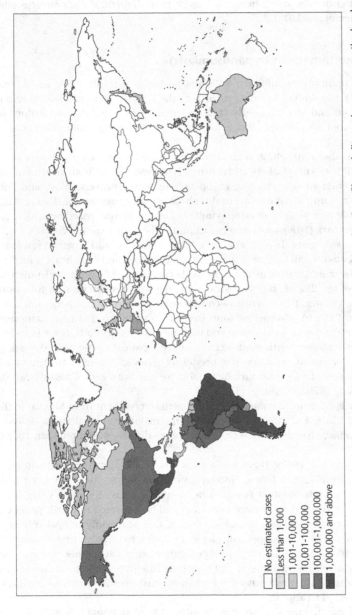

Fig. 29.2 Estimated global population infected by *T. cruzi*, 2009. As a consequence of immigration, Chagas' disease has overcome the borders of the Latin American endemic countries and has settled in North America, Western Europe, and Western Pacific regions. (Reproduced from http://www.treatchagas.org/ with permission from Drugs for Neglected Diseases Initiative (DNDi).)

No estimated cases
Less than 1,000
1,001–10,000
10,001–100,000
100,001–1,000,000
1,000,000 and above

More than 44 million Latin Americans (the majority from Mexico) live in the United States. An estimated 325,000 of these immigrants are infected and more than 65,000 may develop symptoms of the infection. In Canada, there are more than 400,000 Latin Americans: around 5,500 may be infected and 1,100 may be symptomatic.

In Japan, there are 116,000 immigrants from endemic areas: 81,000 of these are from Brazil and up to 3,500 may be infected. In Australia, around 1,400 out of 80,000 immigrants from endemic areas may be infected, and 600 of these may be symptomatic.

Officially, there are 2,600,000 Latin American immigrants in the EU15 (2,090,000 in Spain and 483,000 in the other EU15 countries). Conservative estimates indicate there are more than 121,000 infected immigrants, and 87,000 of these are living in Spain. Infection rates in Spain are around 5% due to the large proportion of Bolivian immigrants from hyperendemic areas such as the mid-altitude valleys of Cochabamba, Chuquisaca, and Santa Cruz. In the other EU15 countries, there are approximately 14,000 infected immigrants (2.9% infection rate). Out of these infected immigrants, more than 20,000 are estimated to be symptomatic (17,400 in Spain alone). Seroprevalence studies of Latin American immigrants in specialized clinics in Spain found rates of 31–41% with a 25% visceral involvement rate (20% with cardiac and 5% with gastrointestinal involvement).

An infected pregnant woman may transmit the parasite to the fetus throughout pregnancy and at delivery. In Spain, the majority of infected immigrants are female Bolivians in their 30s, and therefore of childbearing age. In Spain, seroprevalence in pregnant Latin Americans is 3–4% (18% in Bolivians) and vertical transmission rates vary from 1.3% to 7.3% according to different series. National screening protocols for pregnant women should be established and in an attempt to decrease vertical transmission, chronically infected nonpregnant women of child-bearing age may be offered treatment. Since the treatment of pregnant women with benzni-dazole and nifurtimox is currently contraindicated, early detection (by PCR) and treatment of congenital infections is recommended.

The risk of *T. cruzi* transmission from an infected blood transfusion is estimated to be 20%, and this may vary depending on the concentration of parasites in donor blood, the type of blood product transfused (higher risk of transmission with platelet transfusions), or the parasite strain. Cases of *T. cruzi* infection acquired via blood transfusion have been reported in Europe and in the United States. Since 2005, screening of at risk blood donations for *T. cruzi* has been implemented in Spain and from the year 2007, the CDC recommends screening of all donated blood in the United States. To avoid transfusion-associated *T. cruzi* infections, all countries should develop strategies to identify and exclude those who may pose a transmission risk and refer them for further management.

Severe and fatal cases of *T. cruzi* infection following organ, tissue, and cell transplantation have been reported outside endemic countries, highlighting the need for screening protocols in all transplantation centers. Cardiac transplantation from a donor with chronic Chagas' disease is contraindicated given the high risk of chagasic myocarditis in the recipient following immuno-suppression. There is currently no consensus regarding the use of other organs from infected donors. Severe/fatal reactivation of Chagas' disease has been reported in immigrants with chronic *T. cruzi* infection and immunosuppression (HIV/AIDS associated or drug induced). For the pre-vention of reactivation, screening and treatment of such patients, if appropriate, is recommended.

Cases of acute Chagas' disease have also been reported in western citizens returning from endemic countries. This highlights the need for specific pretravel counseling regarding the risk of vector, oral (food-borne), and transfusion-associated transmission of *T. cruzi* in endemic Latin American countries.

Access to specialized clinics for diagnosis and management of chagasic patients and pre-ventive strategies are essential given the burden of the disease and the potential public health repercussions in nonendemic countries [36].

References

1. International Organization for Migration. Available from http://www.iom.int/jahia/ Jahia/about-migration/facts-and-figures.
2. Barnett ED, Walker PF. Role of immigrants and migrants in emerging infectious diseases. Med Clin North Am 2008;92:1447–58.
3. Wilson ME. Diseases by country of origin. In: Walker PF and Barnett ED (eds). Immigrant Medicine, 1st edn. Philadelphia, USA: Saunders Elsevier, 2007:189–216.
4. Monge-Maillo B, Jiménez BC, Pérez-Molina JA, Norman F, et al. Imported infectious diseases in mobile populations, Spain. Emerg Infect Dis 2009;15:1745–52.
5. Health Protection Agency. Migrant health. Infectious diseases in non-UK born populations in England, Wales and Northern Ireland. 2006. Available from www.hpa.org.uk/publi cations/2006/migrant_health/default.htm.
6. Chen LH, Wilson ME. The role of the traveler in emerging infections and magnitude of travel. Med Clin N Am 2008;92:1409–32.
7. Kremer JR, Brown KE, Jin L, et al. High genetic diversity of measles virus, World Health Organization European Region, 2005–2006. Emerg Infe Dis 2008;14:107–114.
8. Pervanidou D, Horefti E, Patrinos S, et al. Spotlight on measles 2010 ongoing measles outbreak in Greece, January–July 2010. Euro Surveill 2010;15:pii=19629.
9. Martínez-Torres AO, Mosquera MM, Sanz JC, et al. Phylogenetic analysis of Rubella virus strains from an outbreak in Madrid, Spain, from 2004 to 2005. J Clin Microbiol 2009; 47:158–63.
10. Van Steenbergen JE, Tijon G, Van Den A, et al. Two years prospective collection of molecular and epidemiological data shows limited spread of hepatitis A virus outside risk groups in Amsterdam, 2000–2002. J Infect Dis 2004;189: 471–82.
11. Suijkerbuijk AW, Lindeboom R, van Steenbergen JE, et al. Effect of hepatitis A vaccination programs for migrant children on the incidence of hepatitis A in the Netherlands. Eur J Public Health 2009;19:240–4.
12. Pérez-Molina JA, Herrero-Martínez JM, Norman F, et al. Clinical and epidemiological characteristics and indications for liver biopsy and treatment in immigrants with chronic hepatitis B at a referral hospital in Madrid. J Viral Hepatol 2010 (in press).
13. Hurie MB, Mast EE, Davis JP. Horizontal transmission of hepatitis B virus infection to United States-born children of Hmong refugees. Pediatrics 1992;89:269–73.
14. World Health Organization. Global Tuberculosis Control: a short update to the 2009 report. WHO/HTM/TB/2009.426.2009.
15. Cain KP, Benoit SR, Winston CA, Mac Kenzie WR. Tuberculosis among foreign-born persons in the United States. JAMA 2008;300:405–412.
16. CDC. Reported tuberculosis in the United States, 2008. Atlanta, GA: US Department of Health and Human Services, CDC, September 2009.
17. EuroTB and the national coordinators for tuberculosis surveillance in the WHO European Region. Surveillance of tuberculosis in Europe. Report on tuberculosis cases notified in 2006. Institut de veille sanitaire, Saint-Maurice, France, March 2008.
18. World Health Organization. Multidrug and extensively drug-resistant TB (M/XDR-TB): 2010 global report on surveillance and response. WHO/HTM/TB/2010.3. 2010.
19. Djuretic T, Herbert J, Drobniewski F, et al. Antibiotic resistant tuberculosis in the United Kingdom: 1993–1999. Thorax 2002;57:477–82.
20. Banerjee R, Allen J, Westenhouse J, et al. Extensively drug-resistant tuberculosis in california, 1993–2006. Clin Infect Dis 2008;47:450–7.
21. Quinn TC. HIV epidemiology and the effects of antiviral therapy on long-term consequences. AIDS 2008;22(Suppl 3):S7–12.
22. World Health Organization. AIDS epidemic update: November 2009. UNAIDS/09.36E/ JC1700E, 2009.
23. European Centre for Disease Prevention and Control/WHO Regional Office for Europe. HIV/AIDS surveillance in Europe 2007. Stockolm: European Centre for Disease Prevention and Control/WHO Regional Office for Europe, 2008.
24. Pezzoli MC, Hamad IE, Scarcella C, et al. HIV infection among illegal migrants, Italy, 2004–2007. Emerg Infect Dis 2009;15:1802–4.
25. Del Amo J, Broring G, Hamers FF, Infuso A, Fenton K. Monitoring HIV/AIDS in Europe's migrant communities and ethnic minorities. AIDS 2004;18:1867–73.
26. Staehelin C, Rickenbach M, Low N, et al. Migrants from Sub-Saharan Africa in the Swiss HIV Cohort Study: access to antiretroviral

therapy, disease progression and survival. AIDS 2003;17:2237–44.

27. Vigilancia epidemiológica del VIH en España. Valoración de los nuevos diagnósticos de VIH en España a partir de los sistemas de notificación de casos de la CCAA. Periodo 2003–2008. Actualización 30 de junio de 2009. Accessed 9 August, 2010 at http://www.isciii.es/htdocs/pdf/nuevos_diagnosticos_ccaa.pdf.

28. CDC Division of HIV/AIDS Prevention. MMWR Analysis Provides New Details on HIV Incidence in US Populations, September 2008. Available from http://www.cdc.gov/hiv/topics/surveillance/resources/factsheets/pdf/mmwr-incidence.pdf

29. Fakoya I, Reynolds R, Caswell G, Shiripinda I. Barriers to HIV testing for migrant black Africans in Western Europe. HIV Med 2008;9 (Suppl 2):23–5.

30. Perez-Molina J, Mora-Rillo M, Suarez-Lozano I, et al. Do HIV-infected immigrants initiating HAART have poorer treatment-related outcomes than autochthonous patients in Spain? Results of the GESIDA 5808 study. Curr HIV Res 2010 Oct 1;8(7):521–30.

31. Silverberg MJ, Jacobson LP, French AL, Witt MD, Gange SJ. Age and racial/ethnic differences in the prevalence of reported symptoms in human immunodeficiency virus-infected persons on antiretroviral therapy. J Pain Symptom Manage 2009;38:197–207.

32. Tedaldi EM, Absalon J, Thomas AJ, Shlay JC, van den Berg-Wolf M. Ethnicity, race, and gender. Differences in serious adverse events among participants in an antiretroviral initiation trial: results of CPCRA 058 (FIRST Study). J Acquir Immune Defic Syndr 2008;47:441–8.

33. Pérez de Ayala A, Pérez-Molina JA, Norman F, López-Vélez R. Chagasic cardiomyopathy in immigrants from Latin America to Spain. Emerg Infect Dis 2009;15:607–8.

34. Coura JR, Albajar P. Chagas disease: a new worldwide challenge. Nature Outlook, june 2010: S6–S8. The Nature Outlook Chagas Disease suplement: www.nature.com/nature/supplement/outlooks/Chagas.

35. Schmunis GA, Yadon ZE. Chagas disease: a Latin American health problem becoming a world health problem. Acta Tropica 2010;115:14–21.

36. WHO. Control and prevention of Chagas disease in Europe. Report of a WHO Informal Consultation (jointly organized by WHO headquarters and the WHO Regional Office for Europe). Geneva, Switzerland, December 17–18, 2009. WHO/HTM/NTD/IDM/2010.1. Available from http://www.fac.org.ar/1/comites/chagas/Chagas_WHO_Technical%20Report_16_06_10.pdf.

Chapter 30
Climate change and the geographical distribution of infectious diseases

David Harley, Ashwin Swaminathan and Anthony J. McMichael

National Centre for Epidemiology and Population Health, Australian National University, Canberra, Australia

Some infectious agents, cytomegalovirus for example, are ubiquitous in human populations, whereas most are limited in their geographical distribution. Some infectious diseases occur readily all year round; others have a strong seasonal association.

A major limiting influence on these spatial and temporal variations is the climate. Temperature, rainfall, humidity, and consequent physical and ecological characteristics of the environment set limits on the occurrence of a particular infectious disease. However, many other social, cultural, behavioral, technological, biological, and environmental factors act to determine where that infectious disease actually does occur.

A new and potent variable is now entering the equation: namely, climate *change*. Determining the extent to which climate change has altered and will alter the distribution of infectious diseases of humans is therefore a new and important challenge. Answers will often not come easily, but this vital challenge must be addressed.

Human-induced climate change is now regarded, with near-unanimous shared understanding and agreement among climate scientists, as both real and manifestly happening (see http://www.metoffice.gov.uk/corporate/pressoffice/2010/pr20100728.html). Further, on current evidence and trajectories, it seems increasingly likely that global average temperature will increase by about 3°C by later this century [1]. This will inevitably affect the geography and temporality of various infectious diseases, such as airborne, waterborne, food-borne, and vector-borne diseases.

Mechanisms for climate-induced change in infectious disease incidence

Background

Climate influences the biology of hosts, pathogens, and vectors [2]. This framework, rather than the more traditional triadic host, agent, and environment categorization, is useful in considering the effects of climate on infectious disease transmission, and will be used here.

Infectious Diseases: A Geographic Guide, First Edition.
Edited by Eskild Petersen, Lin H. Chen & Patricia Schlagenhauf.
© 2011 John Wiley & Sons, Ltd. Published 2011 by John Wiley & Sons, Ltd.

Pathogen

Viruses and bacteria survive and reproduce only under certain conditions with, for each species, limits in terms of temperature, pH, and so on. Within these limits reproduction and transmission are affected by environmental factors including temperature. Increased temperature often, though not always, increases the likelihood of human disease. Some pathogens (e.g., malaria plasmodium and dengue virus) mature more rapidly at higher temperatures while in the vector organism (mosquito).

Higher temperatures are associated with increased infection of *Culex* mosquitoes with West Nile virus in Illinois [3]. Temperature also influences colonization of chickens with *Campylobacter* [4]. In contrast, rotavirus and respiratory syncytial virus survive better at low than high temperatures [2] and *Cryptosporidium* oocysts maintained at 4°C or 15°C maintain infectivity, but at 20°C or 25°C are completely inactivated after 12 and 8 weeks, respectively [5].

Host

Climatic conditions affect many nonhuman hosts of human infectious diseases. For example, the occurrence of mosquito-borne Ross River virus disease in humans is influenced by the relation between rainfall, vegetation, and, hence, reproduction in kangaroos—a major reservoir species for this virus [2,6]. The water snail *Oncomelania hupensis*, an important host for *Schistosoma japonicum* in China [7], is sensitive to temperature, which affects the proportion of snails hibernating and, indeed, surviving during winter [8].

Vector

Temperature influences mosquito populations. For example, in Kenya the abundance of *Anopheles funestus* is increased at higher temperatures, while for another malaria vector, *Anopheles gambiae*, there is a (nonsignificant) negative correlation [9]. Under experimental conditions, *A. gambiae* and its sibling species *Anopheles arabiensis* demonstrate highest larval survival to adulthood at 25°C, with progressively lower survival at 30°C and 35°C, though for *A. arabiensis* the relation of temperature and survival is modified when reared with *A. gambiae* [10]. Temperature (in combination with humidity) also affects mosquito biting rate, and high temperatures limit mosquito longevity and survival.

Implication

Clearly, there are many, varied, mechanisms whereby climate change can influence the occurrence of infectious diseases. More difficult to determine, though, is whether climate change has changed, and how much it will in future change, the distribution of infectious diseases.

The context: human actions and disease emergence

Human actions

The prevalence and geographic distribution of an infectious disease depends on appropriate conditions for growth, survival, and transmission of pathogens. A suitable climate (i.e., providing optimal temperature, humidity, and rainfall) plays a critical role, as do human activity, behavior and demographics, population movement, and the nature of the built environment.

There are countless examples of public health measures that have contained or eradicated disease in areas once conducive to infection transmission. These measures include mass vaccination (e.g., polio), vector control (e.g., insecticide spraying), early detection (surveillance) and treatment of index cases, and effective public policy (e.g., food safety standards and quarantine measures). Via combinations of these measures countries such as Australia (in 1981) could be declared malaria free, despite a receptive climate in the tropical north and the continuing presence of competent *Anopheles* mosquito vectors [11].

Globalization of travel and trade are also important contributors for infectious disease transmission. The severe acute respiratory syndrome (SARS) epidemic of 2003 [12] and H1N1 influenza (swine flu) pandemic of 2009/2010 [13] dramatically demonstrated how air travel (in particular) can quickly disseminate disease that once may have been contained or slowed by geographic or climatic constraints. There have also been prominent examples where infections or vectors have been spread via trade. *Aedes albopictus* (Asian tiger mosquito), able to carry alpha- and flavi-viruses, is native to Southeast Asia; however, it has been introduced by trade routes to Europe, the Americas, and Africa where it is now endemic [14].

The increasing worldwide trend of urbanization and the development of "megacities" (e.g., Mumbai, Mexico City, and Tokyo) can also contribute to disease propagation, particularly where water, sanitation, and health infrastructure and services have not kept up with increasing population demand [15]. Additionally, the microclimates within cities, such as the urban "heat island" effect wherein the oft-dense built environment is warmer than rural surrounds due to heat retention and lack of vegetation, can alter the distribution of infection [16] and/or make populations more susceptible to infection due to heat stress [17].

Disease emergence

The rate of emergence of apparently new human and animal pathogens has increased over the past four decades, with HIV being the most catastrophic for human health [18]. While pathogen evolution and biology is undoubtedly important in such emergence [19], climate and land use change also play a role [20]. The phenomenon of disease emergence provides an important stimulus for understanding the relation of climate change, often interacting with other global changes, to infectious disease risk. The complex interplay between climate change and social and ecological changes must be understood ecologically and historically if humans are to coexist, as they must, with microbes [21].

Human-induced climate change

Paleoclimatological records show that over the past 2.6 million years of the current ice age, Earth has fluctuated between glacial (cold) and interglacial (warm) periods. These changes at a global level have occurred gradually, over millennia, and have resulted from natural phenomena, such as alterations in Earth's orbit and axial tilt, varying volcanic and solar activity, and changes to marine life distribution and density [22].

However, a sharp rise in average global surface temperature has been observed in recent decades—the rapidity of which is exceptional in the paleoclimatological record. This coincides with a similarly unprecedented increase in the atmospheric concentration of carbon dioxide (CO_2), resulting from the emissions arising from increasingly intensive human industrial activity. The trapping of solar energy by CO_2 and other "greenhouse gases" (GHGs) within the lower atmosphere has led to the range of climatic impacts recently observed (see Box 30.1).

Box 30.1 Observed changes in climate

- Increasing global surface temperature—0.74°C increase over the period 1906–2005; temperatures have increased most rapidly since the mid-1970s.
- The most recent 13 consecutive years (1997–2008) are among the 14 warmest years on record (since 1850 when instrument measurements became available)[a].
- Global average sea level has risen an average 1.8 mm per year over the period 1961–2003; and 3.1 mm per year over the more recent subperiod 1993–2003.
- Extreme weather events have changed in frequency and intensity over the past 50 years— increase in heat waves, hot days and nights, heavy precipitation events; and decrease in cold days, nights, and frosts.
- Changes have not occurred uniformly around the world—there have been significant regional climate differences observed.

Source: IPCC 4AR (2007) [22].
[a]United States National Climate Data Center; www.ncdc.noaa.gov.

The Intergovernmental Panel on Climate Change (IPCC) has developed projections for global average surface temperature based on the emissions that would occur under several future development scenarios (i.e., linking demographic, economic, and technological change with likely resultant GHG emissions). Across the range of internationally agreed scenarios, as inputs to global climate models (GCMs), global temperatures are projected to rise between 1.8°C and 4.0°C by the decade 2090–2099 (compared with the period 1980–1999). Ongoing international negotiations aim to limit global temperature rise to within 2°C by regulating global emissions of GHGs [23].

Future climate change will not occur uniformly across the globe—there will be significant regional differences. It is likely that developing world populations will be most vulnerable due to both significant exposures to the physical elements of climate change and a limited economic and social capacity to positively respond and adapt to change.

A framework for understanding the relation of climate and disease

Modes of infectious disease transmission can be classified in two dimensions: anthroponoses and zoonoses; and direct and indirect modes of transmission, respectively [2]. To understand and analyze climate–disease relations for these different transmission mechanisms, a theoretical framework for climate effects encompassing differing modes of transmission is necessary. Such a framework should account for other factors outlined earlier, including social factors, land use change, pathogen evolution, and so on. Hierarchical conceptual frameworks [24] provide a basis for this (Figures 30.1 and 30.2).

Simple models such as those described earlier, necessarily omitting various lesser influences, are nonetheless sufficiently generalizable to provide a framework for understanding disease causation in different geographical areas and on different timescales.

The present: climate–disease relations

Vector-borne diseases

A key consideration in the theoretical assessment of putative associations between climate change and vector-borne diseases is the basic reproductive number (R_0), which determines

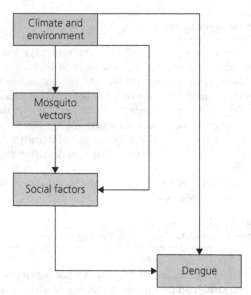

Fig. 30.1 Climate and transmission of dengue virus.

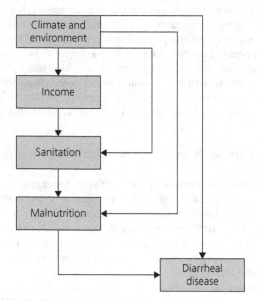

Fig. 30.2 Climate and diarrheal disease [modified after reference 24].

whether disease cases increase or decrease in a population [25]. Because arthropods are sensitive to temperature and other climatic variables, and because all except one (rate of recovery from infection for the vertebrate host) of the parameters that determine R_0 for vector-borne diseases are related to vector biology, one would expect changes in climate to influence the incidence of vector-borne diseases [25].

Several other groups of arthropods as well as mosquitoes transmit human diseases [26]. However, the same general principles apply when considering climate–disease relations among diseases transmitted by all arthropods. Only the mosquito-transmitted diseases, malaria (the most important human disease transmitted by mosquitoes) and dengue (the most significant mosquito-borne arbovirus disease of humans), are considered here.

Malaria   At a global scale malaria has receded in geographical extent in the period 1900–2002, though the population at risk has increased in absolute numbers [27]. While maps may display changes in latitude well, they are less able to show changes in the altitudinal range of infectious diseases. Much of the interest in relation to climate change and malaria is whether the disease will move to higher altitudes—and in some cases impinge on large urban populations currently at low risks (e.g., Nairobi and Harare). Many studies have been done in the eastern African highlands (reviewed in [28]), in mountainous regions of South America, and in parts of South Asia. There are, as yet, no clear-cut instances of climate-attributable changes in the local geography of malaria.

Particular attention has been paid to parts of eastern Africa [29–32]. No scientific consensus has yet emerged as to how best to model and analyze the data. There has been recurring debate over the relevant scale of analysis, the quality of some data sets, the choice of biologically based versus statistical–empirical models (see later), and whether or not the seeming absence of clear-cut climate impacts on malaria in the twentieth century provides an important basis for expectation in the twenty-first century.

Dengue   The geographic range for dengue epidemics is expanding [33]. While Halstead [34] doubts that climate change will increase the incursion of dengue into temperate regions, Hales and others [35], writing in 2002 on the basis of modeling using vapor pressure as a predictor variable for dengue, concluded that "geographical limits of dengue fever transmission are strongly determined by climate" and that climate change will substantially increase the proportion of the global population at risk from dengue.

Food- and water-borne infections

Food- and water-borne disease, usually manifested by diarrheal syndromes, are very sensitive to climate variability. A changing climate can alter the incidence of enteric infections either directly, via effects of climatic variables (e.g., temperature, precipitation, and humidity) on organism proliferation or survival, or indirectly, via effects on sanitation, water and food quality, and outdoor activity patterns (e.g., swimming).

Studies from widely spread geographic locations and including developed and developing world countries have shown a correlation between increasing ambient temperatures and diarrheal disease [36–39]. For example, a European study assessing diarrheal notifications secondary to *Salmonella* spp. infection showed a linear increase in notifications with every 1°C rise in ambient temperature above 6°C, with the maximal effect apparent for temperature 1 week before the onset of illness [40]. A weaker association has been found with *Campylobacter* spp. infection and raised ambient temperature [41]. The effect of temperature can of course be negated by improved food safety practices and public health measures [42].

Indirectly, climate can affect rates of diarrheal disease particularly via extreme events (e.g., severe storms, flooding, and droughts) which can overload the capacity of sanitation systems, contaminate or reduce the availability of safe drinking water, and lead to overcrowded and displaced populations [43]. Increasing sea water temperatures are related to algal blooms which in turn can lead to increased water concentrations of *Vibrio cholerae* and subsequent outbreaks. Outbreaks of cholera have been linked to El Niño events, particularly in South Asia [44].

For the above-mentioned reasons, it is likely that morbidity from diarrheal disease resulting via climate change associated phenomena will be significant, particularly in the developing world. Indeed, the World Health Organization's Global Burden of Disease (2002) [45] report estimated that 47,000 diarrhea-related deaths globally were attributable to climate change in the year 2000 alone.

Respiratory infections

In temperate climates, mortality rates exhibit strong seasonal cycles with winter months associated with higher rates relative to summer months [46]. Infectious respiratory diseases such as influenza and pneumonia play a significant role in this [47]. Aerosol and droplet transmission of respiratory infectious agents may be facilitated by colder conditions, as individuals are more likely to be in closer proximity indoors or in areas with inadequate ventilation. As temperate regions are projected to experience milder (warmer) winters under future climate change conditions, some predict that respiratory infection incidence will decrease [48]. However, as the relationship between ambient temperature and respiratory infectious disease transmission involves complex host–pathogen–environment interactions, the degree to which future climate change may affect rates of infection-related morbidity has not yet been quantified.

Researchers have shown an association between influenza epidemics and the strongest naturally occurring source of interannual climate variability of global consequence—the El Niño Southern Oscillation (ENSO) [49,50]. Zaraket et al. [50] demonstrated that peak influenza activity in Japan over the period 1983–2007 occurred earlier in ENSO years than in non-ENSO years [50]. In France and the United States over the period 1971–1997, deaths from pneumonia and influenza were significantly higher in those years associated with the cold cycle of the ENSO phenomenon [49].

Other environmentally sensitive respiratory infections may also be affected by climate change. Recent reports from Europe and the United States suggest that increased incidence of *Legionella* pneumonia follows humid, warmer weather and heavy precipitation events [51,52]. Also, in a warming climate, reliance on air-conditioning may lead to increased human exposure to *Legionella*-contaminated cooling towers.

Although the direct effect of climate change on the transmission of respiratory infections may be mild, if not slightly beneficial, there may be increased susceptibility to respiratory infections in regions where climate change contributes to increased air pollution (i.e., ground level ozone) or exacerbates underlying comorbidities through increased ambient temperatures [53]. Under more extreme future scenarios of population displacement, due to climate change and its environmental consequences, increased crowding in slums, shanty towns, and temporary settlements would amplify the risk of infection transmission—respiratory, gastrointestinal and, perhaps, sexually transmitted diseases [54].

The future: projections for infectious disease incidence

Projecting likely climate-related changes in disease incidence is fraught with difficulty, both because of uncertainties in predicting future climate variability and the complex interplay between climate and infectious diseases, and the social, ecological, evolutionary, and other changes that are occurring at local, national, and global scales. Nonetheless, projections can provide valuable insights into the likely direction and magnitude of change in infectious disease incidence, which are important for planning future mitigation and adaptation strategies.

Modeling the effect of climate change on infectious disease incidence is a reductionist process—it simulates a highly complex, dynamic process by substitution with simpler, well elucidated and fundamental relationships. The two principal modeling approaches are the biological (or mechanistic) and the empirical (or statistical).

Biological approaches involve the incorporation of knowledge of biological mechanisms of infectious disease transmission into a mathematical model to make projections. For example, formulas describing mosquito reproductive cycles (with parameters including ambient temperature, humidity, and rainfall) have been used to model mosquito population density under various future climate scenarios [55] and transmissibility of mosquito-borne infections by calculation of "vectorial capacity" [47].

Empirical modeling applies the statistical equation derived from the current relationship between climatic exposures and disease outcome to the extrapolation of future disease occurrence under varying projected climate conditions. The strength of this method is that it "captures" and incorporates a host of biological, climatic, ecological, and societal processes—however, the assumption that the relationship will remain static under future climate scenarios is also a major weakness. Examples of this type of modeling include the work of Hales et al. [35] who ascertained that the historic geographic distribution of dengue is statistically related to atmospheric water vapor pressure (a surrogate marker for humidity). Using this knowledge the investigators projected the potential distribution of dengue under future population and climate change projections. Future malaria incidence under varying climate conditions have also been modeled [56], which may serve as potential early warning systems for disease outbreak.

The main limitations of current models—and source of much criticism—is that projections of disease incidence do not allow for changes in the climate exposure–disease relationship due to intervention (i.e., vector clearance and public health measures), evolving ecology, or changes in host immunity (among numerous other factors) [57]. There are valid arguments both for greater sophistication in modeling approaches on the one hand and also for feasible and pragmatic approaches that can provide projections, albeit subject to criticisms, in the present.

Conclusions

Anthropogenic climate change is now accepted by all reputable scientists. Uncertainty persists regarding the magnitude of some effects. Debate will continue on current and future impacts on infectious disease incidence and distribution. While it is implausible that there will be no impacts, determining the magnitude of these impacts is a daunting task—principally because of the difficulty inherent in determining the relation and relative magnitude of climatic and other factors influencing infectious disease epidemiology in the present and the uncertainty in projections for future climate. This uncertainty is compounded by the complex interaction between climate and other factors outlined in this chapter, including interspecific competition between malaria vector species, emerging infectious diseases, and the changing impact of human interventions, resistance to antimalarials being a prime example.

In order to value the future, we must attempt prediction of future disease incidence on the basis of past and current climate–disease associations. Only by making projections can the costs and benefits for mitigation and adaptation strategies be determined, and decisions be made regarding the relative value of mitigation and adaptation by allowing these strategies to be weighed against other health interventions in the present.

References

1. Rockstrom J, Steffen W, Noone K, et al. A safe operating space for humanity. Nature 2009; 461(7263):472–5.

2. McMichael AJ, Woodruff RE. Climate change and infectious diseases. In: Mayer KH, Pizer HF (eds). The Social Ecology of Infectious Diseases. Amsterdam: Elsevier, 2008:378–407.

3. Ruiz MO, Chaves LF, Hamer GL, et al. Local impact of temperature and precipitation on West Nile virus infection in *Culex* species mosquitoes in northeast Illinois, USA. Parasit Vectors 2010;3(1):19; doi:10.1186/1756-3305-3-19.

4. Guerin MT, Martin SW, Reiersen J, et al. Temperature-related risk factors associated with the

colonization of broiler-chicken flocks with *Campylobacter* spp. in Iceland, 2001–2004. Prev Vet Med 2008;86(1–2):14–29.

5. King BJ, Keegan AR, Monis PT, Saint CP. Environmental temperature controls *Cryptosporidium* oocyst metabolic rate and associated retention of infectivity. Appl Environ Microbiol 2005;71(7):3848–57.

6. Harley D, Sleigh A, Ritchie S. Ross River virus transmission, infection and disease: a cross-disciplinary review. Clin Microbiol Rev 2001; 14(4):909–32.

7. Ross AG, Sleigh AC, Li Y, et al. Schistosomiasis in the People's Republic of China: prospects and challenges for the 21st century. Clin Microbiol Rev 2001;14(2):270–95.

8. Zhou X-N, Yang G-J, Yang K, et al. Potential impact of climate change on schistosomiasis transmission in China. Am J Trop Med Hyg 2008;78(2):188–94.

9. Kelly-Hope LA, Hemingway J, McKenzie FE. Environmental factors associated with the malaria vectors *Anopheles gambiae* and *Anopheles funestus* in Kenya. Malar J 2009;8:268; doi:10.1186/1475-2875-8-268.

10. Kirby MJ, Lindsay SW. Effect of temperature and inter-specific competition on the development and survival of *Anopheles gambiae* sensu stricto and *An. arabiensis* larvae. Acta Trop 2009;109(2):118–23.

11. Bryan J, Foley D, Sutherst R. Malaria transmission and climate change in Australia. Med J Aust 1996;164:345–7.

12. Peiris JS, Guan Y, Yuen KY. Severe acute respiratory syndrome. Nat Med 2004;10(12 Suppl.):S88–97.

13. Tang JW, Shetty N, Lam TT. Features of the new pandemic influenza A/H1N1/2009 virus: virology, epidemiology, clinical and public health aspects. Curr Opin Pulm Med 2010; 16(3):235–41.

14. Gratz NG. Critical review of the vector status of *Aedes albopictus*. Med Vet Entomol 2004; 18(3):215–27.

15. Kraas F. Megacities as global risk areas. In: Marzluff J, Shulenberger E, Endlicher W, et al. (eds). Urban Ecology: An International Perspective on the Interaction between Humans and Nature. New York: Springer, 2008:14.

16. Kovats RS, Hajat S. Heat stress and public health: a critical review. Annu Rev Public Health 2008;29:41–55.

17. Bouchama A. The 2003 European heat wave. Intensive Care Med 2004;30(1):1–3.

18. Jones KE, Patel NG, Levy MA, et al. Global trends in emerging infectious diseases. Nature 2008;451(7181):990–3.

19. Antia R, Regoes RR, Koella JC, Bergstrom CT. The role of evolution in the emergence of infectious diseases. Nature 2003;426(6967):658–61.

20. Patz JA, Olson SH, Uejio CK, Gibbs HK. Disease emergence from global climate and land use change. Med Clin North Am 2008;92(6): 1473–91.

21. McMichael AJ. Ecological and social influences on emergence and resurgence of infectious diseases. In: Sleigh AC, Leng CH, Yeo BSA, Hong PK, Safman R (eds). Population Dynamics and Infectious Diseases in Asia. Singapore: World Scientific Publishing, 2006:23–37.

22. IPCC. Climate Change 2007: The Physical Science Basis. Contribution of Working Group I to the Fourth Assessment Report of the Intergovernmental Panel on Climate Change. Cambridge and New York: Cambridge University Press, 2007.

23. UNFCCC (ed). Copenhagen Accord. Conference of the Parties COP-15; 2009 7–18 December 2009. Copenhagen: United Nations Framework Convention on Climate Change, 2009.

24. Victora CG, Huttly SR, Fuchs SC, Olinto MTA. The role of conceptual frameworks in epidemiological analysis: a hierarchical approach. Int J Epidemiol 1997;26(1):224–7.

25. Rogers DJ, Randolph SA. Climate change and vector-borne diseases. Adv Parasitol 2006; 62:345–84.

26. Black WCI, Kondratieff BC. Evolution of arthropod disease vectors. In: Marquardt WC (ed). Biology of Disease Vectors. Burlington, San Diego, and London: Elsevier, 2005:9–23.

27. Hay SI, Guerra CA, Tatem AJ, Noor AM, Snow RW. The global distribution and population at risk of malaria: past, present, and future. Lancet Infect Dis 2004;4(6):327–36.

28. Chaves LF, Koenraadt CJM. Climate change and highland malaria: fresh air for a hot debate. Q Rev Biol 2010;85(1):27–55.

29. Hay SI, Cox J, Rogers DJ, et al. Climate change and the resurgence of malaria in the East African highlands. Nature 2002;415: 905–9.

30. Tanser FC, Sharp B, le Sueur D. Potential effect of climate change on malaria transmission in Africa. Lancet 2003;362(9398):1792–8.

31. Rogers DJ, Randolph SE. The global spread of malaria in a future, warmer world. Science 2000;289(5485):1763–6.

32. Ebi KL, Hartman J, Chan N, McConnell J, Schlesinger M, Weyant J. Climate suitability for stable malaria transmission in Zimbabwe under different climate change scenarios. Clim Change 2005;73(3):375–93.

33. Halstead SB. Dengue. Lancet 2007;370(9599): 1644–52.

34. Halstead SB. Dengue virus–mosquito interactions. Annu Rev Entomol 2008;53(1):273–91.

35. Hales S, de Wet N, Maindonald J, Woodward A. Potential effect of population and climate changes on global distribution of dengue fever: an empirical model. Lancet 2002;360(9336): 830–4.

36. Checkley W, Epstein LD, Gilman RH, et al. Effect of El Nino and ambient temperature on hospital admissions for diarrhoeal diseases in Peruvian children. Lancet 2000;355(9202): 442–50.

37. D'Souza RM, Becker NG, Hall G, Moodie KB. Does ambient temperature affect foodborne disease? Epidemiology 2004;15(1):86–92.

38. Singh RB, Hales S, de Wet N, Raj R, Hearnden M, Weinstein P. The influence of climate variation and change on diarrheal disease in the Pacific Islands. Environ Health Perspect 2001; 109(2):155–9.

39. Zhang Y, Bi P, Hiller JE, Sun Y, Ryan P. Climate variations and bacillary dysentery in northern and southern cities of China. J Infect 2007; 55(2):194–200.

40. Kovats RS, Edward SJ, Hajat S, Armstrong BG, Ebi KL, Menne B. The effect of temperature on food poisoning: a time-series analysis of salmonellosis in ten European countries. Epidemiol Infect 2004;132:443–53.

41. Kovats RS, Edward SJ, Charron D, et al. Climate variability and campylobacter infection: an international study. Int J Biometeorol 2005;49 (4):207–14.

42. Lake IR, Gillespie IA, Bentham G, et al. A re-evaluation of the impact of temperature and climate change on foodborne illness. Epidemiol Infect 2009;137(11):1538–47.

43. Watson JT, Gayer M, Connolly MA. Epidemics after natural disasters. Emerg Infect Dis 2007;13(1):1–5.

44. Pascual M, Rodo X, Ellner SP, Colwell R, Bouma MJ. Cholera dynamics and El Nino-Southern Oscillation. Science 2000;289(5485): 1766–9.

45. McMichael AJ, Campbell-Lendrum D, Kovats S, et al. Global climate change. The World Health Report 2002. Geneva: World Health Organization,2002:1543–649.

46. de Looper M. Seasonality of Death. Bulletin No. 3. Canberra: Australian Institute of Health and Welfare, 2002. Report No.: 3.

47. Martens WJM. Climate change, thermal stress and mortality changes. Soc Sci Med 1998; 46(3):331–44.

48. Morales ME, Ocampo CB, Cadena H, Copeland CS, Termini M, Wesson DM. Differential identification of *Ascogregarina* species (Apicomplexa: Lecudinidae) in *Aedes aegypti* and *Aedes albopictus* (Diptera: Culicidae) by polymerase chain reaction. J Parasitol 2005;91 (6):1352–6.

49. Flahault A, Viboud C, Pakdamana K, et al. Association of influenza epidemics in France and the USA with global climate variability. Int Congr Ser 2004;1263:73–7.

50. Zaraket H, Saito R, Tanabe N, Taniguchi K, Suzuki H. Association of early annual peak influenza activity with El Nino southern oscillation in Japan. Influenza Other Respir Viruses 2008;2(4):127–30.

51. Fisman DN, Lim S, Wellenius GA, et al. It's not the heat, it's the humidity: wet weather increases legionellosis risk in the greater Philadelphia metropolitan area. J Infect Dis 2005;192(12):2066–73.

52. Karagiannis I, Brandsema P, Van der Sande M. Warm, wet weather associated with increased Legionnaires' disease incidence in The Netherlands. Epidemiol Infect 2009;137(2):181–7.

53. Ayres JG, Forsberg B, Annesi-Maesano I, et al. Climate change and respiratory disease: European Respiratory Society position statement. Eur Respir J 2009;34(2):295–302.

54. McMichael AJ, McMichael CE, Berry H, Bowen K. Climate change, displacement and health: Risks and responses. In: McAdam, J. (ed). Climate Change and Population Displacement: Multidisciplinary Perspectives. London: Hart Publishing, 2010.

55. Hopp MJ, Foley JA. Worldwide fluctuations in dengue fever cases related to climate variability. Clim Res 2003;25(1):85–94.

56. Thomson MC, Doblas-Reyes FJ, Mason SJ, et al. Malaria early warnings based on seasonal climate forecasts from multi-model ensembles. Nature 2006;439(7076):576–9.

57. Lafferty KD. The ecology of climate change and infectious diseases. Ecology 2009;90(4): 888–900.

Abbreviations

AIDS	Acquired Immune Deficiency Syndrome
ALT	Alanine aminotransferase
ANA	Anti-nuclear antibodies
ANCA	Anti-neutrophil cytoplasmic antibodies
AST	Aspartate aminotransferase
ATBF	African Tick Bite Fever
BAL	Bronchoalveolar Lavage
BUN	Blood urea nitrogen
CMV	Cytomegalovirus
CCHF	Crimean Congo Haemorrhagic fever
CNS	Central nervous system
COPD	Chronic Obstructive Pulmonary Disease
CRP	C-reactive protein
CRS	Congenital Rubella syndrome
CRPS	Complex regional pain syndrome
CSF	Cerebrospinal fluid
CSOM	Chronic suppurative otitis media
CT	Computerized tomography
DEC	diethylcarbamazine
EAT	East African Trypanosomiasis
EBNA	EBV nuclear antigen
EBV	Epstein-Barr virus
EIA	Enzyme immunosssay (substitute abbreviation for ELISA)
ELISA	Enzyme-linked immunosorbent assay
ESR	Erythrocyte sedimentation rate (Westergren)
ETEC	Enterotoxin producing *Escherichia coli*
EWRS	Early Warning and Response System
FUO	Fever of unknown origin
GAE	Granulomatous amebic encephalitis
GPHIN	Global Public Health Information Network
HAART	Highly active antiretroviral therapy
HACEK	*Haemophilus aphrophilus, H.paraphrophilis, Actinobacillus actinomycetecomitans, Cardiobacterium hominis, Eikenella corrodens, Kingella kingae*
HAV	Hepatitis A virus
HBV	Hepatitis B virus
HCV	Hepatitis C virus
HFRS	Hemorrhagic fever with renal syndrome
HIV	Human immunodeficiency virus
HPA	Health Protection Agency
hMPV	Human Metapneumovirus
HPV	Human Papillomavirus
HSV	Herpes Simplex virus
HTLV	Human T-lymphotropic virus
IDU	Intravenous drug use
IFN	Interferon

iGAS	Invasive group A *Streptococcus*
IHR	International Health Regulations
JE	Japanese encephalitis
LBRF	Louse-borne relapsing fever
MAI	Mycobacterium avium-intracellulare
MDR	Multi drug resistant
MOTT	Mycobacteria other than tuberculosis
MRI	Magnetic resonance imaging
MRSA	Methicillin-resistant *Staphyloccus aureus*
MRSTY	Resistance to ampicillin, trimethoprim, chloramphenicol, streptomycin, sulfonamides, tetracyclines
MS	Member states
MSF	Mediterranean spotted fever
NAR	Nalidixic-acid resistance
NPV	Negative predictive value
PCR	Polymerase chain reaction
PCT	Procalcitonin
PET	Positron emission tomography
PML	Progressive multifocal leukoencephalopathy
PNG	Papua New Guinea
PPV	Positive predictive value
RMSF	Rocky Mountain spotted fever
RVF	Rift Valley fever
RSV	Respiratory syncytial virus
SARS	Severe acute respiratory syndrome
SFG	Spotted fever group (rickettsiosis)
STI	Sexually transmitted infections
TB	Tuberculosis
TBE	Tick borne encephalitis
TBRF	Tick-borne relapsing fever
TEE	Transesophageal echocardiography
TST	Tuberculin skin test
TTE	Transthoracic echocardiography
UTI	Urinary tract infections
VFR	Visiting friends and relatives
VTEC	Verotoxin producing *Escherichia coli*
VZV	Varicella-zoster virus
WAT	West African Trypanosomiasis
WBC	White blood cell count
WNV	West Nile virus

Index